Fragile X Syndrome

The Johns Hopkins Series
in Contemporary Medicine and Public Health

ALSO OF INTEREST IN THIS SERIES

James E. Bowman, M.D., and Robert F. Murray, Jr., M.D., M.S., *Genetic Variation and Disorders in Peoples of African Origin*
Susan E. Folstein, M.D., *Huntington's Disease: A Disorder of Families*
Neil A. Holtzman, M.D., M.P.H., *Proceed with Caution: Predicting Genetic Risks in the Recombinant DNA Era*
Jurg Ott, *Analysis of Human Genetic Linkage, revised edition*
Vincent M. Riccardi, M.D., and June E. Eichner, M.P.H., *Neurofibromatosis: Phenotype, Natural History, and Pathogenesis*
Elizabeth A. Thompson, *Pedigree Analysis in Human Genetics*
Ming T. Tsuang, M.D., Ph.D., D.Sc., and Stephen V. Faraone, Ph.D., *The Genetics of Mood Disorders*
David D. Weaver, M.D., *Catalog of Prenatally Diagnosed Conditions*

Fragile X Syndrome

Diagnosis, Treatment, and Research

EDITED BY

Randi Jenssen Hagerman, M.D.

Associate Professor of Pediatrics
University of Colorado Health Science Center
and Child Development Unit
The Children's Hospital, Denver

AND

Amy Cronister Silverman, M.S.

Genetic Counselor
Fragile X Project
Sewall Child Development Center, Denver

THE JOHNS HOPKINS UNIVERSITY PRESS
Baltimore and London

© 1991 The Johns Hopkins University Press
All rights reserved
Printed in the United States of America

The Johns Hopkins University Press
701 West 40th Street
Baltimore, Maryland 21211–2190
The Johns Hopkins Press Ltd., London

The paper used in this book meets the minimum requirements
of American National Standards for Information Sciences—
Permanence of Paper for Printed Library Materials, ANSI Z39.48-1984.

Library of Congress Cataloging-in-Publication Data

Fragile X syndrome : diagnosis, treatment, and research / edited by
Randi Jenssen Hagerman and Amy Cronister Silverman.
    p. cm. — (The Johns Hopkins series
in contemporary medicine and public health)
    Includes index.
    ISBN 0-8018-4169-0 (alk. paper)
    1. Fragile X syndrome.   I. Hagerman, Randi Jenssen, 1949–
II. Silverman, Amy Cronister, 1957– .   III. Series.
    [DNLM: 1. Fragile X Syndrome.   QS 677 F8115]
RJ506.F7374 1991
616.85′88042—dc 20
DNLM/DLC
for Library of Congress   91-6343

To our families, including Paul, Karin, and Hillary Hagerman
and Howard Silverman, whose support and love are always there,
and to the fragile X families, who have taught us what we know.

CONTENTS

CONTRIBUTORS

J. FERNANDO ARENA, M.D., PH.D., Adjunct Assistant Professor, Division of Genetics, Department of Pediatrics, University of Miami School of Medicine

MARCIA BRADEN, M.S., PH.D., Department of Psychology, University of Denver; Director, Autism Program in El Paso County, Colorado

JOHN BROWN, PH.D., Associated Scientific Staff, Department of Behavioral Sciences, Children's Hospital, Denver

W. TED BROWN, M.D., PH.D., Chief, Division of Human Genetics, Department of Pediatrics, North Shore University Hospital; Professor of Pediatrics, Cornell University Medical College

LOIS HICKMAN, M.S., O.T.R., Occupational Therapy Department, Children's Hospital, Denver

PETER JACKY, PH.D., Director of Cytogenetics/Molecular Biology, Cytogenetics Department, Kaiser Permanente Regional Laboratory, Clackamas, Oregon

CHARLES D. LAIRD, PH.D., Professor, Departments of Zoology and Genetics, Child Development and Mental Retardation Center, University of Washington

MARY M. LAMB, PH.D., Research Scientist, Department of Zoology, University of Washington

HERBERT A. LUBS, M.D., Professor, Division of Genetics, Department of Pediatrics, University of Miami School of Medicine

REBECCA A. O'CONNOR, M.A., Developmental Specialist, Child Development Unit, Children's Hospital, Denver

BRUCE F. PENNINGTON, PH.D., Professor, Department of Psychology, University of Denver

SARAH SCHARFENAKER, M.A., C.C.C., Speech and Language Therapist, Audiology and Speech Department, Children's Hospital, Denver

ix

STEPHANIE SHERMAN, PH.D., Assistant Professor of Pediatrics, Division of Medical Genetics/Pediatrics, Emory University Medical School

WILLIAM SOBESKY, PH.D., Assistant Clinical Professor of Psychology and Director of Clinical Psychology Training, Department of Child Psychiatry, University of Colorado Health Science Center, Denver

VICKI SUDHALTER, PH.D., Research Scientist in Developmental Psycholinguistics, Institute for Basic Research on Developmental Disabilities, Staten Island, New York

JOHN SVED, PH.D., Associate Professor of Genetics, Department of Biological Science, University of Sydney

JEFFREY THORNE, PH.C., Department of Genetics, University of Washington

PREFACE

We created this book because of our concern over the paucity of information on the diagnosis and treatment of fragile X syndrome. Children and adults affected by this disorder are common: the prevalence of fragile X mental retardation approaches 1 per 1000 and the prevalence of milder problems, such as learning disabilities and emotional difficulties, is perhaps far higher. Many professionals in medical specialty areas, behavioral sciences, education, and other fields must deal with fragile X individuals on a daily basis, yet information concerning this disorder is often buried in genetic or cytogenetic specialty journals and is not readily available to them.

We have tried to compile a book with something for everyone. Researchers in the basic sciences will find information on epidemiology, cytogenetics, molecular biology, and theories of inheritance. Clinicians in pediatrics, family practice, neurology, psychiatry, and psychology will find information concerning medical follow-up, medications, and psychotherapy. Geneticists and genetic counselors will find information on the differential diagnosis of fragile X syndrome and other X-linked disorders and practical information on the complexities of genetic counseling. Educators and therapists will find information regarding treatment in the classroom, speech and language therapy, and occupational therapy. Motivated parents who are willing to wade through medical terminology will glean information regarding treatment and insight as to how multiple professionals can work together to give their child optimal care.

Although the chapters are directed to different groups of professionals, we can all learn from each other's work. Most interventions work synergistically, and improved communication among professionals and between parents and professionals is our goal. The diverse information in this volume may raise problems of terminology and may make it difficult for readers to comprehend fully the chapters outside their field. However, the trade-off is worthwhile, in that it promotes an appreciation of the connection between basic science and clinical features. In fragile X syndrome, this connection is uniquely suited for study. What we learn will not only help fragile X children but also will further our understanding of the genetic influences on brain development.

This book is divided into two parts. The chapters in part I describe the phenotype of fragile X syndrome; review its epidemiology, clinical features, and cytogenetic diagnosis; and relate current models that explain its unique pattern of inheritance. Part II reviews treatment and intervention, including genetic counseling, medical follow-up, psychotherapy, and education. To assist selective readers, we summarize the content of each chapter here.

Chapter 1 describes the physical and behavioral phenotype of males and females with fragile X syndrome, emphasizing the broad spectrum of involvement from unaffected carriers to severely retarded and autistic individuals. Chapter 2, by Stephanie Sherman, gives a historical perspective on the recognition of fragile X syndrome and its diagnostic marker. Dr. Sherman summarizes prevalence studies and screening among mentally retarded individuals. In reviewing the large pedigree analyses of 1984 and 1985, she scrutinizes her previous work and tackles the subject of the unusual familial inheritance of the fragile X gene and what has come to be referred to as the "Sherman paradox."

Chapters 3 and 4 concentrate on the diagnostic testing currently available to fragile X families. Ongoing discussion regarding the optimal indications and methods for fragile X analysis has prompted Peter Jacky to outline comprehensively the current requirements and guidelines for eliciting and interpreting the expression of fragile X. Work in the field of molecular biology has further sought to disclose the cryptic relationship between cytogenetic expression and the presence of a mutation responsible for the clinical phenotype. In chapter 4, Ted Brown discusses the current understanding of the molecular basis of the fragile X mutation and the existing methods that will eventually allow the isolation and characterization of the fragile X gene. The applicability of molecular studies to clinical practice, including carrier detection and prenatal diagnosis, is discussed, as is ongoing and future research.

Bruce Pennington, Rebecca O'Connor, and Vicki Sudhalter pose intriguing questions in chapter 5 as they unravel the neuropsychologic phenotype studies of other genetic conditions to provide insight into what we currently observe among fragile X individuals. They also review the fragile X neuropsychologic phenotype as we now understand it, including cognitive and speech and language characteristics, and consider its implications for future research in the areas of genetics and psychiatry.

A better appreciation of other forms of X-linked mental retardation may provide added insight into our current understanding of fragile X syndrome. Chapter 6, by Fernando Arena and Herbert Lubs, reviews other syndromes that serve as differential diagnoses in families who present with X-linked mental retardation. Phenotypic and etiologic similarities are presented in the form of a unique data-entry system to enable the reader to appreciate the interrelationship between these seemingly different entities. In chapter 7, theories that try to explain the unique pattern of inheritance of fragile X syndrome are reviewed. Here, Charles Laird, Mary Lamb, John Sved, and Jeffrey Thorne present a well-developed model of imprinting and discuss its implications for genetic counseling.

We believed that an entire section of this book should be devoted to treatment because this is a critical issue for families and patients. In chapter 8, genetic counseling is reviewed, with an analysis of the risks of recurrence, carrier testing, and prenatal diagnostic techniques, including their applicability and limitations. Information is presented in a practical way to guide counselors through the complexities of an unusual pattern of inheritance. Chapter 9 outlines the medical intervention at each stage in development. Health maintenance and pharmacotherapy for behavior are discussed in detail. Chapter 10, by John Brown, Marcia Braden, and William Sobesky, focuses on behavior management and psychotherapy for both adults and children and covers the spectrum of difficulties present in carrier females and affected males. The education of fragile X children and adults, including individual speech, language, and occupational therapy, is reviewed in chapter 11. Sarah Scharfenaker, Lois Hickman, and Marcia Braden review the unique learning profile in fragile X syndrome and supply the practical information necessary for designing a learning or vocational program.

This book would not have been possible without the support and encouragement of the parents and families of the fragile X individuals we follow. Their enthusiasm and creativity have taught us most of what we know regarding treatment, and we are deeply indebted to them. We also want to thank the Sewall Fragile X Project and its supporters, including the Sewall Foundation, the Colorado Trust, the Children's Hospital Foundation, the Boettcher Foundation, and the Children's Hospital Kempe Research Center, for expanding our knowledge and the knowledge of many others concerning fragile X syndrome. We are grateful for the efforts of many individuals who have made this book possible: the authors, who represent part of a larger international group of researchers noted for their congeniality and dedication to a fascinating field; the hardworking staff of Sewall Child Development Center, including Erin Milne, Keri Harris, and Claire Hull; the Child Development Unit, particularly our always supportive director, Pamela McBogg, M.D., who keeps us focused, and our secretarial staff, Esmeralda Ramirez, Joan Gillis, Vicki Sanudo, and Betty Brown, who make everything possible; the staff of the Children's Hospital library, Anne Klenk, Carol Morgan, and Susan Osborn, who can find any article ever written and have done so thousands of times; Kim Dohren, David Chavez, Tia Brayman, and Steve Kast, of The Children's Hospital photography department, whose artistic excellence is reflected in the figures in this book; the students who have been ever so diligent and supportive, including Jeanette Riddle, Michael Wittenberger, Ari Brunschwig, Anne Salbenblatt, Susan Greenshek, Kahlid Amiri, and Sabrina Jewell-Smart; the professionals who have most recently visited our unit and have provided stimulating discussions and critical review of several chapters, including Drs. Sebíastiano Musumeci, Jeremy Turk, and Vicky Turk; our colleagues and friends who have provided ongoing support and a continuing learning experience, including Drs. Sally

Rogers, Loris McGavran, David Manchester, Rebecca Berry, Ann C. M. Smith; the National Fragile X Foundation and all of the hardworking volunteers who keep it growing; and Walter Koelbel and his wife, Gene, who have given us support for a vision of the future that will lead to ever greater advances in this field.

PART I
Diagnosis and Research

CHAPTER 1

Physical and Behavioral Phenotype

Randi Jenssen Hagerman, M.D.

Physical Phenotype

Recognition of the classic physical phenotype in fragile X [fra(X)] male patients, including large and prominent ears, a long narrow face, and macroorchidism, evolved over a decade. In the early 1970s, Gillian Turner in Australia was impressed with the lack of unusual physical features in this group of patients with X-linked mental retardation (Turner 1983). Escalante (1971), Cantú et al. (1976), and Turner et al. (1975) reported macroorchidism in males with X-linked mental retardation, and Turner et al. (1978) subsequently linked macroorchidism and the marker X or fra(X) chromosome. Approximately 80% of fra(X) patients will have one or more of these features, but their presence varies with age (fig. 1.1). Additional features, including velvetlike skin (Turner et al. 1980), hyperextensible finger joints (Hagerman et al. 1984), a high arched palate, flat feet, and pectus excavatum, stimulated Opitz et al. (1984) to hypothesize the existence of a connective tissue dysplasia in fra(X) syndrome. This hypothesis led to further investigations concerning cardiac abnormalities, and mitral valve prolapse was found in the majority of fra(X) patients (Loehr et al. 1986). A defect in connective tissue has not been proven, but studies by Waldstein et al. (1986) demonstrated abnormal elastin fibers in the skin, aorta, and cardiac valves by light microscopy in fra(X) males. Although the cardiac findings in fra(X) syndrome are not as severe as those in Marfan syndrome, they are typical of the findings in some other heritable disorders of connective tissue (HDCT). There are presently more than 150 HDCT, and Glesby and Pyeritz (1989) recommended the acronym *MASS phenotype* to emphasize the involvement of the *m*itral valve, *a*orta, *s*keleton, and *s*kin in HDCT. An important physical feature in fra(X) syndrome which is not part of the MASS phenotype is macroorchidism.

Facial Features

The classic features of a long narrow face and prominent ears are often not present in the prepubertal child (fig. 1.2) (Chudley and Hagerman 1987).

3

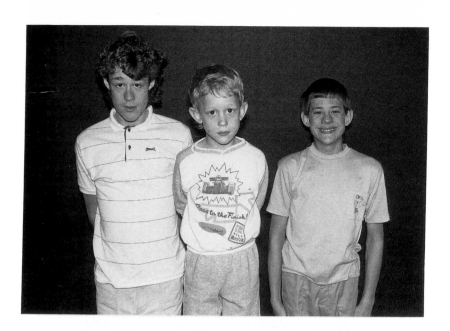
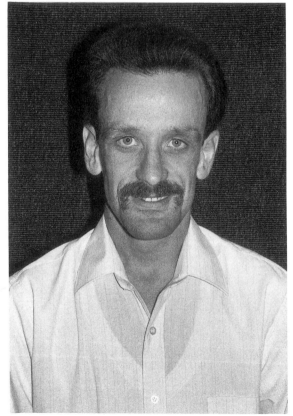

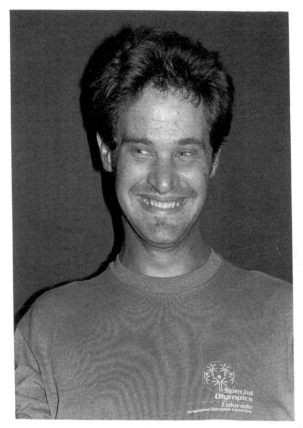

Figure 1.1 Fra(X) males demonstrating typical facial features, including prominent ears and/or a long, narrow face.

However, there exists a gestalt of additional features in the face which are helpful to the experienced clinician in suggesting the diagnosis of fra(X) syndrome. Hockey and Crowhurst (1988) attempted to characterize these features in a retrospective study of photographs from infancy in fra(X) children. Common findings include puffiness around the eyes and narrow palpebral fissures, a large head relative to the body, strabismus, and hypotonia. Epicanthal folds, ptosis, myopia, and skull asymmetry are common but are present in less than 50%. The broad palpebral fissures or long but narrow eye openings are a particularly helpful finding in a subgroup of young fra(X) boys (fig. 1.3), and Butler et al. (1988) showed that this is a significant finding compared to controls. This finding is not seen in all patients and is occasionally associated with epicanthal folds. Simko et al. (1989) found epicanthal folds in 8 of 20 fra(X) boys.

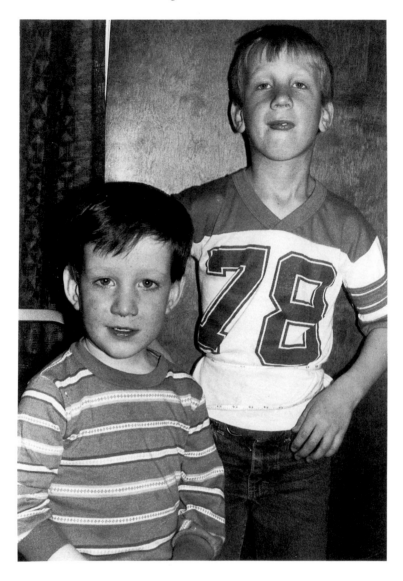

Prominent ears are common in fra(X) males and are present even in pre-pubertal boys. Simko et al. (1989) found long, wide, or protruding ears in 15 of 20 (75%) fra(X) boys. In our experience with 134 fra(X) males, prominent ears were present in 63% (table 1.1). The ears may also be long or wide with the occasional loss of the antihelical fold, so that the upper pinna may be cupped out (fig. 1.4). Surgical pinning of the ear is a treatment option if ear prominence

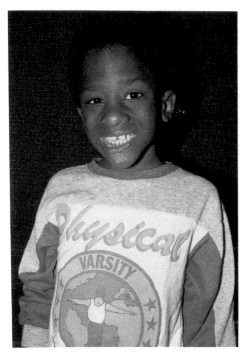 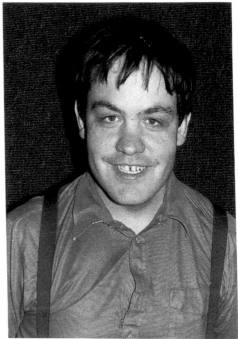

Figure 1.2 Fra(X) boys without remarkably distinguishing physical features. [Reprinted with permission from Hagerman (1987)]

is dramatic and psychologically stressful for the child. Ear width is a more discriminating feature in identifying fra(X) patients than is ear length, and it can be more easily quantified than can ear prominence (Butler et al. 1991). Butler and his colleagues (1991) used a combination of discriminating anthropomorphic variables including testicular volume, ear width, bizygomatic diameter [narrower in fra(X) patients than in controls] and head breadth [wider in fra(X) patients than in controls] and correctly distinguished fra(X) patients from retarded nonfra(X) patients in 95.2% of cases.

A high arched palate has been reported by several authors (Partington 1984; Sutherland and Hecht 1985; Hagerman et al. 1983) and was found in 48% of fra(X) males followed in Denver (table 1.1). This is often seen in association with dental crowding or malocclusion. Partington (1984) reported the presence of cleft palate in 5 of 61 (8%) fra(X) males, and Hagerman (1987) reported a child with Pierre Robin malformation sequence who was subsequently diagnosed with fra(X) syndrome. Four additional cases of Pierre Robin sequence in association with fra(X) were reported by Lachiewicz et al. (1989). This frequency of association suggests that it is not coincidental and that the connective

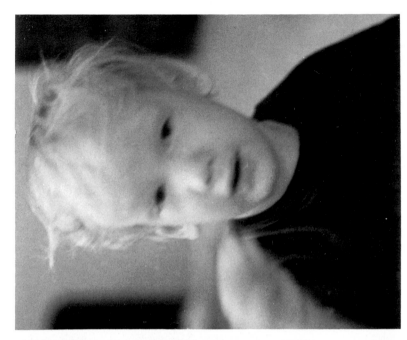

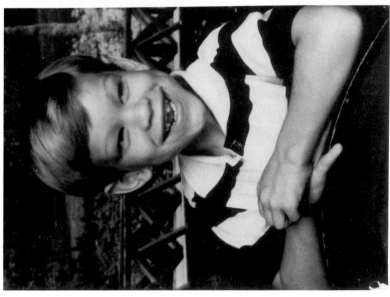

Figure 1.3 Narrow palpebral fissures in fra(X) boys

8

Table 1.1

Physical Features of Fragile X Males Seen at The Children's Hospital in Denver

Feature	No. with Feature/ Total No. of Patients	% of Patients with Feature
Long ears (>2 SD in length)	76/115	66
Prominent ears	85/134	63
High arched palate	62/130	48
Prominent jaw	11/40	28
Long face	60/81	74
Pectus excavatum	47/109	43
Hyperextensible MP joints (MP extension ≥90°)	87/137	64
Hand calluses	43/96	45
Double-jointed thumbs	37/90	41
Single palmar crease (Sydney or simian line)	36/102	35
Flat feet	71/109	65
Macroorchidism	82/111	74
Scoliosis	8/39	20
Strabismus	17/52	33

tissue abnormalities of fra(X) syndrome place these patients at higher risk for the Pierre Robin sequence.

Macroorchidism

Macroorchidism, or large testicles, is present in over 80% of adult fra(X) males (Sutherland and Hecht 1985). Prenatal studies showed abnormalities in the ultrastructure of the fetal fra(X) testicle, including an increase in glycoprotein granules (Shapiro et al. 1986). These findings suggest a primary defect in the structure of the testicle related to the fra(X) mutation. However, evidence also suggests that macroorchidism is secondary to endocrinologic abnormalities associated with fra(X). For instance, macroorchidism is seen in a much smaller percentage of prepubertal boys than postpubertal males, and a dramatic increase in size has been seen in fra(X) boys during early pubertal years, presumably secondary to gonadotropin stimulation. Other endocrine disorders, particularly hypothyroidism, are also associated with macroorchidism when excessive gonadotropin stimulation occurs (Castro-Magana et al. 1988; Roitman et al. 1980). Gonadotropin abnormalities may be associated with hypothalamic dysfunction, which has been postulated in fra(X) and will be discussed below (Fryns et al. 1987; Fryns 1989).

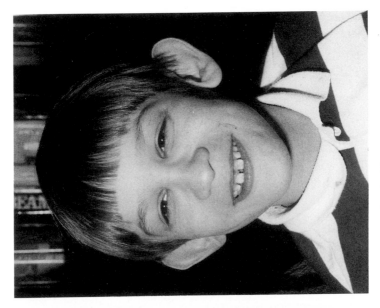

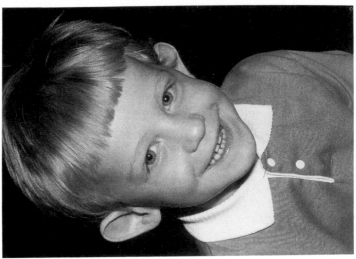

Figure 1.4 Prominent ears that are cupped and wide

10

Macroorchidism is usually measured with an orchidometer, a series of ellipsoid shapes of a known volume which are compared directly with the testicle. The Prader orchidometer, shown in figure 1.5, includes shapes with volumes of 2–25 ml. It can be ordered for a cost of approximately $40.00 from Dr. Andrea Prader, Kinderspital Zurich, Eleonorensiftung, Universitates-Kinderklinik, Steinwiesstrasse 75, 8032 Zurich, Switzerland. The Adelaide orchidometer includes volumes of up to 100 ml (Sutherland and Hecht 1985), which is useful in fra(X) adults. The testicle can also be measured (in centimeters) directly with a tape or calipers and the volume (in milliliters) can be subsequently calculated using the formula $\pi/6$ (length)(width^2). Figure 1.6 demonstrates normal testicular growth through childhood and adolescence. Normative data are sparse for prepubertal patients and a 2-ml volume is considered normal. Approximately 39% of fra(X) boys have a testicular volume of 3 ml or larger (Hagerman et al. 1987). However, our clinical experience indicates that a 3-ml testicular volume is not unusual in normal males. Significant macroorchidism probably begins at 4 ml in young boys and is present in approximately 21% of fra(X) boys (fig. 1.7) (Sutherland and Hecht 1985).

Prader (1966) and Zachman et al. (1974) found that the upper limit of the normal testicular volume was 25 ml in adult normal men. Daniel et al. (1982)

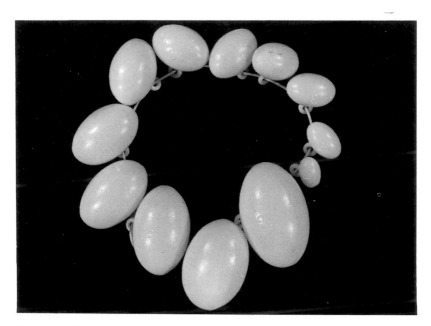

Figure 1.5 The Prader orchidometer shows volumes of 2–25 ml, which are compared to the patient's testicle to measure the volume.

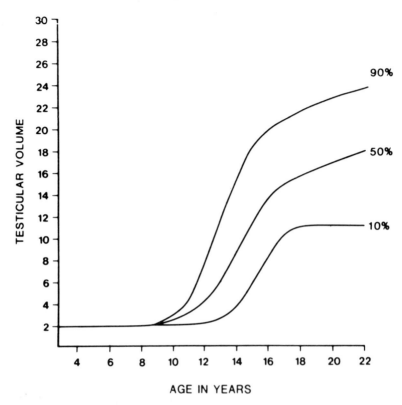

Figure 1.6 Normal testicular volume (in milliliters) throughout childhood and adolescence. [Adapted from Prader (1966) and Zachman et al. (1974); reprinted with permission from Hagerman and Smith (1983)]

and Farkas (1976), however, found larger volumes in normal men. Therefore, significant macroorchidism is probably not present until the testicular volume is larger than 30 ml (fig. 1.8). The usual testicular volume in an adult fra(X) man is 40 to 60 ml. Differences between populations internationally due to racial variation probably account for the discrepancies in the normative data. Sutherland and Hecht (1985) reviewed 22 studies and found the average prevalence of macroorchidism to be 87% in fra(X) adult men. Macroorchidism is not specific to fra(X) syndrome, and studies of institutionalized mentally retarded males have shown that the prevalence of macroorchidism is as high as 29%, whereas only 4–27% of men with macroorchidism are fra(X) positive (Brondum-Nielsen et al. 1982; Primrose et al. 1986; Hagerman et al. 1988a).

Fra(X) men are fertile (Cantú et al. 1976) and offspring have been documented, but those with significant mental retardation rarely reproduce. Ultra-

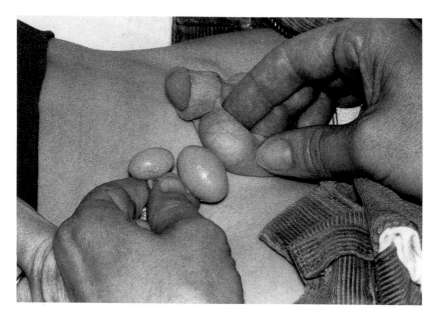

Figure 1.7 Macroorchidism (4- to 5-ml volume) in a four-year-old fra(X) boy

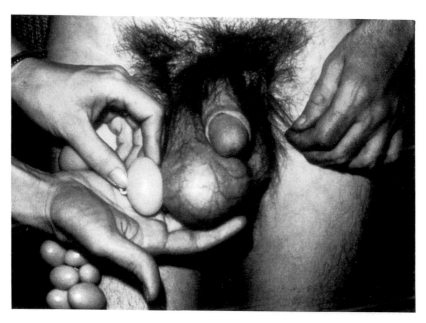

Figure 1.8 Macroorchidism (100-ml volume) in an adult fra(X) man. [Reprinted with permission from Hagerman (1987)]

structural studies of the testicle have documented an increased ground substance (Shapiro et al. 1986), interstitial fibrosis, edema (Cantú et al. 1976; Johannisson et al. 1987), and abnormal tubular morphology (Rudelli et al. 1985). Reduced spermatogenesis coupled with an excessive number of malformed spermatids suggest decreased fertility in fra(X) males (Johannisson et al. 1987).

Two cases of testicular tumors in fra(X) males have been reported, although it is unclear whether they are related to the fra(X) gene or to macroorchidism. The first report was of a benign testicular tumor similar to a sperm granuloma in a 34-year-old man with macroorchidism (del Pozo and Millard 1983). In the second case, a classic seminoma in the left testis of a 45-year-old man was removed, but at 50 years of age the patient developed a spermatocystic seminoma in the right testis (Phelan et al. 1988). Three other cancers have been reported in fra(X) males: a malignant ganglioma (Rodewald et al. 1987), an adenocarcinoma of the colon in a 14-year-old boy (Phelan et al. 1988), and a case of acute lymphocytic leukemia (Cunningham and Dickerman 1988), but there is not sufficient evidence to support an increased rate of cancer associated with the fra(X) gene.

Ophthalmologic Findings

Ophthalmologic problems in fra(X) syndrome include strabismus (lazy eye), which was reported in 56% of 16 males (Schinzel and Largo 1985) and in 6 of 15 fra(X) patients (40%), including both exotropia and esotropia (fig. 1.9) (Storm et al. 1987). Strabismus is a common problem in many developmental disorders and requires early diagnosis and treatment to avoid amblyopia (Maino et al. 1990). Storm et al. (1987) and Flood and Sanner (1985) found frequent refractive errors in fra(X) patients, including one case with high myopia and others with hyperopia. Nystagmus was seen in 2 of 15 fra(X) patients but was not coincidental with strabismus. All fra(X) children should be evaluated by an ophthalmologist by 4 years of age or sooner if obvious problems are present. Surgery and/or patching are often necessary to treat strabismus. Ptosis (lid lowering) is also occasionally seen and may require surgery for cosmetic reasons or to avoid amblyopia. Perhaps some of the ophthalmologic findings, particularly high myopia, may be related to connective tissue problems.

Otitis

A frequent complaint of fra(X) children is recurrent otitis media (middle ear infections) in early childhood. Although this is a common disorder of all children (Teele et al. 1983), the frequency of infection is excessive in a subgroup of fra(X) boys. Hagerman et al. (1987) studied 30 fra(X) boys and 63%

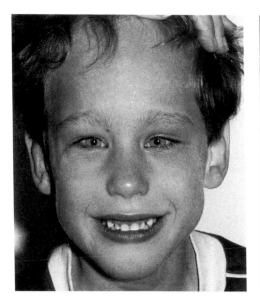 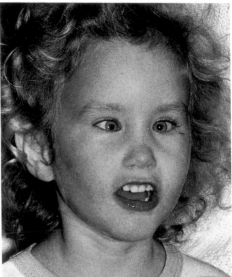

Figure 1.9 Esotropia in a fra(X) boy and his sister

had recurrent otitis compared to 15% of their normal male siblings and 38% of developmentally disabled nonfra(X) children. Forty-three percent of the fra(X) children required the insertion of one or more sets of polyethylene (PE) tubes in the tympanic membranes. Simko et al. (1989) also found recurrent otitis in 45% of 20 fra(X) children.

Recurrent otitis media is associated with a fluctuating conductive hearing loss and subsequent language and articulation deficits (Rapin 1979). Evidence also exists for cognitive sequelae affecting the verbal IQ (Zinkus et al. 1978) and behavior problems including hyperactivity (Hagerman et al. 1987) in otherwise normal children. In the retarded population, abnormal tympanograms secondary to serous otitis have also been associated with a lower IQ compared to those without ear problems (Saxon and Witriol 1976; Libb et al. 1985). Fra(X) children usually have significant language and cognitive deficits that can be worsened by the sequelae of recurrent otitis. It is therefore imperative that fra(X) children be vigorously monitored and treated for recurrent otitis media so that hearing is always optimal and sequelae are avoided. This often means the insertion of PE tubes when a hearing loss is documented or the use of prophylactic antibiotics to avoid otitis media when a child has a history of recurrent infections.

Why fra(X) children are predisposed to recurrent otitis media infections is unknown. The facial structure, including a long face and a high arched palate, may affect the angle of the eustachian tube and prevent appropriate drainage of the middle ear. The looseness of connective tissue and hypotonia may lead to a collapsible eustachian tube, which would also affect drainage. A transient hypogammaglobulinemia was documented in one young boy (Hagerman et al. 1987), and a second fra(X) child had an immunoglobulin G (IgG) subclass 1 and 3 deficiency with recurrent otitis and sinusitis. Other cases of hypogammaglobulinemia in fra(X) syndrome have not been reported, so a consistent immunodeficiency is unlikely in this syndrome.

Orthopedic Problems

The most common musculoskeletal manifestations in fra(X) syndrome include flexible pes planus (flat feet), excessive joint laxity, and scoliosis (figs. 1.10 and 1.11). Davids et al. (1990) reviewed the orthopedic problems of 150 fra(X) males. Fifty percent demonstrated significant pes planus, which was not associated with pain or disability but was usually associated with uneven shoe wear. Thirty-nine percent of the children with pes planus were seen by an orthopedist before the diagnosis of fra(X) syndrome was made, and almost all were treated with a foot orthosis or with orthopedic shoes. This usually improved the gait

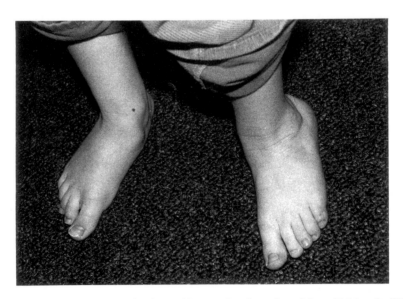

Figure 1.10 Pes planus, or flat feet, with pronation (inturning of the ankle) in a fra(X) boy.

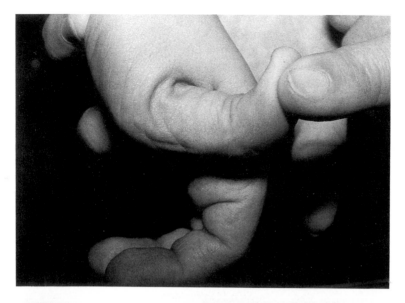

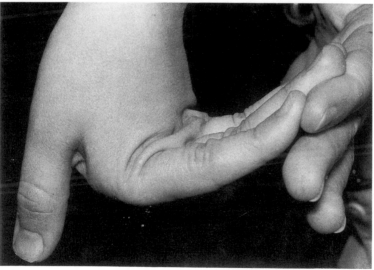

Figure 1.11 *Top*, double-jointed thumbs in a fra(X) boy; *bottom*, hyperextensible finger joints with metacarpophalangeal extension of >90° in a fra(X) boy.

pattern and shoe wear. In only one case was foot surgery done, specifically an extra-articular subtalar arthrodesis.

Davids et al. (1990) also evaluated joint laxity and found that 73% of fra(X) children younger than 11 years had joint laxity with hyperextensible metacarpophalangeal (MP) joints (MP extension ≥90°), whereas 56% of those 11–19 years old and 30% of those older than 20 had this finding. This suggests that the ligaments tighten with age.

Theoretically, fra(X) patients should be at risk for joint dislocations. Although double-jointed thumbs are common in both males and females (fig. 1.11), joint dislocations are rare. We followed one fra(X) patient with recurrent patellar dislocation that eventually required patellectomy (Davids et al. 1990) and a second patient with congenital hip dislocation. Looseness of the connective tissue may also predispose patients to positional malformations in utero. We have seen 3 cases of clubfoot deformity in 150 fra(X) males (fig. 1.12). Mild pectus excavatum is also common and was seen in 43% of fra(X) males in Denver (table 1.1).

Skin Manifestations

The most notable feature of the skin in fra(X) patients is its softness and smoothness. This is particularly noticeable on the hands. The palms may occasionally appear wrinkled, a callus is often present on the hand from hand biting, and a single palmar crease, either a simian crease or a Sydney line (fig. 1.13), is seen in 51% of males (Simpson et al. 1984).

The microscopic correlate of smooth, soft skin was studied by Waldstein et al. (1986) in the skin biopsies of five fra(X) males. There was incomplete or absent arborization of elastin in the papillary dermis and a decreased number of elastin fibrils in the deep dermis when compared to controls. These findings were also seen in a subsequent patient at autopsy (Waldstein and Hagerman 1988). Abnormal elastin fibrils were also present in the aorta and in cardiac valves, and there were hypoplasia of the aorta and mitral valve prolapse. It is uncertain whether the elastin abnormality represents the connective tissue dysplasia in fra(X) syndrome, and further studies are necessary.

The rare occurrence of cutis verticis gyrata (CVG), which is the development of furrows or folds in the skin of the scalp, giving it a convoluted appearance, has been reported in fra(X) syndrome. Musumeci et al. (1989) described a single case. In a subsequent survey of 20 unrelated institutionalized males with CVG, 5 were found to be fra(X) positive (Schepis et al. 1989).

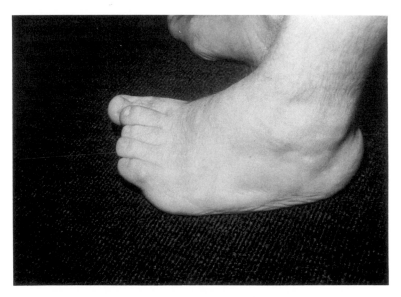

Figure 1.12 Clubfoot deformity in a fra(X) boy

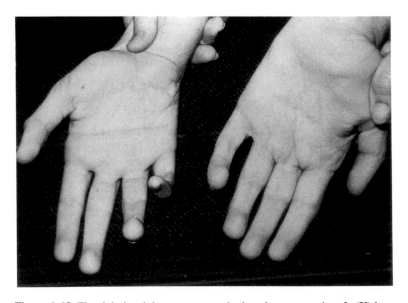

Figure 1.13 The right hand demonstrates a single palmar crease in a fra(X) boy

Dermatoglyphics

A characteristic pattern of dermatoglyphic findings has been described in fra(X) by several investigators (Simpson 1986; Rodewald et al. 1986; Hagerman et al. 1983; Steinbach et al. 1986; Milone et al. 1988). This pattern in males includes an increased frequency of radial loops, whorls, and arches on the fingertips, a lower total ridge count, abnormal palmar creases, and a hallucal crease on the sole (fig. 1.14). Two index systems for males have shown excellent specificity and sensitivity (Simpson 1986; Rodewald et al. 1986). However, the technical aspects of dermatoglyphic analysis and the utilization of an index system are beyond the efforts of most clinicians. Langenbeck et al. (1988) evaluated the usefulness of the Rodewald index in screening 160 institutionalized males for fra(X). An abnormal index score was seen in 32 men, and 14 were fra(X) positive (predictive value, 44%). This predictive value is similar to that of other screening tools that combine physical and behavioral features to assess the risk for fra(X) (Turner et al. 1989; Hagerman et al. 1991a).

Cardiac Involvement

Concern for a possible connective tissue dysplasia in fra(X) syndrome led to further studies of cardiac function. Loehr et al. (1986) evaluated 40 fra(X) patients, including 6 females, and found mitral valve prolapse (MVP) in 55% diagnosed by echocardiographic findings in combination with clinical findings of a click or systolic murmur. An occasional male demonstrated significant mitral regurgitation that required more frequent follow-up. MVP was also seen in 3 heterozygous females. Seven males (18%) also had mild dilatation of the base of the aorta, but this did not seem to be progressive. These findings were corroborated by Sreeram et al. (1989), who found dilatation of the aortic root in 12 of 23 (52%) fra(X) men and MVP in 5 of 23 (22%).

If a click or murmur is present in a fra(X) patient, a cardiac evaluation that includes an echocardiogram is recommended. If MVP is documented, prophylaxis for subacute bacterial endocarditis is warranted during dental procedures or operations that could contaminate the bloodstream with bacteria. MVP is usually a benign finding, although it can predispose a patient to cardiac arrhythmias. There have been no complaints of arrhythmias in affected males, although palpitations occur in 31% of normal IQ heterozygotes (Cronister et al. 1991a), and in several MVP has been diagnosed. However, MVP is also common in the general population, and we do not know whether its occurrence is increased in heterozygotes compared to controls. It is interesting that MVP is also associated with panic disorder (Hartman et al. 1982), which is a problem for some otherwise unaffected heterozygous females.

Fra(X) males do not seem to have a shortened life-span, but one case of

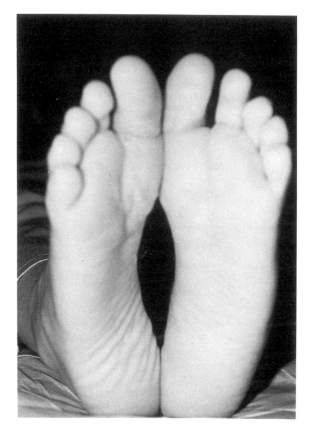

Figure 1.14 A hallucal crease on the sole consists of a deep line in the skin between the first and second toes in a fra(X) boy.

sudden death was reported in an 18-year-old fra(X) male (Waldstein and Hager-man 1988). This teenager presumably died from an arrhythmia precipitated by a viral myocarditis. His autopsy demonstrated a diffuse tubular hypoplasia of the aorta and a mild postductal coarctation. This malformation has not been found previously in fra(X) syndrome, but the finding in this case of abnormal elastin fibers in the wall of the aorta and in the cardiac valves suggests a relationship to abnormal connective tissue.

Hypertension is not uncommon in fra(X) men, although it has never been studied in detail nor in comparison to other retarded males. The elevated blood pressure is often blamed on the anxiety experienced by fra(X) men in the clinician's office during an examination. Persistent hypertension is experienced by some patients, however, and it requires a more thorough work-up and subsequent antihypertensive medication. Perhaps connective tissue problems, such as abnormal elastin fibers, affect the resiliency of the vessel walls and predispose fra(X) males to hypertension. Further studies are necessary to document the prevalence of hypertension and anatomic or connective tissue correlates in fra(X) patients.

Growth

Several authors have commented on unusual growth patterns in fra(X) syndrome, including increased birth weights, macrocephaly, increased or decreased height, and an acromegalic appearance in many adults (Turner et al. 1980, 1986; Fryns 1984; Meryash et al. 1984; Sutherland and Hecht 1985; Brondum-Nielsen 1988; Borghgraef et al. 1990).

Partington (1984) evaluated 61 fra(X) males and found a mean birth weight close to the fiftieth percentile and evenly spread height and weight growth percentiles. He found that 6.5% were at or below the fifth percentile for height and that no one was significantly increased over the ninety-fifth percentile. Sutherland and Hecht (1985) summarized data in several studies and found that 21 of 29 boys who were younger than 15 had growth percentiles above the fiftieth percentile and that 9 (31%) were at or above the ninety-fifth percentile. The adults, on the other hand, tended to be short, with 23 of 87 (26%) measuring at or below the fifth percentile. Loesch et al. (1988) confirmed the finding of a tendency for short stature in fra(X) men and women compared to controls.

Prouty et al. (1988) reported that fetal growth, including head circumference and birth weight, were normal. They also found a mild increase in head circumference growth during childhood, which persisted into adult life. This was similar to the findings of Sutherland and Hecht (1985), who reported that the head circumference data demonstrated a mild tendency for an increased size, even in adulthood, when 70% were at or above the fiftieth percentile and 7% were above the ninety-seventh percentile. Individuals with fra(X) syndrome have been misdiagnosed as having Soto syndrome or cerebral gigantism because of the association of developmental delay and a large head circumference (Beemer et al. 1986; Fryns 1984). Greenberg (Dr. Frank Greenberg, Houston, personal communication, 1989) studied 15 patients with Soto syndrome; 3 were fra(X) positive on cytogenetic studies. On the other hand, an occasional fra(X) male will demonstrate microcephaly (Partington 1984; Wisniewski et al. 1991), although this is less common than mild macrocephaly. In general, the majority of fra(X) patients do not demonstrate somatic overgrowth; however, evidence is accumulating for endocrine dysfunction in fra(X) syndrome.

Endocrine Dysfunction

The focus of early work has been on macroorchidism. In an effort to find the cause of macroorchidism, the levels of testosterone, luteinizing hormone (LH), follicle-stimulating hormone (FSH), and thyroid hormone were measured and reported to be normal (Bowen et al. 1978; Cantú et al. 1978; Brondum-Nielsen et al. 1982). However, mild elevations in gonadotropin levels (FSH and LH) were reported by Turner et al. (1975), Ruvalcaba et al. (1977), and McDermitt et al. (1983). This finding is consistent with an elevated gonadotropin etiology for the macroorchidism seen in some hypothyroid patients (Castro-Magana et al. 1988). Further studies by Berkovitz et al. (1986) in fra(X) males demonstrated a normal testosterone response to human chorionic gonadotropin stimulation and normal 5-alpha-reductase activity and androgen receptor binding in genital skin fibroblasts, but mild elevations of androstenedione, 17-hydroxyprogesterone, and progesterone. Additional evidence for abnormal hypothalamic-pituitary function includes a blunted thyroid-stimulating hormone response to thyrotropin-releasing hormone stimulation (Wilson et al. 1988).

Clinically, Fryns et al. (1987) identified a subgroup of fra(X) males with extreme obesity, short stature, stubby hands and feet, and diffuse hyperpigmentation. This phenotype is somewhat similar to that of Prader-Willi syndrome, which is associated with hypothalamic dysfunction, and Fryns et al. postulated hypothalamic problems in fra(X) syndrome. We have also seen a fra(X) boy with a phenotype similar to that of Prader-Willi syndrome but without short stature (fig. 1.15). His obesity seemed to be related to the behavioral phenotype in fra(X) syndrome, which includes perseverative eating, instead of to endocrine dysfunction, although the behavioral phenotype may certainly be influenced by hormonal problems.

Further evidence of hypothalamic dysfunction is seen in the precocious puberty reported in an $8^{1}/_{2}$-year-old mentally retarded fra(X) girl (Butler and Najjar 1988) and in a 2-year and 8-month-old developmentally delayed fra(X) girl (Moore et al. 1990). Both had an advanced bone age, a mature response to gonadotropin-releasing hormone stimulation, and a normal computed tomographic (CT) scan. Further support for hypothalamic dysfunction as a cause of the fra(X) phenotype comes from the report by Fryns et al. (1986) of three fra(X)-negative males with acquired lesions of the central nervous system (CNS), including one with a hypothalamic tumor. All three patients had macroorchidism and facial features typical of fra(X) syndrome.

Cronister et al. (1991a) reported premature ovarian failure in 13% of normal heterozygotes compared to 5% of controls. This finding is unusual because it is not associated with the phenotype of affected females but instead occurs in otherwise unaffected carriers. The region Xq26-Xq28 appears to be important

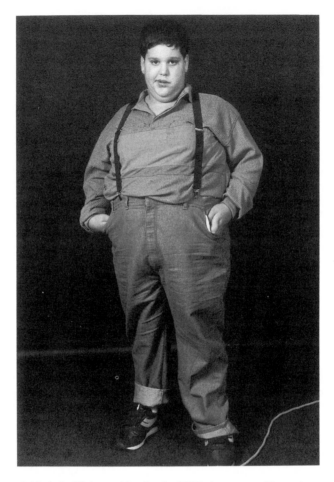

Figure 1.15 A fra(X) boy with a Prader Willi phenotype without short stature

for the maintenance of ovarian function, and women with deletions in this region have been reported to have premature menopause (Krauss et al. 1987). Perhaps this locus is affected by the fra(X) mutation in the carrier state only. Fryns et al. (1988) also reported increased fertility and an increase in the twinning rate in fra(X) females.

Heterozygotes

Physical Features

Escalante (1971) was the first to report mental retardation in females in association with the marker X chromosome. His clinical descriptions included a high palate, genu valgum, and flat feet, which are suggestive of the connective tissue problems in fra(X) males (Vianna-Morgante et al. 1982). Years later, Sherman et al. (1985) reported a penetrance of approximately 35% for mental impairment (IQ $<$ 85) in females who carry the fra(X) gene. The recognition of physical involvement in females, however, has evolved somewhat more slowly than has the recognition of cognitive involvement.

Fryns (1986) analyzed the physical features in 135 heterozygotes. He found facial stigmata, which were similar to those in males, including a long face, a prominent forehead, and mandibular prognathism in 28%. These findings were present in 14% of the subjects with normal intelligence and in 55% of those with mental retardation. Loesch and Hay (1988) subsequently studied 90 adult and 20 prepubertal heterozygotes. Typical facial features were seen in 37% of adults but only 14% of girls. Additionally, hypermobility of the finger joints was seen in 40% of adults and 52% of the girls. Flat feet were seen in 19% of both groups. All of the features were more prevalent in mentally impaired heterozygotes compared to normal IQ heterozygotes. Cronister et al. (1991a) compared the physical features of 105 heterozygotes to those of 90 controls but found a paucity of statistical differences, although hyperextensible MP joints and double-jointed thumbs were seen twice as frequently in impaired heterozygotes as in impaired controls. Although less pronounced, there seems to be evidence of a connective tissue dysplasia in affected heterozygotes which has manifestations similar to those of the male. Occasionally, more significant malformations, such as a cleft palate, have also been reported in heterozygotes (Loesch and Hay 1988).

Macrocephaly was a significant finding in 7 prepubertal fra(X)-positive girls reported by Borghgraef et al. (1990). They postulated an overgrowth phenomenon similar to that proposed for males. However, Hagerman et al. (1991b) compared 32 fra(X)-positive prepubertal girls to 18 fra(X)-negative sisters and found no significant differences in height, weight, and head circumference. Significant differences were seen in ear prominence, face length, and the presence of shyness, poor eye contact, hand flapping, and hand biting. The fra(X)-positive girls had more physical and behavioral features typical of the syndrome than had their fra(X)-negative sisters.

Approximately 40 to 50% of all heterozygotes are fra(X) negative cytogenetically (see chapter 3). Of the fra(X)-positive females, three-quarters usually show some degree of mental impairment ranging from learning dis-

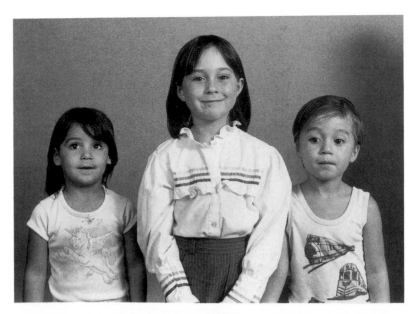

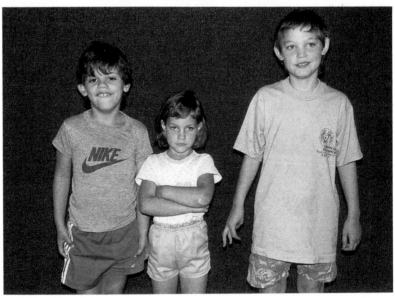

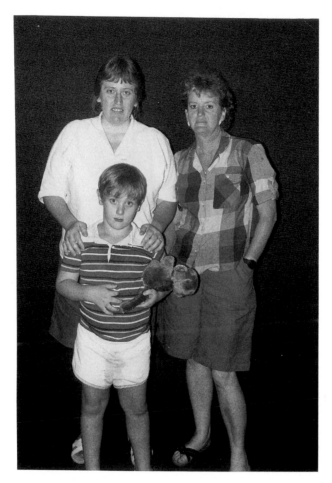

Figure 1.16 *Left,* a fra(X)-positive, learning-disabled sister is flanked by her fra(X)-positive brothers in each picture. *Right,* three generations in a family: the unaffected carrier grandmother on the *right,* her daughter with mild learning disabilities on the *left,* and her grandson with fra(X) syndrome.

abilities to mental retardation (Cronister et al. 1991b; Hagerman et al. 1991b). These individuals usually demonstrate a few typical physical features; mildly prominent ears are the most common finding in prepubertal girls (fig. 1.16). Enlargement of the ovaries has been seen in two affected women who were evaluated by ultrasound (Turner et al. 1986) and in a young fra(X)-positive girl who presented with precocious puberty (Moore et al. 1990).

Cronister et al. (1991a) showed a significant correlation between the number of typical physical features, transformed into a physical index score, and the percentage of fragility in heterozygotes. This suggests that a heterozygote's degree of involvement from the syndrome is reflected in her percentage of fragility. This has been reported previously in regard to cognitive abilities (Chudley et al. 1983) and is discussed in chapter 5. However, Cronister's studies also demonstrate that both cognitive and physical features do not correlate with percentage of fragility above 2%. Therefore, higher-expressing females are affected by the syndrome, but the degree of involvement may then be determined by X inactivation. That is, if an affected female inactivates her fragile X chromosome instead of her normal X chromosome in the majority of her cells, she will have a higher IQ than a female who inactivates her normal X chromosome in the majority of her cells and is utilizing her fragile X chromosome. Several studies support this hypothesis (Wilhelm et al. 1988; Knoll et al. 1984; Rocchi et al. 1990).

Neurological Features

Young fra(X) boys are often described as hypotonic with poor motor tone (Hagerman et al. 1983; Wisniewski et al. 1991). The cause of the hypotonia seems to be a general effect of the CNS dysfunction in fra(X) syndrome, and the consequences may be significant. Fryns suggested that the facial features in fra(X) syndrome, particularly a long narrow face and joint laxity, may be a consequence of hypotonia and be unrelated to connective tissue abnormalities (Brown et al. 1991). Hypotonia, however, has also been reported in other known connective tissue disorders and was present to a severe degree in all children with Ehlers-Danlos type VI with lysyl hydroxylase deficiency reported by Wenstrup et al. (1989). Hypotonia may affect joint stability, fine and gross motor coordination, and sensory integration. These problems should be treated with early occupational therapy. Intervention techniques are described in chapter 11.

Wisniewski et al. (1989, 1991) described a lack of focal or hard neurologic findings in fra(X) syndrome. The most common findings on examination were soft neurologic signs indicative of motor incoordination. An occasional patient, however, has cerebral palsy involving unilateral spasticity or spastic diplegia, which may be secondary to birth asphyxia (Dunn et al. 1963) in some cases, although in others there is no such history (Fryns 1984; Gillberg 1983). These findings may simply be coincidentally associated with fra(X) syndrome.

Finnelli et al. (1985) described hyperreflexia in fra(X) syndrome, but this is not a consistent finding. The palmomental reflex is often positive in fra(X) males, suggesting frontal lobe dysfunction. This reflex is elicited by scraping the thumb across the palm of the patient; the patient's chin will twitch if the sign is positive (S. A. Musumeci, 1990, personal communication).

Fryns et al. (1988) also reported an unexpectedly high incidence of sudden infant death in fra(X) boys and girls. Seventeen deaths before the age of 18 months occurred in 219 male offspring (8%) and 6 of 169 female offspring (4%) of obligate carrier women. The authors attributed this finding to CNS disturbances in affected offspring, although hypotonia leading to an obstructed airway or seizures may have been contributing features. In general, fra(X) patients have a normal life-span, and hypotonia is significantly improved by adulthood.

Seizures and Electroencephalographic (EEG) Findings

The most common neurologic abnormality in fra(X) syndrome is seizures. Sanfilippo et al. (1986) reported an EEG pattern in three epileptic fra(X) males which included medium to high voltage unilateral or bilateral spikes in the temporal area during sleep. Musumeci et al. (1988a) subsequently reported this finding as characteristic of fra(X) syndrome but not other causes of mental retardation. The temporal or central spikes were sometimes multifocal with two or more independent, occasionally alternating foci that also occurred during sleep but rarely were seen in the waking record (fig. 1.17). This pattern was present in 7 of 12 fra(X) males (58%) and in 4 of 88 (4.5%) retarded males without fra(X) syndrome, suggesting significant specificity for fra(X). The pattern was mainly present in children, and it could be identified in epileptic and nonepileptic fra(X) males. Musumeci et al. (1988b) noted the similarities between this pattern and benign rolandic spikes, which are a common cause of benign rolandic epilepsy (BRE) (Aicardi 1986) in childhood.

Wisniewski et al. (1991) reported the follow-up of 14 fra(X) patients with seizures. All were well controlled with anticonvulsants, usually carbamazepine (Tegretol). All of the seizures began in childhood or adolescence, they were usually infrequent, and, in 10 of the 14 patients, the seizures were outgrown before adulthood. The rolandic spikes were present in 17% of 26 fra(X) patients who had an EEG, and patients with these spikes included some with and some without seizures. In two patients with follow up EEGs, the spikes disappeared at a later age, suggesting a benign, age-related effect similar to BRE (Wisniewski et al. 1991). In BRE, the spikes are more commonly present in the sleep EEG than in the awake EEG, as in fra(X) syndrome.

The 14 fra(X) patients in the study by Wisniewski et al. (1991) usually had generalized seizures. In a review of 169 fra(X) males, however, Musumeci et al. (1991) found a high frequency of partial complex seizures. Of 29 patients with seizures, 26 demonstrated partial complex seizures and 14 demonstrated generalized tonic-clonic or grand mal seizures. Of those with partial motor

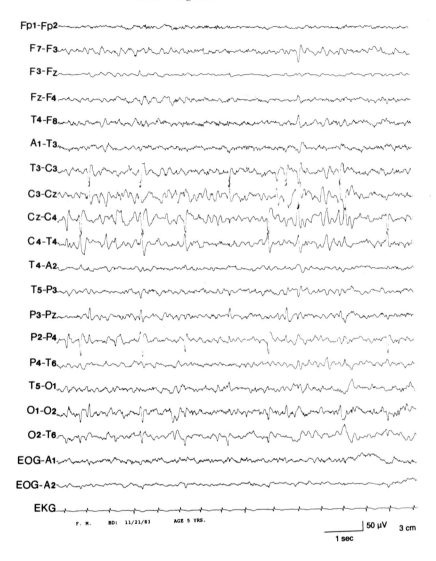

Fp1-Fp2
F7-F3
F3-Fz
Fz-F4
T4-F8
A1-T3
T3-C3
C3-Cz
Cz-C4
C4-T4
T4-A2
T5-P3
P3-Pz
P2-P4
P4-T6
T5-O1
O1-O2
O2-T6
EOG-A1
EOG-A2
EKG

F. M.   BD: 11/21/83   AGE 5 YRS.

50 µV   3 cm
1 sec

seizures, 31% later developed grand mal seizures. Although most seizures were well controlled by anticonvulsants, a few were poorly controlled, and in two cases status epilepticus occurred. In one case, status epilepticus was precipitated by a diphtheria-pertussis-tetanus (DPT) shot that caused fever. In another case, the patient was withdrawn from his anticonvulsants after approximately two seizure-free years, and status epilepticus then occurred. Not all fra(X)

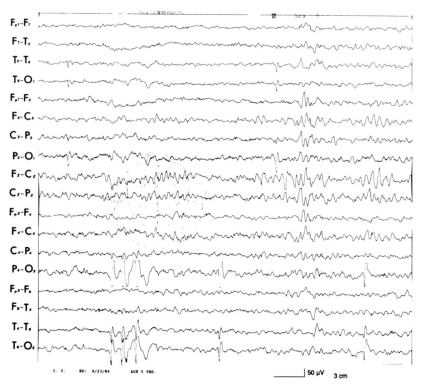

Figure 1.17 *Left,* bilateral asynchronous central-temporal or rolandic spikes with extension to the occipital area on the right in a five-year-old fra(X) boy with complex partial seizures; *right,* asynchronous spike and spike wave discharges in the right occipital area in a young fra(X) boy without seizures.

patients outgrow their seizures, and at least 17% of epileptic fra(X) patients continue to have seizures in adulthood.

The prevalence of seizures in fra(X) males has varied depending on the referral basis for each clinic. Musumeci et al. (1988a) found a rate of 50% (6 of 12 males studied); however, their center specializes in epilepsy and their patient population has an ascertainment bias in favor of epilepsy. Other investigators found seizures in 4 of 27 males (15%) (Brondum-Nielsen et al. 1983), 8 of 61 (13%) (Partington 1984), 4 of 20 (20%) (Harvey et al. 1977), 14 of 62 (23%) (Wisniewski et al. 1991), and 4 of 29 (14%) (Vieregge and Froster-Iskenius 1989). Loesch and Hay (1988) studied seizures in heterozygotes and found them in 7.8% of adults and 5.0% of girls. The overall prevalence of clinical seizures in males is approximately 17%; however, this may be a low estimate. Many individuals may have had one or two episodes of partial complex seizures that were brief and not recognized as seizures because the majority of fra(X) males are not able to accurately describe unusual sensory sensations that are part of complex seizures. On the other hand, Vieregge and Froster-Iskenius (1989) suggested that seizures are not part of the fra(X) syndrome and may instead be nonspecific or linked to other familial forms of epilepsy. The cause of epilepsy in fra(X) syndrome is not known. As previously mentioned, the gene(s) for BRE may be associated with the genetic dysfunction in fra(X) syndrome, but it is not known why the spikes occur. Vieregge and Froster-Iskenius (1989) suggested that the dendritic spine abnormalities observed in fra(X) syndrome may cause excessive neuronal excitation and spiking.

Another possible cause of seizures in fra(X) syndrome relates to the cerebellar vermal deficits in fra(X). The main neurotransmitter from the cerebellum is gamma-aminobutyric acid (GABA), and the pathophysiology of some seizures is dependent on a lack of inhibition from GABA neurons (Christensen and Krogsgaard-Larsen 1984). Perhaps seizures in fra(X) syndrome are a manifestation of a lack of appropriate inhibition secondary to the cerebellar abnormality reported by Reiss et al. (1988b). Bell et al. (1989) cloned a gene for a subunit of the $GABA_A$ receptor which is closely linked to the fragile site at the Xq27.3 region. Perhaps the fra(X) mutation causes dysfunction in this gene either directly or through imprinting, as described by Laird et al. (chapter 7). Although the seizures seem to be related to the fra(X) syndrome, their clinical occurrence may be exacerbated by environmental factors. In our population, many fra(X) patients had their first seizure after a significant stimulus, such as a febrile illness, encephalitis, meningitis, or a DPT vaccination. If the seizures were also associated with brain trauma, such as meningitis, the seizure disorder was likely to be prolonged and not to disappear at puberty.

Neuroanatomic Findings

Only four postmortem neuropathologic studies have been performed on fra(X) males. Dunn et al. (1963) reported findings in a 28-year-old retarded man who died from bronchopneumonia. The family was later identified as being fra(X) positive. This man demonstrated mildly dilated ventricles and islands of small numbers of nerve cells (heterotopia) scattered throughout the subcortical white matter. Heterotopia was also seen in an autopsy performed on a 41-year-old retarded fra(X) man who died of amyotrophic lateral sclerosis (ALS) (Desai et al. 1990). This patient had significant abnormalities associated with ALS including marked neuronal loss and degeneration of the corticospinal tracts. A small olivary heterotopia present beneath the right inferior cerebellar peduncle was unrelated to ALS. Heterotopia has been identified in many other disorders and represents arrested migration of neuronal cells (Musumeci et al. 1985). Dunn et al. (1963) also found marked siderosis of the globus pallidus and loss of myelin in the centrum semiovale and in the pyramidal tracts of the brain stem.

The third postmortem study was performed by Rudelli et al. (1985), who autopsied a 62-year-old fra(X) man with moderate retardation who died from chronic lymphocytic leukemia treated with prednisone. Malformations of the CNS were not present, but a mild degree of atrophy was seen in the frontal and parietal lobes. Rapid Golgi dendritic spine patterns were analyzed from the third and fifth layers of the cortex and the pyramidal layer. The spine morphology was abnormal, with long, thin, tortuous spines; irregular dilatations were also seen in prominent terminal heads. Synaptic vesicle density was normal; however, the synaptic length was reduced, with a resulting mean synaptic contact area that was 35% less than that in controls (Rudelli et al. 1985).

The fourth study, reported by Fryns et al. (1988), was performed on a 3.5-month-old fra(X) child who died from sudden infant death. Microscopic examination showed that all organs, including the brain, were normal.

Neuroimaging procedures have also demonstrated mild ventricular enlargement in approximately 39% of cases, suggesting mild frontal and parietal atrophy (Wisniewski et al. 1991; Fryns 1984). An occasional additional abnormality may relate to factors other than fra(X). One 18-year-old fra(X) male followed in Denver had a history of hypoxia secondary to birth trauma and focal seizures in childhood. His magnetic resonance imaging (MRI) scan demonstrated a cystic area in the basal ganglia, most probably secondary to his birth trauma. Wisniewski et al. (1991) described an arteriovenous malformation in the left temporal area, and Rodewald et al. (1987) reported the occurrence of a malignant ganglioma in a fra(X) male.

Reiss et al. (1988b) described cerebellar abnormalities in four fra(X) males compared to controls on MRI testing with planimetric analysis in the midsagittal plane. They found a significantly decreased size of the posterior cerebellar vermis (fig. 1.18), which is similar to the findings of Courchesne et al. (1987) in autistic males. The vermis has connections with many areas of the brain, including the brain stem reticular formation, pontine vestibular nuclei, thalamus, hypothalamus, limbic system, and cortex. Lesions in the vermis cause abnormalities in behavior activity level, motor control, and social interactions in both animal studies (Bemtson and Schumacher 1980) and human case studies. The vermis seems to be important for modulation of sensory motor integration, which has been postulated to be dysfunctional in autism (Ornitz and Ritvo 1968; Ornitz 1989). Hirst et al. (1991) reported that the gene for a cerebellar degeneration-related protein is tightly linked but on the distal side of the fra(X) locus. Perhaps this gene is partially inactivated in the imprinted form of the fra(X) mutation (chapter 7) and is related to the cerebellar findings. A recent report by Vincent et al. (1991) demonstrated methylation changes at the fragile site in affected individuals but not in carriers, which supports the imprinting theory. Bell et al. (1991) also demonstrated evidence of methylation in

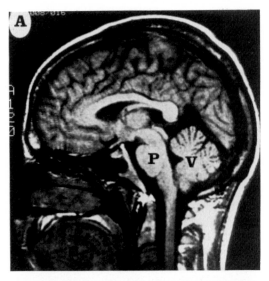

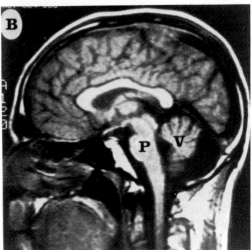

Figure 1.18 *A*, an MRI scan of the brain of a normal male; *B*, an MRI scan of the brain of a fra(X) male. *P* identifies the pons. Note the decrease in size of the posterior cerebellar vermis (*V*). [Reprinted with permission from Reiss et al. (1988b)]

fra(X)-affected individuals, but the extent of methylation did not consistently correlate with clinical involvement.

Further studies by Reiss (1989) found no significant correlation between the severity of autism and the size of the posterior vermis. Reiss (1989) also found the vermal abnormality in a learning-disabled heterozygous female. Reiss et al. (1988b) noted a smaller size of the pons and a larger fourth ventricle in fra(X) patients compared to controls. These findings may be secondary effects of the vermal abnormality. Previous reports of frontal and parietal atrophy on CT or MRI scan may also be secondary to a lack of appropriate vermal connections. Many findings in the cognitive and behavioral area suggest a lack of appropriate inhibition (perhaps from the vermal inhibitory fibers to the frontal area), causing hyperactivity, poor impulse control, tangential speech, and difficulty in making transitions. These findings are usually considered frontal deficits, but perhaps they may arise from faulty connections to the frontal area.

Evoked Potentials

A limited number of studies of evoked potentials have been done. Gillberg et al. (1986) reported that 6 of 7 autistic fra(X) boys demonstrated prolonged transmission times in auditory brain stem responses (ABRs). Wisniewski et al. (1991) found prolonged latencies in waves III–V in 4 of 12 fra(X) patients. Ferri et al. (1988) also found variable prolonged latencies in ABRs and slight but significantly prolonged latencies in visual pattern-evoked potentials in fra(X) males. Arinami et al. (1988) confirmed the ABR findings in 12 fra(X) men compared to controls. For the group data, interpeak latencies were prolonged in fra(X) syndrome for waves III–V but not for waves I–III, suggesting a central rather than a peripheral lesion. Individually, 5 of the 12 fra(X) patients had interpeak latencies longer than 2.5 standard deviations above the control mean. Arinami et al. (1988) postulated that recurrent otitis media, which is common in fra(X) syndrome (Hagerman et al. 1987), may have altered the development of the brain stem portion of the auditory nervous system, as reported in nonfra(X) patients (Folsom et al. 1983). Waves III to V represent the pathway from the superior olivary nucleus (III) to the pontine lateral lemniscus (IV) to the inferior colliculus in the midbrain (V). Slower conduction through the pons relates to the MRI scan results showing a smaller pons, suggesting more global dysfunction in this area. Prolongation of ABRs is more common in white matter diseases, such as leukodystrophies or multiple sclerosis, than in grey matter diseases. This suggests that white matter abnormalities, as reported by Dunn et al. (1963), are significant in some fra(X) patients, although the magnitude of the prolongation is slight in fra(X) syndrome compared to other diseases. Arinami et al. (1988) postulated that minimal prolongation of ABRs in fra(X) syndrome is consistent with synaptic transmission deficits, as reported by Rudelli et al. (1985).

Behavioral Phenotype

The behavior of fra(X) males represents a phenotype that has some rather consistent features and may often be more helpful diagnostically than the physical phenotype. This is particularly true for young fra(X) males, who usually do not demonstrate macroorchidism or a long narrow face. They typically present to their physician in early childhood because they are not speaking in sentences by two years of age and are temperamentally difficult children. Tantrums are frequent problems, and hyperactivity is seen in the majority. Hypotonia, irritability, and perseveration in speech and behavior are usually complicating features. Autistic-like features, such as poor eye contact, hand flapping, and hand biting, are often seen by four or five years of age. The following case history illustrates several typical features.

Case History

P.B. is a five-year-old boy who was diagnosed with the fra(X) syndrome after cytogenetic studies demonstrated the fra(X) chromosome in 29% of his lymphocytes. He was born after a normal pregnancy and full-term delivery, his birth weight was 9 pounds 10 ounces, and he did well during the newborn period. In his early development, he cried frequently, nursed poorly, and had difficulty with lactose intolerance. He rolled over at 6 months, crawled at 14 months, and began walking at 17 months. He was somewhat slow in smiling and cooing, and he was unable to say several words until four years of age. He has had difficulty with hand flapping and rare hand biting, but he more frequently bites his shirt. He has problems with poor eye contact, although this has improved recently. He is fascinated by glass, running water, loud noises, vacuum cleaners, and books. He is particularly interested in sharks and whales.

PB has had frequent otitis media infections, although PE tubes have not been placed. He dislikes many foods and he reacts adversely to the texture of foods so he has failed to thrive in the past. He requires the addition of a liquid protein supplement to maintain weight and growth. He is hypotonic, and his occupational therapist in his developmental preschool program has worked on improving motor coordination and on increasing food tolerance with oral motor stimulation. He has a short attention span, particularly for preacademic work, and a high activity level related to restlessness and impulsivity. In school, he has frequently been noted to laugh abruptly or inappropriately. Perseveration and echolalia have also been problems, and he is receiving speech and language therapy. Cognitive testing using the Kaufman Assessment Battery for Children demonstrates a mental processing composite score of 60, with a significant difference between his sequential processing (56) and simultaneous processing (69) scores.

Physical examination shows that his growth is at the fiftieth percentile for height, weight, and head circumference. His face is mildly narrow with a ptosis involving the left eye and a mild strabismus. His palate is narrow, his cardiac examination is normal, and his extremities demonstrate bilateral single palmar creases and MP joint extension to 80°. Hallucal creases are seen bilaterally, and his feet are not flat. His testicles demonstrate a volume of 3–4 ml bilaterally.

Hyperactivity

Hyperactivity was a notable problem in early reports of fra(X) males (Mattei et al. 1981; Turner et al. 1980) and was further documented in 47% of 17 fra(X) boys by Finnelli et al. (1985). Largo and Schinzel (1985) reported the onset of hyperactivity by two years of age, whereas Fryns (1985) emphasized the disappearance of hyperactivity after puberty. Fryns et al. (1984) reported attentional problems in all 21 fra(X) boys who underwent a detailed psychologic profile. Hyperactivity and attention deficits can be the presenting complaint of even high-functioning fra(X) boys with a borderline or normal IQ (Hagerman et al. 1985). Hyperactivity was documented by a Conners rating score (Conners 1973; Werry et al. 1975) of 15 or higher in 73% of prepubertal fra(X) boys, although all demonstrated concentration difficulties (Hagerman 1987). Bregman et al. (1988) also found attentional or concentration problems in 100% of 14 fra(X) males, although only 71% fulfilled criteria of the *Diagnostic and Statistical Manual*, third edition (DSM III) for attention deficit disorder with hyperactivity (ADHD). The residual state of ADHD was seen in a further 21%, suggesting that many of the older patients had outgrown their hyperactivity, a result similar to the report by Fryns (1985). Borghgraef et al. (1987) also emphasized the improvement with age, in that 80% of young fra(X) boys and 54% of school-aged boys had ADHD. They studied 23 fra(X) males compared to 17 nonfra(X) retarded males and found twice the incidence of hyperactivity in fra(X) males. Although attentional problems are common in mentally retarded populations (Crosby 1972), there seems to be an increased incidence in fra(X) patients at all IQ levels compared to controls.

The cause of ADHD in fra(X) syndrome seems to be related to the neuropsychologic effect of the fra(X) gene. Even mildly affected heterozygotes can demonstrate significant attentional problems, although hyperactivity is less severe than in males. Perhaps the frequent otitis media infections in young fra(X) boys (Hagerman et al. 1987) further exacerbate their predisposition to ADHD. Recurrent otitis media infections during the first three to five years of life have been associated with language deficits, auditory processing problems (Rapin 1979), attentional problems, distractibility (Roberts et al. 1989), and even hyperactivity (Hagerman and Falkenstein 1987) in normal nonfra(X) children. The influences of recurrent otitis media infections on behavior and cognitive development in fra(X) syndrome requires further study; however, such infections should be treated vigorously in fra(X) patients to avoid possible sequelae (see chapter 9).

The presence of ADHD in the majority of prepubertal fra(X) boys has important implications for treatment. ADHD has been successfully treated with stimulants since the 1950s (Bradley 1950), and more recent studies suggest that mildly retarded patients with ADHD can also benefit from stimulants (Gadow and Kalachnik 1981; Gadow 1985; Varley and Trupin 1982). Hagerman et al. (1988b) performed a double-blind crossover trial of methylphenidate, dextroamphetamine, and placebo in 15 prepubertal fra(X) patients with ADHD and found a 75% response rate. A more detailed discussion of stimulants and other drugs used in the treatment of ADHD can be found in chapter 9.

Autism

Several early reports of fra(X) syndrome included cases of autism in males (Meryash et al. 1982; Proops and Webb 1981; Turner et al. 1980), but Brown et al. (1982) pointed out the association between fra(X) syndrome and autism when 5 of 27 (18.5%) fra(X) males were diagnosed with autism. Subsequently, several authors confirmed this report (Levitas et al. 1983; Brondum-Nielsen et al. 1983; August and Lockhart 1984; Kerbeshian et al. 1984; Varley et al. 1985), which stimulated the screening of autistic males for fra(X) syndrome. Table 1.2 summarizes these studies through 1990 and demonstrates an overall prevalence of 6.5 fra(X) males in the autistic population. The smaller studies may show no association, but the larger studies demonstrate a significant prevalence, with a high of 15.7% in Sweden (Blomquist et al. 1985; Fisch et al. 1988).

Variability among studies is probably related to several factors. Autism can be defined by a variety of criteria, although the one most commonly used in the past is DSM III (American Psychiatric Association 1980). The diagnosis in DSM III includes a "pervasive lack of relatedness," which may have a variable interpretation among researchers. Levitas et al. (1983) first suggested that fra(X) patients represent a unique behavioral subgroup in autism because of common features including hyperactivity, perseverative speech, hand biting (fig. 1.19), hand flapping (fig. 1.20), and a higher functioning level in relatedness compared to other autistics. Although social interactional deficits are very common in fra(X) syndrome, a pervasive lack of relatedness is only occasionally present. Table 1.3 documents the number of fra(X) males who fulfill DSM III criteria for infantile autism in comparison to other criteria. The two largest studies by Brown et al. (1986) and Hagerman et al. (1986b) document infantile autism in 16–17% of fra(X) males.

Hagerman et al. (1986b) showed that, within the same group of 50 fra(X) males, the use of different diagnostic tools for autism will yield different results. The Autism Behavior Checklist (ABC) yielded 31% with autism because the diagnosis is dependent on a large number of autistic features involving

Table 1.2

Prevalence of Fragile X in Autistic Males

Author	Diagnostic Criteria	No. with Fra(X)/Total No. of Autistic Males	%
Venter et al. (1984)	Not specified	0/40	0
Goldfine et al. (1984)	DSM III	0/34	0
McGillivray et al. (1986)	DSM III	3/33	10
In Opitz and Sutherland (1984)			
Leckman		0/25	0
Turner		1/70	1.4
Mikkelsen		1/20	5
Chudley		1/16	6.3
White		0/6	0
Jorgensen et al. (1984)	Not specified	1/11	9
Pueschel et al. (1985)	DSM III	0/18	0
Jayakar et al. (1986)	CARS or DSM III	0/20	0
Wright et al. (1986)	DSM III	1/31	3
Watson et al. (1984)	Autism or autistic features	4/76	5.3
Blomquist et al. (1985)	DSM III	13/83	15.7
Mandokoro et al. (1986)	DSM III	2/38	5
Brown et al. (1986)	DSM III	24/183	13.1
Matsuishi et al. (1987)	DSM III	2/39	5
Crowe et al. (1988)	DSM III	2/20	10
Payton et al. (1989)	DSM III	2/85	2.4
Ho et al. (1989)	DSM III	1/41	2.4
Total		**58/889**	**6.5**

Source: Adapted from Brown et al. (1986) and Hagerman (1990).

unusual responses to the environment combined with sensory and communication problems. A similar behavior rating for autism used by Borghgraef et al. (1987) yielded 39% with autism, which again is higher than the 16–17% yield with DSM III criteria. Hagerman et al. (1986b) pointed out that the percentage with autism is not as important an issue as are the autistic features seen among almost all fra(X) patients. Poor eye contact was noted in 90% of fra(X) males (fig. 1.21) and has been a consistent finding in studies comparing fra(X) with other retarded patients (Cohen et al. 1988; Payton et al. 1989). The eye contact difficulty seems to be unique to fra(X) patients when compared to nonfra(X) autistic males. Cohen et al. (1989b) showed that fra(X) males are more sensitive to an adult's initiation of social gaze and demonstrate a subsequent greater aversion to mutual gaze than do nonfra(X) autistics. In addition, Sudhalter et al. (1990) showed that the speech of fra(X) patients demonstrated more persevera-

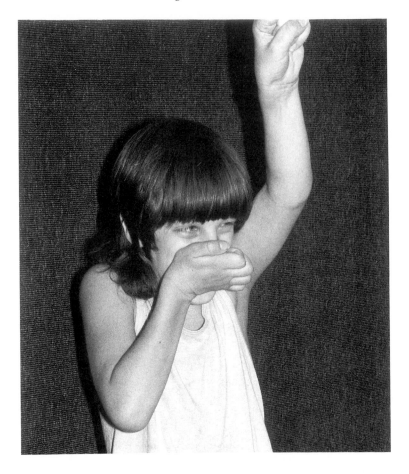

tion of words and phrases and less echolalia than that of nonfra(X) autistic patients and cognitively matched retarded patients. Fra(X) individuals have unique behavioral and language features compared with other groups of retarded or autistic patients.

Fra(X) males usually do not show a disinterest in social interaction but instead demonstrate an approach-withdrawal behavior that is affected by the excessive anxiety that some experience with social contact. Bregman et al. (1988) found that anxiety is a problem for approximately one-third of fra(X) males. Wolff et al. (1989) described the greeting behavior of fra(X) males, which is influenced by anxiety. These patients want to relate, but they demonstrate avoidant behavior by avoiding eye contact and turning their body away from the person they are greeting while they shake hands. This approach-withdrawal behavior or the combination of friendliness and a desire to relate

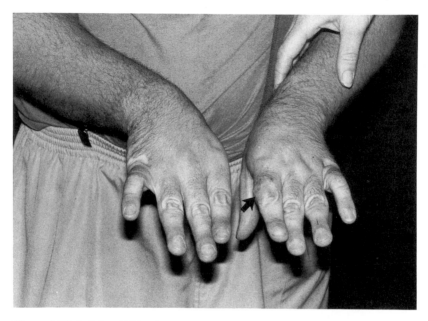

Figure 1.19 *Left,* hand biting in a fra(X) boy; *right,* hand calluses secondary to repetitive hand biting.

with avoidant behaviors and unusual interactional styles has stimulated a significant amount of controversy concerning the association of fra(X) syndrome and autism (Payton et al. 1989; Hagerman 1989; Einfeld et al. 1989; Dykens and Leckman 1990; Hagerman 1991).

It is helpful to clarify the spectrum of autistic features in fra(X) males. The more severely retarded males are most likely to demonstrate a pervasive lack of relatedness and to fulfill DSM III criteria for autism, but this occurs in less than 20% (Borghgraef et al. 1987; Hagerman et al. 1986b). The less retarded fra(X) males, however, still demonstrate a variety of autistic features including perseverative speech, tactile defensiveness, hand mannerisms, poor eye contact, and limited avoidant behavior. The majority fulfill criteria for a pervasive developmental disorder (PDD) using DSM III terminology (Hagerman 1987). See table 1.4 for a summary of behavioral features in fra(X) males.

In 1987, the DSM III-R (American Psychiatric Association 1987) revised the definition of infantile autism to autistic disorder. The DSM III-R lists 16 criteria in three main categories and requires that 8 of these criteria be present to fulfill the diagnosis of autism disorder (table 1.5). A "pervasive lack of relatedness" is replaced by a "qualitative impairment in reciprocal social interaction." The other categories include "impairment in verbal and nonverbal communica-

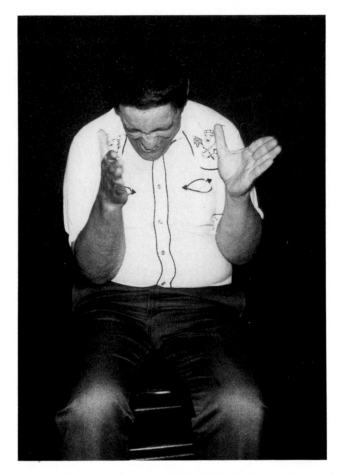

Figure 1.20 Adult fra(X) man demonstrating hand flapping in association with squinting and eye avoidance.

tion" and a "markedly restricted repertoire of activities and interests." The detailed criteria in each category allow further descriptive studies of various subtypes of autism.

Reiss and Freund (1990) evaluated DSM III-R criteria in 17 noninstitutionalized fra(X) males and confirmed the distinct behavioral profile previously reported. Over 50% of the fra(X) males met criteria A4 and A5, although over 80% met criterion B2, mainly because of gaze aversion (table 1.5). Criteria B4 and B5 were met by over half of the fra(X) males because of speech problems, including echolalia and perseveration. Over 80% also met criterion C1 because of stereotyped body movements, and more than half also demonstrated unusual

Table 1.3

Frequency of Autism in Fragile X Males

Author	Diagnostic Criteria	No. with Autism/Total No. of Fra(X) Males	%
Jacobs et al. (1983)		2/9	22.2
Brondum-Neilsen et al. (1983)		9/27	33.3
Rhoads (1984)		3/17	17.6
Fryns et al. (1984)		3/21	14.3
Partington (1984)		3/61	5
Benezech and Noel (1985)	Psychotic & DSM III features	15/28	53.6
Hagerman et al. (1986a)	DSM III	8/50	16
	ABC criteria	15/48	31
Brown et al. (1986)	DSM III	24/150	17.3
Borghgraef et al. (1987)	Autistic behavior	9/23	39
Bregman et al. (1988)	DSM III	1/14	7
Reiss and Freund (1990)	DSM III-R	3/17	18

Source: Adapted from Brown et al. (1986) and Hagerman (1990).

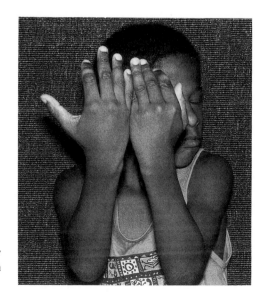

Figure 1.21 A young fra(X) boy covering his eyes in association with eye avoidance.

Table 1.4

Behavioral Features of Fragile (X) Males Seen at The Children's Hospital
in Denver

Feature	No. with feature/ Total No.	% of Patients with Feature
Hand flapping	101/136	74
Hand biting	81/145	56
Tactile defensiveness	66/89	74
Poor eye contact	108/124	87
Hyperactivity	84/128	66
Perseverative speech	80/88	91

Table 1.5

DSM III-R Criteria for Autistic Disorder

A. Qualitative impairment in reciprocal social interaction as manifested by the following:
   1. Marked lack of awareness of the existence or feelings of others
   2. No or abnormal seeking of comfort at times of distress
   3. No or impaired imitation
   4. No or abnormal social play
   5. Gross impairment in ability to make peer friendships
B. Qualitative impairment in verbal and nonverbal communication and in imaginative activity, as manifested by the following:
   1. No mode of communication, such as communicative babbling, facial expression, gesture, mime, or spoken language
   2. Markedly abnormal nonverbal communication, as in the use of eye-to-eye gaze, facial expression, body posture, or gestures to initiate or modulate social interaction
   3. Absence of imaginative activity (such as playacting of adult roles, fantasy characters, or animals), lack of interest in stories about imaginary events
   4. Marked abnormalities in the production of speech, including volume, pitch, stress, rate, rhythm, and intonation
   5. Marked abnormalities in the form or content of speech, including stereotyped and repetitive use of speech; use of "you" when "I" is meant; idiosyncratic use of words or phrases; or frequent irrelevant remarks
   6. Marked impairment in the ability to initiate or sustain a conversation with others, despite adequate speech
C. Markedly restricted repertoire of activities and interests, as manifested by the following:
   1. Stereotyped body movements, e.g., hand flicking or twisting, spinning, head banging, complex whole-body movements
   2. Persistent preoccupation with parts of objects or attachment to unusual objects
   3. Marked distress over changes in trivial aspects of environment
   4. Unreasonable insistence on following routines in precise detail
   5. Markedly restricted range of interests and a preoccupation with one narrow interest
D. Onset during infancy or childhood.

Eight items are necessary for diagnosis, including two from A, one from B, and one from C.

responses to sensory stimuli, item C2. However, most of the fra(X) males did not show a significant impairment in reciprocal interactions with care givers, and those who did improved over time. In contrast to the relationship with care givers, significant problems existed with peer interactions, and this required a more detailed history to document. Only 3 of 17, or 18%, fulfilled full DSM III-R criteria, but 10 of 17, or over half of the study population, fulfilled PDD criteria. Reiss and Freund (1990) did not find a correlation with IQ, and their consistency in the behavioral phenotype supports the theory of a core neurobiologic phenotype caused by the fra(X) gene.

Autism has also been reported in fra(X) females in both mildly and severely retarded cases (Hagerman et al. 1986a; Edwards et al. 1988; Le Couteur et al. 1988; Gillberg et al. 1988; Bolton et al. 1989). Autism is not a common finding in females, but it represents the most severe end of the spectrum of social anxiety and social withdrawal, which are common in even mildly affected heterozygotes. Usually these symptoms present as shyness, which is discussed in more detail below.

Several studies have screened autistic females for fra(X) syndrome, but the numbers have been limited with usually negative results. Cohen et al. (1989a) screened the largest number and found that 12.1% were fra(X) positive (table 1.6). The overall yield for screening autistic females is 4%, which is similar to the frequency in autistic males (table 1.2). The same recommendations concerning cytogenetic testing of mentally retarded or autistic males also apply to females.

Table 1.6
Prevalence of Fragile X in Autistic Females

Author	Diagnostic Criteria	No. with Fra(X)/Total No. of Autistic Females	%
Venter et al. (1984)	Not specified	0/17	0
Jorgensen et al. (1984)	Not specified	0/4	0
Goldfine et al. (1985)	DSM III	0/3	0
Blomquist et al. (1985)	DSM III	0/19	0
Wright et al. (1986)	DSM III	0/9	0
McGillivray et al. (1986)	DSM III	0/8	0
Matsuishi et al. (1987)	DSM III	0/8	0
Cohen et al. (1989a)	DSM III	4/33	12.1
Total		**4/101**	**4**

Source: Adapted from Hagerman (1989).

Stereotypies and Tics

Fra(X) syndrome has been identified in several patients who had previously been diagnosed with Tourette syndrome. Kerbeshian et al. (1984) were the first to report this association in an 11-year-old boy, who developed both simple and complex motor tics in early childhood. Vocal tics included barking, throat clearing, and repetitive swearing or coprolalia. The boy also demonstrated compulsive mannerisms and automatic vocalizations or perseverative statements. This patient had an older brother with fra(X) syndrome and an atypical tic disorder. Hagerman (1987) subsequently reported a 9-year-old boy who was diagnosed with Tourette syndrome and autism before fra(X) syndrome was recognized. He demonstrated both simple and complex motor tics and vocal tics including coprolalia, which was greatly exacerbated when he was placed in a self-contained setting where other children used foul language. In our clinic, another fra(X) boy developed eye-blinking and facial grimacing while taking stimulant medication for his hyperactivity.

Although only an occasional fra(X) patient demonstrates both motor and vocal tics that are simple and typical of Tourette syndrome (TS) patients, there exists a spectrum of TS-related problems in many fra(X) males. Coprolalia, or repetitive bursts of swearing, are rather common in fra(X) syndrome in our experience, particularly when individuals are exposed to foul language in their educational or social environment. There is a propensity to imitate such language, frequently manifested by a burst of pressured speech which is perhaps a complex vocal tic. Other statements previously described as automatic verbalizations, such as "you're to blame" or "let's get out of here," are said in a perseverative, compulsive, and sometimes pressured fashion reminiscent of a complex vocal tic. These statements have also been termed palilalia (Newall et al. 1983) and are thought to be a language deficit. However, the neurologic dysfunction responsible for tics may also contribute to these vocalizations.

Complex stereotypies involving the hands and arms are also similar to complex motor tics exhibited by TS patients. Kano et al. (1988) tried to differentiate the two by pointing out that tics have a spasmodic nature, usually involving the face, and are affected by psychosocial factors, whereas stereotypies do not have these qualities. In our experience, however, complex hand stereotypies, such as hand flapping or other mannerisms (figs. 1.20 and 1.22), can dramatically increase when the fra(X) patient is anxious or afraid. Burd et al. (1987) found that 12 of 59 PDD patients manifested TS and that tic symptoms were frequently misclassified as stereotyped movements.

Obsessive-compulsive behavior is a significant part of TS and is also seen in approximately 20% of first degree relatives (Pauls et al. 1986). Compulsive or ritualistic behavior is also common in fra(X) syndrome, but this has been ascribed to the autistic features in fra(X) (Levitas et al. 1983). Hyperactivity is also common in TS, and a controversy exists as to whether it simply coexists

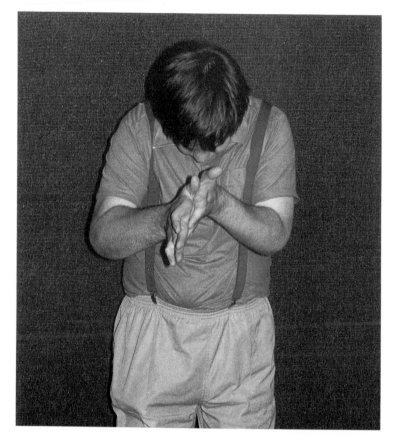

Figure 1.22 A hand mannerism or stereotypy that involves rubbing the hands together

with TS or whether it is etiologically part of TS. There seem to be many similarities between TS and fra(X) syndrome, although the two syndromes have far more differences, including mental retardation. The overlap of findings, however, suggests some similarities in the neurologic dysfunction, probably at a neurochemical level. Tourette syndrome has also been reported in other cases of mental retardation, autism, and Down syndrome (Golden and Greenhill 1981; Barabas et al. 1986; Burd et al. 1987).

Asperger Syndrome

High-functioning fra(X) males, including those with a normal or borderline IQ, have been described (Hagerman et al. 1985; Goldfine et al. 1987; Loesch et al. 1987; Theobald et al. 1987) (see chapter 5). Although a borderline IQ is common in fra(X) boys less than five years old (Hagerman et al. 1985), the usual course of IQ change is down (Lachiewicz et al. 1987; Hagerman et al. 1989; Dykens et al. 1989), so that, in our experience, normal or borderline IQ adult men are infrequent. They usually present as severely learning disabled with attentional deficits, math difficulties, and social withdrawal (Goldfine et al. 1987). These individuals have an interest in relating socially, but they are awkward in interactions and may feel more comfortable when alone. Hagerman (1989) reported the occurrence of Asperger syndrome (Asperger 1944; Wing 1981) in two high-functioning fra(X) men, and one case is described in depth below.

Case History

CD is a 25-year-old man who was diagnosed with fra(X) syndrome when his cytogenetic studies demonstrated 8 of 100 lymphocytes with the fra(X) chromosome. He was diagnosed after his brother was identified with fra(X) syndrome. He was born after a normal pregnancy, and his birth weight was seven pounds. His developmental milestones included crawling at 7 months, walking at 13 months, and riding a tricycle at 3 and a bicycle by 8 years of age. He said words in the first year and complete sentences at 1½ years of age. He was thought to be verbally precocious at that time. He was identified in school as learning disabled because of math deficits and handwriting problems. He received remediation for these deficits, but he was also found to have exceptional strengths in reading and spelling. He continued to receive special education help throughout high school, and after graduation he spent two years at a community college, where he received a humanities degree.

He has been in psychiatric counseling since six years of age, when he was treated for anxiety, hyperactivity, and learning disabilities. He was treated with methylphenidate for approximately five years in early childhood to reduce his hyperactivity. Because of significant social anxiety and unusual behaviors, he was diagnosed as having schizoid personality disorder in late adolescence. He has exhibited mild obsessive-compulsive behavior; for instance, he would insist on lining up his shoes and placing his shoe laces inside each shoe. He is also compulsive about body cleanliness and about cleaning, and he vacuums every other day.

As an adult, he became very interested in religion and joined a monastery. He had difficulty, however, with monastic life, including an aversion to body odor related to infrequent bathing. He left the monastery after several months and subsequently joined the army at age 23. He liked the structure and discipline of the army but had difficulty with the technical aspects of guns and the anxiety they caused. He subsequently left boot camp. At present he works as a volunteer in a community center. He works with a nurturing group of women, and he attends church daily. He is followed by the local mental health center, and he has received a diagnosis of schizophreniform disorder and social phobia in addition to his schizoid personality syndrome. He was hospitalized at 25 years of age for psychiatric treatment because of intermittent delusions and hallucinations in addition to significant anxiety. His anxiety was manifested by constant pacing, agitation, pressured speech, and poor interpersonal judgment. He was treated with thioridazine, 100 mg three times a day. The response was elimination of his hallucinations and delusions and a decrease in his excessive preoccupations of a religious nature. He was subsequently discharged and maintained in outpatient therapy with a continuation of his thioridazine treatment.

His physical examination at age 25 at the time of his diagnosis with fra(X) demonstrated weight in the fortieth percentile for age, height in the fiftieth percentile for age, and head circumference at the ninetieth percentile for age. His face is not dysmorphic, although his ears are very mildly prominent, with the right ear slightly more cupped than the left. His palate is mildly high, and his chest examination is normal. He demonstrates a mild degree of macroorchidism with a testicular volume of 35 ml bilaterally. His MP joints on the right extend to 60°, but on the left they hyperextend to 90°. His cognitive testing using the Weschler Adult Intelligence Scale, Revised (WAIS-R), included a verbal IQ of 93, a performance IQ of 73, and a full-scale IQ of 83. His lowest subtest scores were 2 on arithmetic and 5 on digit span, in contrast to 12 on comprehension and 13 on similarities. In the performance area, the lowest test score was 4 on block design, with a high of 7 on picture arrangement.

This patient is an adult who is mildly affected with fra(X) syndrome and has cognitive abilities within the broad range of normal. His greatest area of deficit is in the social and emotional arena, and he has had difficulty in his adult life maintaining a job and establishing a close or intimate relationship. He is significantly disabled because of his psychiatric problems. This individual has fulfilled the diagnostic features for Asperger syndrome as restated by Gillberg (1985) including (1) inability to relate normally to other people (social isolation); (2) pedantic and perseverative speech; (3) nonverbal communication that is deviant, including reduced facial expression, monotonous intonation and limited or inappropriate gestures; (4) repetitive activities and strong attachment to certain possessions; and (5) clumsy and poorly coordinated gross motor movements. Work can often be overwhelming or overstimulating, and occasional outbursts, both verbal and physical, are seen when frustration or stress is excessive. Long-term intimate relationships are also difficult because of social cognitive deficits. Psychotherapy may be helpful in both of these areas.

Gillberg et al. (1987) screened 14 high-functioning autistic or Asperger syndrome boys and found 4 with fra(X). Although the original description by

Asperger (1944) identified exceptional verbal abilities as a feature of Asperger syndrome (AS), Wing (1981) expanded the diagnostic features to include language deficits. Her description is more typical of fra(X) males. Tourette syndrome has also been described in AS (Kerbeshian and Burd 1986), but there was no mention of fra(X) testing in this report. DeLong and Dwyer (1988) reported a correlation between AS and bipolar affective disease and suggested an etiologic link. This is an intriguing finding in view of the correlation between fra(X) syndrome, depression, and schizotypal features (Reiss et al. 1988a). Also of note in AS is a significant incidence of psychosis. Tantam (1988) reported that 11.7% of 60 males with lifelong social isolation and eccentricity demonstrated psychosis.

Psychosis

Although psychosis is occasionally mentioned as a manifestation of adult fra(X) in men, these features have never been systematically studied. When psychosis was recognized in fra(X) syndrome, most clinicians and researchers ascribed the unusual behavior to autistic-like characteristics. In the past the diagnosis of childhood schizophrenia (DSM II) encompassed autism and psychosis together. Using these criteria, an early study of severely mentally retarded patients in Denmark by Haracopos and Kelstrup (1978) found a high incidence of psychosis, which included bizarre behavior and autistic characteristics. Subsequently, DSM III (American Psychiatric Association 1980) subdivided childhood schizophrenia and identified infantile autism as a separate diagnosis. DSM III-R (1987) further clarified the distinction between autistic disorder and schizophrenia by requiring prominent delusions or hallucinations for schizophrenia (Kendler et al. 1989). Although these features are not typical of fra(X) patients, they can occasionally occur and they are important to recognize because antipsychotic medication can be helpful. It is often difficult to identify delusions or hallucinations among the usual fra(X) behavior, which may include perseverative mumbling, tangential associations, and stereotypies (see previous case history). The psychotic process will usually involve deterioration in life skills and level of functioning; such a history should key the clinician into further investigation (Russell and Tanguay 1981; Petty et al. 1984).

Aggressive Outbursts

Periodic aggressive outbursts have been a problem for approximately 30% of fra(X) men followed in Denver. For a few, aggression is a problem on a daily basis, but for many it is a periodic difficulty that occurs after a reasonable period (weeks to months) of appropriate behavior. The outburst is often precipitated by excessive stimuli in the environment, such that the patient is overwhelmed and cannot maintain control. Fra(X) men may misperceive social approaches or confrontations by others as threatening, and their response is aggressive. Anxiety, tactile defensiveness, and a low frustration tolerance further exacerbate aggressive behavior. The treatment of aggressive or violent outbursts often includes psychotherapy and medication (discussed in chapters 9 and 10).

Nonpenetrant and Not So Nonpenetrant (Mildly Affected) Males

The spectrum of cognitive involvement in fra(X) males is broad and ranges from a normal IQ and learning disabilities to profound mental retardation (see chapter 5). Nonpenetrant males have been identified beginning with the Martin and Bell pedigree (1943) and subsequently documented by many others (Dunn et al. 1963; Fryns 1984; Sherman et al. 1985). Nonpenetrant or transmitting males are typically fra(X) negative and cognitively and physically unaffected. However, the boundary between nonpenetrant males and high-functioning or learning-disabled fra(X) males can sometimes become obscure. For instance, Loesch et al. (1987) studied four large fra(X) pedigrees and carefully evaluated the three living grandfathers, who were considered nonpenetrant, transmitting males. Two of these men were fra(X) positive at 26% and 5%, and all three had a mentally deficient score for the block design subtest of the WAIS-R, although their overall IQ was not assessed. All three men had facial features typical of fra(X) syndrome, including a long narrow face, and two had large prominent ears. Other problems noted were explosive speech, blurred speech, nervous breakdown, and an excitable, impatient personality. These men seemed to be not so nonpenetrant or mildly affected and were similar to learning-disabled fra(X) males.

Learning-disabled fra(X) males with normal IQ and both physical and cognitive features typical of syndrome have been reported (Goldfine et al. 1987; Hagerman et al. 1985; Hagerman et al. 1989). They are usually identified in further work up of a pedigree because they do not present as a proband with mental retardation. Cytogenetic testing should be performed on all males in a fra(X) pedigree with learning problems or suggestive physical features, regardless of a normal IQ. As more individuals with fra(X) syndrome are identified, we will have a better understanding of the number of individuals who fit this high functioning category (see previous case history).

Many authors have reported fra(X)-positive transmitting or nonpenetrant males (Daker et al. 1981; Webb et al. 1986; Voelckel et al. 1988), although cognitive testing was not included in the reports. A thorough cognitive and physical assessment is warranted, with an analysis of behavior features, before one can state that an individual is truly nonpenetrant and unaffected by the fra(X) gene. Nonpenetrant males are usually fra(X) negative, so a cytogenetically expressing male is clearly suspect for at least learning disabilities or emotional/behavioral problems related to the fra(X) gene.

Voelckel et al. (1989) reported a large family with multiple members who express the fragile site at Xq27.3 but do not show any evidence of cognitive or physical impairment from fra(X). This is the only example of a large pedigree demonstrating a dissociation between the expression of the fra(X) gene and mental or physical involvement, although other examples of fra(X)-negative but mentally impaired men in a fra(X)-positive pedigree have been reported (for review, see Nussbaum and Ledbetter 1989). Since the expression of the fragile site is one of many manifestations of the abnormal gene(s), this is theoretically possible if the mutation was altered somewhat.

Heterozygotes

In contrast to the literature on behavioral and emotional problems of fra(X) males, relatively little has been written about the behavioral and emotional difficulties of females affected with the fra(X) syndrome. Although some females seem to be completely unaffected emotionally and cognitively, the range of problems among the affected is broad. Schizophrenic (Hagerman et al. 1983; Fryns et al. 1986) and autistic fra(X) females (Hagerman et al. 1986a; Edwards et al. 1988; Le Couteur et al. 1988; Gillberg et al. 1988; Bolton et al. 1989) have been described, but these cases are rare and represent only one end of the spectrum of involvement. More typically affected fra(X) females are learning disabled or mildly retarded and present with shyness and social anxiety (Hagerman and Sobesky 1989; Cronister et al. 1991a; Borghgraef et al. 1990; Hagerman et al. 1991b). Approximately 30% of school-age fra(X)-positive girls have attention deficit disorder and 60% have poor eye contact (Hagerman et al. 1991b). The emotional problems seem to be related to the neurocognitive deficits, although the subtlest form of the phenotype may be in the emotional area. A limited number of heterozygotes without obvious neurocognitive deficits have complained of social anxiety and panic attacks; however, it is unclear whether this is secondary to the stress of raising a developmentally disabled child or secondary to the fra(X) gene(s).

The work of Reiss et al. (1988a, 1989) has made valuable contributions to our understanding of potential emotional and behavioral difficulties of fra(X) females. Reiss et al. (1988a) studied 38 fra(X) females and 26 adult female controls. On the basis of standardized interviews utilizing Research Diagnostic Criteria (RDC), they found that 34% of the fra(X) females as opposed to 7.7% of the controls met diagnostic criteria for schizotypal features. The most common RDC inclusion criteria met were (1) inadequate rapport due to constricted or inappropriate affect, (2) poor communication, and (3) social isolation, undue social anxiety, or hypersensitivity to criticism. They also found that 39.5% of the fra(X) females met criteria for either intermittent depressive disorder or recurrent/chronic major depressive disorder. Reiss et al. (1988a) found that the overlap between fra(X) subjects with chronic affective disorders and those with schizotypal features was not significant, suggesting two relatively independent groups. Reiss et al. (1988a) did not find that cognitive impairment was related to the incidence of psychopathology within the fra(X) group. Based on a retrospective report, they found a moderate incidence of attention deficit disorder (15.8%), but this was not significantly different from the incidence in controls (11.5%). Additionally, they found that problems in interpersonal relations in adolescence were more prevalent for the fra(X) group than for controls.

In a more recent paper, Reiss et al. (1989) reanalyzed the same data to assess whether fra(X) females who had inherited the condition from their fathers showed a different pattern of emotional or behavioral difficulties than did fra(X) females who inherited the gene from their mothers. This distinction was suggested by Laird in his imprinting hypothesis (chapter 7); that is, females who inherit the gene from a nonpenetrant male, their father, should be unaffected and unimprinted. Reiss found few differences in psychopathology between maternal and paternal inheritance groups. However, when females with positive fragility and maternal inheritance were compared with fra(X)-negative heterozygotes and controls, there was a significant increase in schizotypal features. There was also a trend toward an increased frequency of depression in fra(X)-negative heterozygotes with paternal inheritance.

Hagerman and Sobesky (1989) also described areas of difficulty for affected fra(X) females, which include problems in focusing and attending, tangential thinking, and difficulties with introspection. In the social area, problems including social anxiety, passivity and a sense of helplessness, and extreme social sensitivity were described. In the emotional domain, feelings of isolation, low self-esteem, difficulties experiencing and expressing feelings, and depression were noted. It was found that depression may occur more frequently in less cognitively impaired females. Hagerman and Sobesky (1989) also noted a number of strengths demonstrated by heterozygotes, including creativity, a high energy level, an ability to elicit structure, and an interest in people. Emotional problems often coexist with cognitive deficits, but it is unclear whether they are present without cognitive deficits. In a recent report by Mazzocco et al. (1990), frontal lobe deficits were documented in mildly affected heterozygotes compared to controls. These deficits may be responsible for aspects of the emotional/behavioral phenotype, which includes perseveration and impulsivity.

Differential Diagnosis

Before the diagnosis of fra(X) syndrome is made, many patients have been diagnosed with general terms, such as hyperactivity, autism, nonspecific or X-linked mental retardation, pervasive developmental disorder, learning disability, or emotional impairment. Any child or adult who presents with autism or autistic-like features and/or mental retardation without a specific cause should undergo a cytogenetic evaluation for the fra(X) chromosome, which must also include an assessment of all other chromosomes (see chapter 3). Screening such patients yields a 2–10% positive rate for fra(X) and for other cytogenetic abnormalities (Hagerman et al. 1988a).

Not all hyperactive patients should have cytogenetic testing for fra(X);

Table 1.7
Fragile X Checklist

	Not Present	*Borderline or Present in the Past*	*Definitely Present*
Score:	*0*	*1*	*2*
Mental retardation			
Hyperactivity			
Short attention span			
Tactile defensiveness			
Hand-flapping			
Hand-biting			
Poor eye contact			
Perseverative speech			
Hyperextensible MP joints			
Large or prominent ears			
Large testicles			
Simian crease or Sydney line			
Family history of mental retardation			
Total Score: _____			

however, individuals with additional features typical of PDD, such as poor eye contact, hand flapping, hand biting, or perseverative speech, should be tested. These behavioral features and additional physical features typical of the syndrome have been compiled in a fra(X) checklist (table 1.7), which can be scored similarly to the Apgar score: give 2 points if the feature is present, 1 point if the feature was present in the past or is present to a borderline degree, and no points if the feature is absent (Hagerman 1987). Preliminary studies screening 107 males show that 45% of those with a score of 16 or higher are fra(X) positive and 60% of those with a score of 19 or higher are fra(X) positive (Hagerman et al. 1991a).

Because fra(X) syndrome has been found in those with a previous diagnosis of Soto, Asperger, Prader Willi, and Pierre Robin syndromes, individuals with these diagnoses should be reevaluated for fra(X) syndrome. Other chromosomal disorders, including Down syndrome, Klinefelter syndrome (XXY), and XXX may occur with fra(X) (Brondum-Nielsen 1986; Sutherland and Hecht 1985; Fryns and Van den Berghe 1988; Fuster et al. 1988; Watson et al. 1988), suggesting an increased rate of nondisjunction in heterozygotes. Therefore, individuals with these disorders but with physical and behavioral features typical of fra(X) syndrome should be retested cytogenetically for fra(X).

There are a variety of X-linked disorders with physical features reminiscent of fra(X) syndrome, such as Coffin-Lowry syndrome with prominent ears, coarse features, and hypotonia; Lujan syndrome with marfanoid habitus and macrocephaly; and Atkin syndrome with large ears and macroorchidism. The differential diagnosis is complex, and chapter 6 is devoted to a discussion of X-linked disorders other than fra(X) syndrome. The important point is that cytogenetic testing will differentiate these other syndromes from the fra(X) syndrome.

This work was supported in part by National Institutes of Mental Health Grant MH 45916.

References

Aicardi, J. 1986. *Epilepsy in children: The international review of child neurology.* New York: Raven Press, pp. 119–129.

American Psychiatric Association. 1980. *Diagnostic and statistical manual of mental disorders (DSM III)*, 3rd ed. Washington, D.C., pp. 87–90.

American Psychiatric Association. 1987. *Diagnostic and statistical manual of mental disorders, revised (DSM III R)*, 4th ed. Washington, D.C.

Arinami, T., M. Sato, S. Nakajima, and I. Kondo. 1988. Auditory brain-stem responses in the fragile X syndrome. *Am. J. Hum. Genet.* 43:46–51.

Asperger, H. 1944. Die autistischen psychopathen im kindersalter. *Arch. Psychisbue Nervenkrankh.* 117:76–136.

August, G. J., and L. H. Lockhart. 1984. Familial autism and the fragile X chromosome. *J. Autism Dev. Disord.* 14:197–204.

Barabas, G., B. Wardell, M. Sapiro, et al. 1986. Coincident Down's and Tourette syndromes: Three case reports. *J. Child Neurol.* 1:358–360.

Bell, M. V., J. Bloomfield, M. McKinley, M. N. Patterson, M. G. Darlinson, E. A. Barnard, and K. E. Davies. 1989. Physical linkage of $GABA_A$ receptor subunit gene to the DXS 374 locus in human Xq28. *Am. J. Hum. Genet.* 45:883–889.

Bell, M. V., M. C. Hirst, Y. Nakahori, R. N. MacKinnon, A. Roche, T. J. Flint, P. A. Jacobs, N. Tommerup, L. Tranebjaerg, U. Froster-Is'Kenius, B. Kerr, G. Turner, R. H. Lindenbaum, R. Winter, M. Pembrey, S. Thibodeau, and K. E. Davies. 1991. Physical mapping across the fragile X: Hypermethylation and clinical expression of the fragile X syndrome. *Cell* 64:861–866.

Beemer, F. A., H. Veenema, and J. M. de Pater. 1986. Cerebral gigantism (Sotos syndrome) in two patients with fra X chromosomes. *Am. J. Med. Genet.* 23:221–226.

Bemtson, G. G., and K. M. Schumacher. 1980. Effects of cerebellar lesions on activity, social interactions and other motivated behaviors in the rat. *J. Comp. Physiol. Psychol.* 94:707–717.

Benezech, M., and B. Noel. 1985. Fragile X syndrome and autism. *Clin. Genet.* 28:93.

Berkovitz, G. D., D. P. Wilson, N. J. Carpenter, T. R. Brown, and C. J. Migeon. 1986. Gonadal function in men with the Martin-Bell (fragile-X) syndrome. *Am. J. Med. Genet.* 23:227–239.

Blomquist, M. K., M. Bohman, S. O. Edvinsson, C. Gillberg, K. H. Gustavson, G. Holmgren, and J. Wahlstrom. 1985. Frequency of the fragile X syndrome in infantile autism. A Swedish multicenter study. *Clin. Genet.* 27:113–117.

Bolton, P., M. Rutter, L. Butler, and D. Summers. 1989. Females with autism and the fragile X. *J. Autism Dev. Disord.* 19:473–476.

Borghgraef, M., J. P. Fryns, A. Dielkens, K. Dyck, and H. Van den Berghe. 1987. Fragile (X) syndrome: A study of the psychological profile in 23 prepubertal patients. *Clin. Genet.* 32:179–186.

Borghgraef, M., J. P. Fryns, and H. Van den Berghe. 1990. The female and the fragile X syndrome: Data on clinical and psychological findings in fragile X carriers. *Clin. Genet.* 37:341–346.

Bowen, P., B. Biederman, and K. A. Swallow. 1978. The X-linked syndrome of macroorchidism and mental retardation: Further observations. *Am. J. Med. Genet.* 2:409–414.

Bradley, C. 1950. Benzedrine and dexedrine in the treatment of children's behavior disorders. *Pediatrics* 5:116–121.

Bregman, J. D., J. F. Leckman, and S. I. Ort. 1988. Fragile X syndrome: Genetic predisposition to psychopathology. *J. Autism Dev. Disord.* 18:343–354.

Brondum-Nielsen, K. 1986. Sex chromosome aneuploidy in fragile X carriers. *Am. J. Med. Genet.* 23:537–544.

———. 1988. Growth pattern in boys with fragile X. *Am. J. Med. Genet.* 30:143–147.

Brondum-Nielsen, K., N. Tommerup, H. V. Dyggve, and C. Schou. 1982. Macroorchidism and fragile X in mentally retarded males: Clinical, cytogenetic and some hormonal investigations in mentally retarded males, including two with the fragile site at Xq28, fra (X) (q28). *Hum. Genet.* 61:113–117.

Brondum-Nielsen, K., N. Tommerup, B. Frilis, K. Hjelt, and E. Hippe. 1983. Diagnosis of the fragile X syndrome (Martin-Bell syndrome): Clinical findings in 27 males with the fragile site at Xq28. *J. Ment. Defic. Res.* 27:211–226.

Brown, W. T., E. C. Jenkins, E. Friedman, J. Brooks, K. Wisniewski, S. Raguthu, and J. French. 1982. Autism is associated with the fragile X syndrome. *J. Autism Dev. Disord.* 12:303–308.

Brown, W. T., E. C. Jenkins, I. L. Cohen, G. S. Fisch, E. G. Wolf-Schein, A. Gross, L. Waterhouse, D. Fein, A. Mason-Brothers, E. Ritvo, B. A. Rittenberg, W. Bentley, and S. Castells. 1986. Fragile X and autism: A multicenter survey. *Am. J. Med. Genet.* 23:341–352.

Brown, W. T., E. C. Jenkins, G. Neri, H. Lubs, L. R. Shapiro, K. E. Davies, S. Sherman, R. J. Hagerman, and C. Laird. 1991. Conference report: 4th International Workshop on the Fragile X and X-linked Mental Retardation. *Am. J. Med. Genet.* 38:158–172.

Burd, L., W. W. Fisher, J. Kerbeshian, and M. E. Arnold. 1987. Is development of Tourette disorder a marker for improvement in patients with autism and other pervasive developmental disorders? *J. Am. Acad. Child Psychiatry* 26:162–165.

Butler, M. G., and J. L. Najjar. 1988. Do some patients with fragile X syndrome have precocious puberty? *Am. J. Med. Genet.* 31:779–781.

Butler, M. G., A. Allen, D. Slingh, N. J. Carpenter, and B. D. Hall. 1988. Preliminary communication: Photoanthropometric analysis of individuals with the fragile X syndrome. *Am. J. Med. Genet.* 30:165–168.

Butler, M. G., G. A. Allen, J. L. Haynes, D. N. Singh, M. S. Watson, and W. R. Breg. 1991. Anthropometric comparison of mentally retarded males with and without the fragile X syndrome. *Am. J. Med. Genet.* 38:260–268.

Cantú, J. M., H. E. Scaglia, M. Medina, M. Gonzalez-Diddi, T. Morato, M. E. Moreno, and G. Perez-Palacios. 1976. Inherited congenital normofunctional testicular hyperplasia and mental deficiency. *Hum. Genet.* 33:23–33.

Cantú, J. M., H. E. Scaglia, M. Gonzalez-Diddi, P. Hernandez-Jauregui, T. Morato, M. E. Moreno, J. Giner, A. Alcantar, D. Herrera, and G. Perez-Palacios. 1978. Inherited congenital normofunctional testicular hyperplasia and mental deficiency. A corroborative study. *Hum. Genet.* 41:331–339.

Castro-Magana, M., M. Angulo, A. Canas, A. Sharp, and B. Fuentes. 1988. Hypothalamic-pituitary gonadal axis in boys with primary hypothyroidism and macroorchidism. *J. Pediatr.* 112:397–402.

Christensen, A. V., and P. Krogsgaard-Larsen. 1984. GABA agonists: Molecular and behavioral pharmacology. In R. G. Fariello (ed.), *Neurotransmitters, seizures and epilepsy II*. New York: Raven Press, pp. 109–126.

Chudley, A. E., and R. J. Hagerman. 1987. Fragile X syndrome. *J. Pediatr.* 110:821–831.

Chudley, A. E., J. Knoll, J. W. Gerrard, L. Shepel, E. McGahey, and J. Anderson. 1983. Fragile(X) X-linked mental retardation. I: Relationship between age and intelligence and the frequency of expression of fragile(X)(q28). *Am. J. Med. Genet.* 14:699–712.

Cohen, I. L., G. S. Fisch, E. G. Wolf-Schein, V. Sudhalter, D. Hanson, R. J. Hagerman, E. C. Jenkins, and W. T. Brown. 1988. Social avoidance and repetitive behavior in fragile X males: A controlled study. *Am. J. Ment. Retard.* 92:436–446.

Cohen, I. L., W. T. Brown, E. C. Jenkins, J. H. French, S. Raguthu, E. G. Wolf-Schein,

V. Sudhalter, G. Fisch, and K. Wisniewski. 1989a. Fragile X syndrome in females with autism. Letter to the editor. *Am. J. Genet.* 34:302–303.

Cohen, I.L., P. M. Vietze, V. Sudhalter, E. C. Jenkins, and W. T. Brown. 1989b. Parent-child dyadic gaze patterns in fragile X males and in nonfragile X males with autistic disorder. *J. Child Psychol. Psychiatry* 30:845–856.

Conners, C.K. 1973. Rating scales for use in drug studies with children. *Psychopharmacol. Bull. (special issue)*, pp 24–84, 219–222.

Courchesne, E., J. R. Hesselink, T. L. Jemigan, and R. Young-Courchesne. 1987. Abnormal neuroanatomy in a nonretarded person with autism. *Arch. Neurol.* 44:335–341.

Cronister, A., R. Schreiner, M. Wittenberger, K. Amiri, K. Harris, and R. J. Hagerman. 1991a. The heterozygous fragile X female: Historical, physical, cognitive and cytogenetic features. *Am. J. Med. Genet.* 38:269–274.

Cronister, A., K. Amiri, and R. J. Hagerman. 1991b. Mental impairment in fragile X positive girls. *Am. J. Med. Genet.* 38:503–504.

Crosby, K.G. 1972. Attention and distractability in mentally retarded and intellectually average children. *Am. J. Ment. Defic.* 77:46–53.

Crowe, R. R., L. Y. Tsai, J. C. Murray, S. R. Patil, and J. Quinn. 1988. A study of autism using X chromosome DNA probes. *Biol. Psychol.* 24:473–479.

Cunningham, M., and J. D. Dickerman. 1988. Fragile X syndrome and acute lymphoblastic leukemia. *Cancer* 62:2383–2386.

Daker, M. G., P. Chidiac, C. N. Fear, and A. C. Berry. 1981. Fragile X in a normal male: A cautionary tale. *Lancet* 1:780.

Daniel, W. A., R. A. Feinstein, P. Howard-Peebles, and W. D. Baxley. 1982. Testicular volumes of adolescents. *J. Pediatr.* 101:1010–1012.

Davids, J. R., R. J. Hagerman, and R. E. Eilert. 1990. The orthopaedist and fragile X syndrome. *J. Bone Joint Surg. [Br.]* 72:889–896.

del Pozo, B. C., and P. R. Millard. 1983. Demonstration of the fra(X) in lymphocytes, fibroblasts, and bone marrow in a patient with testicular tumor. *J. Med. Genet.* 20:225–227.

DeLong, R.G., and J. Dwyer. 1988. Correlation of family history with specific autistic subgroups: Asperger's syndrome and bipolar affective disease. *J. Autism Dev. Disord.* 18:593–600.

Desai, H.B., J. Donat, M. H. K. Shokeir, and D. G. Munoz. 1990. Amyotrophic lateral sclerosis in a patient with fragile X syndrome. *Neurology* 40:378–380.

Dunn, H. G., H. Renpenning, J. W. Gerrard, J. R. Miller, T. Tabata, and S. Federoff. 1963. Mental retardation as a sex-linked defect. *Am. J. Ment. Defic.* 67:827–848.

Dykens, E., and J. Leckman. 1990. Developmental issues in fragile X syndrome. In R. M. Hodapp, J. A. Burack, and E. Zigler (eds.), *Issues in the developmental approach to mental retardation*. New York: Cambridge University Press, pp. 226–245.

Dykens, E., R. Hodapp, S. Ort, B. Finucane, L. Shapiro, and J. Leckman. 1989. The trajectory of cognitive development in males with fragile X syndrome. *J. Am. Acad. Child Adolesc. Psychiatry* 28:422–426.

Edwards, D. R., L. D. Keppen, J. D. Ranells, and S. M. Gollin. 1988. Autism in association with fragile X syndrome in females: Implications for diagnosis and treatment. *Neurotoxicology* 9:359–366.

Einfeld, S., H. Molony, and W. Hall. 1989. Autism is not associated with the fragile X syndrome. *Am. J. Med. Genet.* 34:187–193.

Escalante, J. A. 1971. Estudo genetico da deficiencia mental. Ph.D. thesis presented to the University of São Paulo.

Escalante, J. A., H. Grunspun, and O. Frota-Pessoa. 1971. Severe sex-linked mental retardation. *J. Genet. Hum.* 19:137–140.

Farkas, L. G. 1976. Basic morphological data of external genitals in 177 healthy Central European men. *Am. J. Phys. Anthropol.* 34:325–328.

Feingold, M., and W. H. Bossert. 1974. Normal values for selected physical parameters: An aid to syndrome delineation. *Birth Defects* 10:1–15.

Ferri, R., R. M. Colognola, S. Falsone, S. A. Musumeci, M. A. Petrella, S. Sanfilippo, A. Viglianesi, and P. Bergonzi. 1988. Brainstem auditory and visual evoked potentials in subjects with fragile X mental retardation syndrome. In C. Barber and T. Blum (eds.), *Evoked potentials. III: The Third International Evoked Potentials Symposium.* Boston: Butterworths, pp. 167–169.

Finnelli, P. F., S. M. Pueschel, T. Padre-Mendoza, and M. M. O'Brien. 1985. Neurological findings in patients with the fragile X syndrome. *J. Neurol. Neurosurg. Psychiatry* 48:150–153.

Fisch, G. S., I. L. Cohen, E. C. Jenkins, and W. T. Brown. 1988. Screening developmentally disabled male populations for fragile X: The effect of sample size. *Am. J. Med. Genet.* 30:655–663.

Flood, A., and G. Sanner. 1985. Refractive errors in the fragile X syndrome. *Acta Pediatr. Scand.* 74:974.

Folsom, R. C., B. R. Weber, and G. Thompson. 1983. Auditory brainstem responses in children with early recurrent middle ear disease. *Ann. Otol. Rhinol. Laryngol.* 92:249–253.

Fryns, J. P. 1984. The fragile X syndrome: A study of 83 families. *Clin. Genet.* 26:497–528.

———. 1985. X-linked mental retardation. In *Medical genetics: Past, present and future.* New York: Alan R. Liss, pp. 309–319.

———. 1986. The female and the fragile X: A study of 144 obligate female carriers. *Am. J. Med. Genet.* 23:157–169.

———. 1989. X-linked mental retardation and the fragile X syndrome: A clinical approach. In K. Davies (ed.), *The fragile X syndrome.* Oxford: Oxford University Press, pp. 1–39.

Fryns, J. P., and H. Van den Berghe. 1988. The concurrence of Klinefelter syndrome and fragile X syndrome. *Am. J. Med. Genet.* 30:109–113.

Fryns, J. P., J. Jacobs, A. Kleczkowska, and H. Van den Berghe. 1984. The psychological profile of the fragile X syndrome. *Clin. Genet.* 25:131–134.

Fryns, J. P., A. M. Dereymaeker, M. Hoefnagels, P. Volcke, and H. Van den Berghe. 1986. Partial fra(X) phenotype with megalotestes in fra(X) negative patients with acquired lesions of the central nervous system. *Am. J. Med. Genet.* 23:213–219.

Fryns, J. P., M. Haspeslagh, A. M. Dereymaeker, P. Volcke, and H. Van den Berghe. 1987. A peculiar subphenotype in the fra(X) syndrome: Extreme obesity, short stature, stubby hands and feet, diffuse hyperpigmentation. Further evidence of disturbed hypothalamic function in the fra(X) syndrome? *Clin. Genet.* 32:388–392.

Fryns, J. P., P. Moerman, F. Gilis, L. d'Espallier, and H. Van den Berghe. 1988. Suggestively increased incidence of infant death in children of fra(X) positive mothers. *Am. J. Med. Genet.* 30:73–75.

Fuster, C., C. Templado, R. Miro, L. Barrios, and J. Egozcue. 1988. Concurrence of the triple-X syndrome and expression of the fragile site Xq27.3. *Hum. Genet.* 78:293.

Gadow, K. D. 1985. Prevalence of efficacy of stimulant drug use with mentally retarded children and youth. *Psychopharmacol. Bull.* 21:291–303.

Gadow, K. D., and J. Kalachnik. 1981. Prevalence and pattern of drug treatment for behavior and seizure disorders of TMR students. *Am. J. Ment. Defic.* 85:588–595.

Gillberg, C. 1983. Identical triplets with infantile autism and the fragile-X syndrome. *Br. J. Psychiatry* 143:256–260.

———. 1985. Asperger's syndrome and recurrent psychosis—a case study. *J. Autism Dev. Disord.* 15:389–396.

Gillberg, C., and J. Wahlstrom. 1985. Chromosome abnormalities in infantile autism and other childhood psychoses: A population study of 66 cases. *Dev. Med. Child Neurol.* 27:293–304.

Gillberg, C., E. Persson, and J. Wahlstrom. 1986. The autism-fragile X syndrome (AFRAX): A population based study of ten boys. *J. Ment. Defic. Res.* 30:27–39.

Gillberg, C., S. Steffenburg, and G. Jakobsson. 1987. Neurobiological findings in 20 relatively gifted children with Kanner-type autism or Asperger syndrome. *Dev. Med. Child Neurol.* 29:641–649.

Gillberg, C., V. A. Ohlson, J. Wahlstrom, S. Steffenburg, and K. Blix. 1988. Monozygotic female twins with autism and the fragile-X syndrome (AFRAX). *J. Child Psychol. Psychiatry* 29:447–451.

Glesby, M. J., and R. E. Pyeritz. 1989. Association of mitral valve prolapse and systemic abnormalities of connective tissue. *JAMA* 262:523–528.

Golden, G. S., and L. Greenhill. 1981. Tourette syndrome in mentally retarded children. *J. Ment. Retard.* 19:17–19.

Goldfine, P. E., P. M. McPherson, G. A. Heath, V. A. Hardesty, L. J. Beauregard, and B. Gordon. 1985. Association of fragile X syndrome with autism. *Am. J. Psychiatry* 142:108–110.

Goldfine, P. E., P. M. McPherson, V. A. Hardesty, G. A. Heath, L. J. Beauregard, and A. A. Baker. 1987. Fragile-X chromosome associated with primary learning disability. *J. Am. Acad. Child Adolesc. Psychiatry* 26:589–592.

Hagerman, R. J. 1987. Fragile X syndrome. *Curr. Probl. Pediatr.* 17:627–674.

———. 1989. Behavior and treatment of the fragile X syndrome. In K. E. Davies (ed.), *The fragile X syndrome.* New York: Oxford University Press, pp. 56–75.

———. 1990. Chromosomes, genes, and autism. In C. Gillberg (ed.), *Autism—diagnosis and treatment: The state of the art.* New York: Plenum Press, pp. 105–131.

———. 1991. The association between autism and the fragile X syndrome. *Brain Dysfunction.* In press.

Hagerman, R. J., and A. Falkenstein. 1987. The association between recurrent otitis media in infancy and later hyperactivity. *Clin. Pediatr.* 26:253–257.

Hagerman, R. J., and A. C. M. Smith. 1983. The heterozygous female. In R. J. Hagerman and P. McBogg (eds.), *The fragile X syndrome: Diagnosis, biochemistry and intervention.* Dillon, Colo.: Spectra Publishing, pp. 83–94.

Hagerman, R. J., and W. E. Sobesky. 1989. Psychopathology in fragile X syndrome. *Am. J. Orthopsychiatry* 59:142–152.

Hagerman, R. J., A. C. M. Smith, and R. Mariner. 1983. Clinical features of the fragile X syndrome. In R. J. Hagerman and P. McBogg (eds.), *The fragile X syndrome: Diagnosis, biochemistry, and intervention.* Dillon, Colo.: Spectra Publishing, pp. 17–53.

Hagerman, R. J., K. Van Housen, A. C. M. Smith, and L. McGavran. 1984. Consideration of connective tissue dysfunction in the fragile X syndrome. *Am. J. Med. Genet.* 17:111–121.

Hagerman, R. J., M. Kemper, and M. Hudson. 1985. Learning disabilities and attentional problems in boys with the fragile X syndrome. *Am. J. Dis. Child.* 139:674–678.

Hagerman, R. J., A. E. Chudley, J. H. Knoll, A. W. Jackson, M. Kemper, and R. Ahmad. 1986a. Autism in fragile X females. *Am. J. Med. Genet.* 23:375–380.

Hagerman, R. J., A. W. Jackson, A. Levitas, B. Rimland, and M. Braden. 1986b. An analysis of autism in 50 males with the fragile X syndrome. *Am. J. Med. Genet.* 23:359–370.

Hagerman, R. J., D. Altshul-Stark, and P. McBogg. 1987. Recurrent otitis media in boys with the fragile X syndrome. *Am. J. Dis. Child.* 141:184–187.

Hagerman, R. J., R. Berry, A. W. Jackson III, J. Campbell, A. Smith, and L. McGavran. 1988a. Institutional screening for the fragile X syndrome. *Am. J. Dis. Child.* 142:1216–1221.

Hagerman, R. J., M. A. Murphy, and M. D. Wittenberger. 1988b. A controlled trial of stimulant medication in children with the fragile X syndrome. *Am. J. Med. Genet.* 30:377–392.

Hagerman, R. J., R. A. Schreiner, M. B. Kemper, M. D. Wittenberger, B. Zahn, and K. Habicht. 1989. Longitudinal IQ follow-up in fragile X males. *Am. J. Med. Genet.* 33:513–518.

Hagerman, R. J., K. Amiri, and A. Cronister. 1991a. The fragile X checklist. *Am. J. Med. Genet.* 38:283–287.

Hagerman, R. J., C. Jackson, K. Amiri, A. Cronister, M. Wittenberger, R. Schreiner, and W. Sobesky. 1991b. Fragile X girls: Physical and neurocognitive status and outcome. *Pediatrics.* In press.

Haracopos, D., and A. Kelstrup. 1978. Psychotic behavior in children under the institutions for the mentally retarded. *J. Autism Child. Schizo.* 8:1–12.

Hartman, N., R. Kramer, W. T. Brown, and R. B. Devereaux. 1982. Panic disorder in patients with mitral valve prolapse. *Am. J. Psychiatry* 139:669–670.

Harvey, J., C. Judge, and S. Weiner. 1977. Familial X-linked mental retardation with an X chromosome abnormality. *J. Med. Genet.* 14:46–50.

Hirst, M. C., M. V. Bell, R. N. MacKinnon, J. E. V. Watson, D. Callen, G. Sutherland, N. Dahl, M. N. Patterson, C. Schwartz, D. Ledbetter, S. Ledbetter, and K. E. Davies. 1991. Mapping of a cerebellar degeneration related protein and DXS304. *Am. J. Med. Genet.* 38:354–356.

Ho, H. H., and D. K. Kalousek. 1989. Brief report: Fragile X syndrome in autistic boys. *J. Autism Dev. Disord.* 19:343–347.

Hockey, A., and J. Crowhurst. 1988. Early manifestations of the Martin-Bell syndrome based on a series of both sexes from infancy. *Am. J. Med. Genet.* 30:61–71.

Jacobs, P. A., M. Mayer, J. Matsuura, F. Rhoades, and S. C. Yu. 1983. Cytogenetic study of a population of mentally retarded males with special reference to the marker X chromosome. *Hum. Genet.* 63:139–148.

Jayakar, P., A. E. Chudley, M. Ray, J. Evans, J. Perlov, and R. Wand. 1986. Fra(2)(q13) and inv(9) (p11q12) in autism: Causal relationship? *Am. J. Med. Genet.* 23:381–392.

Johannisson, R., H. Rehder, V. Wendt, and E. Schwinger. 1987. Spermatogenesis in two patients with fragile X syndrome. *Hum. Genet.* 76:141–147.

Jorgensen, O. S., K. Brondum-Nielsen, T. Isager, and S. E. Mouridsen. 1984. Fragile X-chromosome among child psychiatric patients with disturbances of language and social relationships. *Acta Psychiatr. Scand.* 70:510–514.

Kano, Y., M. Ohta, Y. Nagai, K. Yokota, and Y. Shimizu. 1988. Tourette's disorder coupled with infantile autism: A prospective study of two boys. *Jpn. J. Psychiatry Neurol.* 42:49–57.

Kendler, K. S., R. L. Spitzer, and J. B. W. Williams. 1989. Psychotic disorders in DSM-III-R. *Am. J. Psychiatry* 146:953–962.

Kerbeshian, J., and L. Burd. 1986. Asperger's syndrome & Tourette syndrome: The case of the pinball wizard. *Br. J. Psychiatry* 148:731–736.

Kerbeshian, J., L. Burd, and J. T. Martsoff. 1984. Fragile X syndrome associated with Tourette symptomatology in a male with moderate mental retardation and autism. *J. Dev. Behav. Pediatr.* 5:201–203.

Knoll, J. H., A. E. Chudley, and J. W. Gerrard. 1984. Fragile(X) X-linked mental retardation. II. Frequency and replication pattern of fragile(X)(q28) in hetero-zygotes. *Am. J. Hum. Genet.* 36:640–645.

Krauss, C. M., N. Turksoy, L. Atkins, C. McLaughlin, L. Brown, and D. C. Page. 1987. Familial premature ovarian failure due to an interstitial deletion of the long arm of the X chromosome. *N. Engl. J. Med.* 317:125–131.

Lachiewicz, A. M., C. Gullion, G. Spiridigliozzi, and A. Aylsworth. 1987. Declining IQs of young males with the fragile X syndrome. *Am. J. Ment. Retard.* 92:272–278.

Lachiewicz, A. M., S. F. Hoegerman, G. Holmgren, E. Holmberg, A. Westerlund, and K. Arinbjarnarson. 1989. Association of the Robin sequence with the fragile X syndrome. Presented at the 4th International Workshop for Fragile X and X-linked Mental Retardation. July 4–9, 1989. New York.

Langenbeck, U., I. Varga, and I. Hansmann. 1988. The predictive value of der-matoglyphic anomalies in the diagnosis of fra X-positive Martin-Bell syndrome (MBS). *Am. J. Med. Genet.* 30:169–175.

Largo, R. H., and A. Schinzel. 1985. Developmental and behavioral disturbances in 13 boys with fragile X syndrome. *Eur. J. Pediatr.* 143:269–275.

Le Couteur, A., M. Rutter, D. Summers, and L. Butler. 1988. Fragile X in female autistic twins. *J. Autism Dev. Disord.* 18:458–460.

Levitas, A., R. J. Hagerman, M. Braden, B. Rimland, P. McBogg, and I. Matus. 1983. Autism and the fragile X syndrome. *J. Dev. Behav. Pediatr.* 4:151–158.

Libb, J. W., A. Dahle, K. Smith, F. P. McCollister, and C. McLain. 1985. Hearing disorder and cognitive function of individuals with Down syndrome. *Am. J. Ment. Defic.* 90:353–356.

Loehr, J. P., D. P. Synhorst, R. R. Wolfe, and R. J. Hagerman. 1986. Aortic root dilatation and mitral valve prolapse in the fragile-X syndrome. *Am. J. Med. Genet.* 23:189–194.

Loesch, D. Z., and D. A. Hay. 1988. Clinical features and reproductive patterns in fragile X female heterozygotes. *J. Med. Genet.* 25:407–414.

Loesch, D. Z., D. A. Hay, G. R. Sutherland, J. Halliday, C. Judge, and G. C. Webb. 1987. Phenotypic variation in male transmitted fragile X: Genetic inferences. *Am. J. Med. Genet.* 27:401–417.

Loesch, D. Z., M. Lafranchi, and D. Scott. 1988. Anthropometry in Martin-Bell syndrome. *Am. J. Med. Genet.* 30:149–164.

Maino, D. M., D. Schlange, J. H. Maino, and B. Caden. 1990. Ocular anomalies in fragile X syndrome. *J. Am. Optom. Assoc.* 61:316–323.

Mandokoro, H., S. Ohdo, T. Sonoda, and K. Ohba. 1986. Frequency of the fragile X syndrome in infantile autism. *Acta Pediatr. Jpn.* 90:719.

Martin, J. P., and J. Bell. 1943. A pedigree of mental defect showing sex-linkage. *J. Neurol. Psychiatry* 6:154–157.

Matsuishi, T., Y. Shiotsuki, N. Nikawa, Y. Katafuchi, E. Otaki, and H. Ando. 1987. Fragile X syndrome in Japanese patients with infantile autism. *Pediatr. Neurol.* 3:284–287.

Mattei, J. F., M. G. Mattei, C. Aumeras, M. Auger, and F. Giraud. 1981. X-linked mental retardation with the fragile X: A study of 15 families. *Hum. Genet.* 59:281–289.

Mazzocco, M. M. M., B. F. Pennington, A. E. Cronister, and R. J. Hagerman. 1990. The neurocognitive phenotype of women with fragile X. Presented at the American Society of Human Genetics, October 1990, Cincinnati, Ohio.

McDermott, A., R. Walters, R. T. Howell, and A. Gardner. 1983. Fragile X-chromosome: Clinical and cytogenetic studies on cases from 7 families. *J. Med. Genet.* 20:169–178.

McGillivray, B. C., D. S. Herbst, F. J. Dill, H. J. Sandercock, and B. Tischler. 1986. Infantile autism: An occasional manifestation of fragile X mental retardation. *Am. J. Med. Genet.* 23:353–358.

Meryash, D. L., L. S. Szymanski, and P. S. Gerald. 1982. Infantile autism associated with the fragile X syndrome. *J. Autism Dev. Disord.* 12:295–301.

Meryash, D. L., C. E. Cronk, B. Sachs, and P. S. Gerald. 1984. An anthropometric study of males with the fragile-X syndrome. *Am. J. Med. Genet.* 17:159–174.

Milone, G., L. Conti, R. Rizzo, S. Sanfilippo, V. Sammito, and C. Romano. 1988. A dermatoglyphic study of a group of Sicilian children with fragile X syndrome. *Am. J. Med. Genet.* 30:177–183.

Moore, P. S. J., A. E. Chudley, and S. D. Winterf. 1990. True precocious puberty in a girl with the fragile X syndrome. *Am. J. Med. Genet.* 37:265–267.

Musumeci, S. A., P. Bergonzi, and G. L. Gigli. 1985. Patologia malformativa come fattore eziopatogenetico dell 'epilessia nel bambino. *Boll. Lega Ital. Epilessia* 51/52:55–57.

Musumeci, S. A., R. Ferri, R. M. Colognola, G. Neri, S. Sanfilippo, and P. Bergonzi. 1988a. Prevalence of a novel epileptogenic EEG pattern in the Martin-Bell syndrome. *Am. J. Med. Genet.* 30:207–212.

Musumeci, S. A., R. M. Colognola, R. Ferri, G. L. Gigli, M. A. Petrella, S. San Filippo, P. Bergonzi, and C. A. Tassinari. 1988b. Fragile-X syndrome: A particular epileptogenic EEG pattern. *Epilepsia* 29:41–47.

Musumeci, S. A., R. Ferri, M. Viglianesi, M. Elia, R. M. Colognola, R. M. Ragusa, and P. Bergonzi. 1989. Cutis verticis gyrata in subjects with chromosomal fragile sites: An occasional observation? Poster presented at the 4th International Workshop for Fragile X and X-linked Mental Retardation. July 4–9, 1989, New York.

Musumeci, S. A., R. J. Hagerman, K. Amiri, and A. Cronister. 1991. Epilepsy, EEG findings and associated complaints in fragile X syndrome. Submitted for publication.

Newell, K., B. Sanborn, and R. Hagerman. 1983. Speech and language dysfunction in the fragile X syndrome. In R. J. Hagerman and P. M. McBogg (eds.), *The fragile X syndrome*. Dillon, Colo.: Spectra Publishing, pp. 175–200.

Nussbaum, R. L., and D. H. Ledbetter. 1989. The fragile X syndrome. In C. Scriver, A. L. Beaudet, W. S. Sly, and D. Valle (eds.), *The metabolic basis of inherited disease,* 6th edition. New York: McGraw-Hill, pp. 327–341.

Opitz, J. M., and G. R. Sutherland. 1984. Conference report: International workshop on the fragile X and X-linked mental retardation. *Am. J. Med. Genet.* 17:5–94.

Opitz, J. M., J. M. Westphal, and A. Daniel. 1984. Discovery of a connective tissue dysplasia in the Martin-Bell syndrome. *Am. J. Med. Genet.* 17:101–109.

Ornitz, E. M. 1989. Autism at the interface between sensory and information processing. In G. Dawson (ed.), *Autism: Nature, diagnosis and treatment*. New York: Guilford Press, pp. 174–207.

Ornitz, E. M. and E. R. Ritvo. 1968. Perceptual inconstancy in early infantile autism. *Arch. Gen. Psychiatry* 18:76–98.

Partington, M. W. 1984. The fragile X syndrome: Preliminary data on growth and development in males. *Am. J. Med. Genet.* 17:175–194.

Pauls, D. L., K. E. Towbin, J. F. Leckman, E. P. Zahner, and D. J. Cohen. 1986. Gilles de la Tourette syndrome and obsessive-compulsive disorder. *Arch. Gen. Psychiatry* 43:1180–1182.

Payton, J. B., M. W. Steele, S. L. Wenger, and N. J. Minshaw. 1989. The fragile X marker and autism in perspective. *J. Am. Acad. Child Adolesc. Psychiatry* 28:417–421.

Petty, L. K., E. M. Ornitz, J. D. Michelman, and E. G. Zimmerman. 1984. Autistic children who become schizophrenic. *Arch. Gen. Psychiatry* 41:129–135.

Phelan, M. C., R. E. Stevenson, J. L. Collins, and H. E. Trent. 1988. Fragile X syndrome and neoplasia. *Am. J. Med. Genet.* 30:77–82.

Prader, A. 1966. Testicular size: Assessment and clinical importance. *Triangle* 7:240–243.

Primrose, D. A., R. El-Matmati, E. Boyd, C. Gosden, and M. Newton. 1986. Prevalence of the fragile X syndrome in an institution for the mentally handicapped. *Br. J. Psychiatry* 148:655–657.

Proops, R., and T. Web. 1981. The fragile X chromosome in the Martin-Bell-

Renpenning syndrome and in males with other forms of familial mental retardation. *J. Med. Genet.* 18:366–373.

Prouty, L. A., R. C. Rogers, R. E. Stevenson, J. H. Dean, K. K. Palmer, R. J. Simensen, G. N. Coston, and C. E. Schwartz. 1988. Fragile X syndrome: Growth development and intellectual function. *Am. J. Med. Genet.* 30:123–142.

Pueschel, S. M., R. Herman, and G. Groden. 1985. Brief report: Screening children with autism for fragile-X syndrome and phenylketonuria. *J. Autism Dev. Disord.* 15:335–338.

Rapin, I. 1979. Conductive hearing loss effects on children's language and scholastic skills: A review of the literature. *Ann. Otol. Rhinol. Laryngol.* 88:3–12.

Reiss, A. L. 1989. Neuroanatomical abnormalities in fragile X syndrome. Presented at the 2nd International Fragile X Conference, April 1989, Denver, Colo.

Reiss, A. L., and L. Freund. 1990. Fragile X syndrome, DSM III-R and autism. *J. Am. Acad. Child Psychiatry.* 29:885–891.

Reiss, A. L., R. J. Hagerman, S. Vinogradov, M. Abrams, and R. J. King. 1988a. Psychiatric disability in female carriers of the fragile X chromosome. *Arch. Gen. Psychiatry* 45:25–30.

Reiss, A. L., S. Patel, A. J. Kumar, and L. Freund. 1988b. Preliminary communication: Neuroanatomical variations of the posterior fossa in men with the fragile X (Martin-Bell) syndrome. *Am. J. Med. Genet.* 31:407–414.

Reiss, A. L., L. Freund, S. Vinogradov, R. Hagerman, and A. Cronister. 1989. Parental inheritance and psychological disability in fragile X females. *Am. J. Hum. Genet.* 45:697–705.

Rhoads F. A. 1984. Fragile-X syndrome in Hawaii: A summary of clinical experience. *Am. J. Med. Genet.* 17:209–214.

Roberts, J. E., M. R. Burchinal, A. M. Collier, C. T. Ramey, M. A. Koch, and F. W. Henderson. 1989. Otitis media in early childhood and cognitive, academic, and classroom performance of the school aged child. *Pediatrics* 83:477–485.

Rocchi, M., N. Archidiacono, A. Rinaldi, G. Filippi, G. Bartolucci, G. S. Fancello, and M. Sininscalo. 1990. Mental retardation in heterozygotes for the fragile-X mutation: Evidence in favor of an X inactivation-dependent effect. *Am. J. Hum. Genet.* 46:738–743.

Rodewald, A., U. Froster-Iskenius, E. Kab, U. Langenbeck, A. Schinzel, A. Schmidt, E. Schwinger, P. Stembech, T. T. Veenema, R. D. Wegner, A. Wirtz, H. Zankl, and M. Zankl. 1986. Dermatoglyphic pecularities in families with X-linked mental retardation and fragile Xq27: A collaborative study. *Clin. Genet.* 30:1–13.

Rodewald, L., D. C. Miller, L. Sciovra, G. Barabas, and M. Lee. 1987. Central nervous system neoplasm in a young man with Martin-Bell syndrome/fra(X) X-linked mental retardation. *Am. J. Med. Genet.* 26:7–12.

Roitman, A., S. Assa, R. Kauli, and Z. Laron. 1980. Prolactin deficiency, obesity and enlarged testes—a new syndrome? *Arch. Dis. Child.* 55:647–649.

Rudelli, R. D., W. T. Brown, and H. M. Wisniewski. 1985. Adult fragile X syndrome. *Acta Neuropathol. (Berl.)* 67:289–295.

Russell, A. T., and P. E. Tanguay. 1981. Mental illness and mental retardation: Cause or coincidence? *Am. J. Ment. Defic.* 85:570–574.

Ruvalcaba, R. H. A., S. A. Myhre, E. C. Roosen-Runge, and J. B. Beckwith. 1977. X-linked mental deficiency megalotestes syndrome. *JAMA* 238:1646–1650.

Sanfilippo, S., R. M. Ragusa, S. Musumeci, and G. Neri. 1986. Fragile X mental retardation: Prevalence in a group of institutionalized patients in Italy and description of a novel EEG pattern. *Am. J. Med. Genet.* 23:589–595.

Saxon, S. A., and E. Witriol. 1976. Down's syndrome and intellectual development. *J. Pediatr. Psychol.* 1:45–47.

Schepis, C., R. Palazzo, R. M. Ragusa, E. Spina, and E. Barletta. 1989. Association of cutis verticis gyrata with fragile X syndrome and fragility of chromosome 12. *Lancet* 2:279.

Schinzel, A., and R. H. Largo. 1985. The fragile X syndrome (Martin-Bell syndrome): Clinical and cytogenetic findings in 16 prepubertal boys and in 4 of their 5 families. *Helv. Paediatr. Acta* 40:133–152.

Shapiro, L. R., P. L. Wilmot, R. A. Omar, M. M. Davidian, and P. N. Chander. 1986. Prenatal onset of macroorchidism in the fragile X syndrome: Significance in prenatal diagnosis. *Am. J. Hum. Genet.* 39:A265.

Sherman, S. L., P. A. Jacobs, N. E. Morton, U. Froster-Iskenius, P. N. Howard-Peebles, K. B. Nielsen, M. W. Partington, G. R. Sutherland, G. Turner, and M. Watson. 1985. Further segregation analysis of the fragile X syndrome with special reference to transmitting males. *Hum. Genet.* 69:289–299.

Simko, A., L. Hornstein, S. Soukup, and N. Bagamery. 1989. Fragile X syndrome: Recognition in young children. *Pediatrics* 83:547–552.

Simpson, N. E. 1986. Dermatoglyphic indices of males with the fragile X syndrome and of the female heterozygotes. *Am. J. Med. Genet.* 23:171–178

Simpson, N. E., B. J. Newman, and M. W. Partington. 1984. Fragile X syndrome: III. Dermatoglyphic studies in males. *Am. J. Med. Genet.* 17:195–207.

Sreeram, N., C. Wren, M. Bhate, P. Robertson, and S. Hunter. 1989. Cardiac abnormalities in the fragile X syndrome. *Br. Heart J.* 61:289–291.

Steinbach, P., H. Veenema, R. D. Wegner, A. Wirtz, H. Zankl, and M. Zanke. 1986. Dermatoglyphic peculiarities in families with X-linked mental retardation and fragile site Xq27: A collaborative study. *Clin. Genet.* 30:1–13.

Storm, R. L., R. De Benito, and C. Ferretti. 1987. Ophthalmologic findings in the fragile X syndrome. *Arch. Ophthalmol.* 105:1099–1102.

Sudhalter, V., I. L. Cohen, W. Silverman, and E. G. Wolf-Schein. 1990. Conversational analyses of males with fragile X, Down syndrome and autism: A comparison of the emergence of deviant language. *Am. J. Ment. Retard.* 94:431–441.

Sutherland, G. R., and F. Hecht. 1985. *Fragile sites on human chromosomes.* New York: Oxford University Press.

Tantam, D. 1988. Lifelong eccentricity and social isolation. *Br. J. Psychiatry* 153:777–782.

Teele, D. W., J. O. Klein, B. Rosner, L. Bratton, G. Fisch, O. R. Mathieu, P. J. Porter, S. G. Starobin, L. D. Tarlin, and R. P. Younes. 1983. Middle ear disease and the practice of pediatrics: Burden during the first five years of life. *JAMA* 249:1026–1029.

Theobald, T. M., D. A. Hay, and C. Judge. 1987. Individual variation and specific cognitive deficits in the fra(X) syndrome. *Am. J. Med. Genet.* 28:1–11.

Turner, G. 1983. Historical overview of X-linked mental retardation. In R. J. Hagerman and P. M. McBogg (eds.), *The fragile X syndrome: Diagnosis, biochemistry and intervention.* Dillon, Colo.: Spectra Publishing, pp. 1–16.

Turner, G., C. Eastman, J. Casey, A. McLeary, P. Procopis, and B. Turner. 1975. X-linked mental retardation associated with macro-orchidism. *J. Med. Genet.* 12:367–371.

Turner, G., R. Till, and A. Daniel. 1978. Marker X chromosomes, mental retardation and macro-orchidism. *N. Engl. J. Med.* 299:1472.

Turner, G., A. Daniel, and M. Frost. 1980. X-linked mental retardation, macroorchidism, and the Xq27 fragile site. *J. Pediatr.* 96:837–841.

Turner, G., J. M. Opitz, W. T. Brown, K. E. Davies, P. A. Jacobs, E. C. Jenkins, M. Mikkelsen, M. W. Partington, and G. R. Sutherland. 1986. Conference report: Second International Workshop on the Fragile X and on X-linked Mental Retardation. *Am. J. Med. Genet.* 23:11–67.

Turner, G., J. M. Opitz, W. T. Brown, K. E. Davies, P. A. Jacobs, E. C. Jenkins, M. Mikkelsen, G. Turner, H. Robinson, S. Laing, and M. Partington. 1989. A clinical score for use in screening for the fragile X syndrome. Poster presented at the 17th Annual Meeting of the Human Genetics Society of Australasia, July 4–7, 1989, Alice Springs, Australia.

Varley, C. K., and E. W. Trupin. 1982. Double blind administration of methylphenidate to mentally retarded children with attention deficit disorder: A preliminary study. *Am. J. Ment. Defic.* 86:560–566.

Varley, C. K., V. A. Holm, and M. O. Eren. 1985. Cognitive and psychiatric variability in 3 brothers with fragile X syndrome. *Dev. Behav. Pediatr.* 6:87–90.

Venter, P. A., J. Op't Hof, D. J. Coetzee, C. A. Van der Walt, and A. E. Retief. 1984. No marker (X) syndrome in autistic children. *Hum. Genet.* 67:107–111.

Vianna-Morgante, A. M., I. Armando, and O. Frota-Pessoa. 1982. Escalante syndrome and the marker X chromosome. *Am. J. Med. Genet.* 12:237–240.

Vieregge, P., and U. Froster-Iskenius. 1989. Clinico-neurological investigations in the fra X form of mental retardation. *J. Neurol.* 236:85–92.

Vincent, A., D. Heitz, C. Petit, C. Kretz, I. Oberlé, J.-L. Mandel. 1991. Abnormal pattern detected in fragile-X patients by pulse-field gel electrophoresis. *Nature* 349:624–626.

Voelckel, M. A., M. G. Mattei, C. N'Guyen, N. Philip, F. Birg, and J. F. Mattei. 1988. Dissociation between mental retardation and fragile site expression in a family with fragile X-linked mental retardation. *Hum. Genet.* 80:375–378.

Voelckel, M. A., N. Philip, C. Piquet, M. C. Pellissier, I. Oberle, F. Birg, M. G. Mattei, and J. F. Mattei. 1989. Study of a family with a fragile site of the X chromosome at Xq27–28 without mental retardation. *Hum. Genet.* 81:353–357.

Waldstein, G., and R. Hagerman. 1988. Aortic hypoplasia and cardiac valvular abnormalities in a boy with fragile X syndrome. *Am. J. Med. Genet.* 30:83–98.

Waldstein, G., G. Mierau, R. Ahmad, S. N. Thibodeau, R. J. Hagerman, and S. Caldwell. 1986. Fragile X syndrome: Skin elastin abnormalities. In E. F. Gilbert and J. M. Opitz (eds.), *Genetic aspects of developmental pathology.* New York: Alan R. Liss, pp. 103–114.

Watson, M. S., J. F. Leckman, B. Annex, W. R. Breg, D. Boles, F. R. Volkmar, D. J.

Cohen, and C. Carter. 1984. Fragile X in a survey of 75 autistic males. Letter to the editor. *N. Engl. J. Med.* 310:1462.

Watson, M. S., W. R. Breg, D. Pauls, W. T. Brown, A. J. Carroll, P. N. Howard-Peebles, D. Meryash, and L. R. Shapiro. 1988. Aneuploidy and the fragile X syndrome. *Am. J. Med. Genet.* 30:115–121.

Webb, T. P., A. Thake, and J. Todd. 1986. Twelve families with fragile Xq27. *J. Med. Genet.* 23:400–406.

Wenstrup, R. J., S. Murad, and S. R. Pinnelli. 1989. Ehlers-Danlos syndrome type VI: Clinical manifestations of collagen lysyl hydroxylase deficiency. *J. Pediatr.* 115:405–409.

Werry, J. S., R. L. Sprague, and M. N. Cohen. 1975. Conners' Teacher Rating Scale for use in drug studies with children: An empirical study. *J. Abnorm. Child Psychol.* 3:217–229.

Wilhelm, P. L., U. Froster-Iskenius, J. Paul, and E. Schwinger. 1988. Fra(X) frequency on the active X-chromosome and phenotype in heterozygous carriers of the fra(X) form of mental retardation. *Am. J. Med. Genet.* 30:407–415.

Wilson, D. P., N. J. Carpenter, and G. Berkovitz. 1988. Thyroid function in men with fragile X-linked MR. *Am. J. Med. Genet.* 31:733–734.

Wing, L. 1981. Asperger's syndrome: A clinical account. *Psychol. Med.* 11:115–129.

Wisniewski, K. E., J. H. French, W. T. Brown, E. C. Jenkins, and C. M. Miezejeski. 1989. The fragile X syndrome and developmental disabilities. In J. French and C. P. Harels (eds.), *Child neurology and developmental disabilities: Selected proceedings of the Fourth International Child Neurology Congress*. Baltimore: Paul H. Brookes Publishing, pp. 11–20.

Wisniewski, K. E., S. M. Segan, C. M. Miezejeski, E. A. Sersen, and R. D. Rudelli. 1991. The fragile X syndrome: Neurological, electrophysiological and neuropathological abnormalities. *Am. J. Med. Genet.* 38:476–480.

Wolff, P. H., J. Gardner, J. J. Paccia, and J. Lappen. 1989. The greeting behavior of fragile X males. *Am. J. Ment. Retard.* 93:406–411.

Wright, H. H., S. R. Young, J. G. Edwards, R. K. Abramson, and J. Duncan. 1986. Fragile X syndrome in a population of autistic children. *J. Am. Acad. Child Psychiatry* 25:641–644.

Zachman, M., A. Prader, H. P. Kind, H. Halliger, and H. Budliger. 1974. Testicular volume during adolescence: Cross sectional and longitudinal studies. *Helv. Paediatr. Acta* 29:61–72.

Zinkus, P. W., M. I. Gottlieb, and M. Shapiro. 1978. Developmental and psychoeducational sequelae of chronic otitis media. *Am. J. Dis. Child.* 132:1100–1104.

CHAPTER 2

Epidemiology

Stephanie Sherman, Ph.D.

Recognition of the Fragile X or Martin-Bell Syndrome

It has long been known that there is a large preponderance of males among mentally retarded people. In 1897, Johnson briefly mentioned that there were 24% more retarded males than females according to the U.S. census figures but gave no explanation for this excess. In 1938, Penrose noted the high male:female ratio in the Colchester survey of institutionalized individuals and suggested that the male majority was due to biases in ascertainment. Males were more often identified as mentally retarded because of the higher expectation for males than for females, and males exhibited aggressive behavior more often than females and therefore were more likely to be institutionalized. No genetic explanation for the excess of males was considered at this time or for many years. Lehrke, in his Ph.D. thesis written in 1969, was the first to argue persuasively that the preponderance of mentally retarded males was due to X-linked genes and that X-linked mental retardation (XLMR) may be responsible for a large proportion of mental retardation (MR). He suggested that the contribution of XLMR had gone largely unnoticed because of the lack of obvious clinical symptoms (Lehrke 1974).

In 1971, Turner et al. suggested that XLMR in individuals with no other clinical signs should be considered a distinct diagnostic category. They suggested that one of the earliest XLMR pedigrees published by Martin and Bell (1943) as well as others (Renpenning et al. 1962; Dunn et al. 1963; Losowsky 1961; Snyder and Robinson 1969) fit into this category. Thus, by the mid-1970s, the importance of nonspecific XLMR had been recognized but it was appreciated that this group was etiologically heterogeneous.

In 1969, Lubs reported a unique cytogenetic marker on the X chromosome which was seen in four retarded males in a family with XLMR. However, this was thought to be an isolated finding and was not considered relevant to the diagnosis of XLMR. It was not until 1973 that a second XLMR family with a cytogenetic marker was reported, but the report was written in Portuguese and published in Brazil (Escalante and Frota-Pessoa 1973) and, unfortunately, largely went unnoticed. However, by the late 1970s, it was realized that non-specific XLMR associated with a cytogenetic marker located on the end of the long arm of the X chromosome was not uncommon (Giraud et al. 1976; Harvey et al. 1977) and, moreover, that the cytogenetic marker may be a useful diagnostic tool. Confirmation of the original observation was delayed primarily because expression of the marker depends on culturing cells under particular conditions. In 1977, Sutherland showed that the cell medium must be deficient in folic acid or thymidine to stimulate expression. This marker is now known as the fragile X site (fra[X] site) because of its appearance as a gap or break in the chromosome arm.

Macroorchidism was shown to be associated with some forms of XLMR in 1971 by Escalante et al. and subsequently by others (Turner et al. 1975; Cantú et al. 1976). Endocrine and germinal functions of the large testes were shown to be normal (Ruvalcaba et al. 1977). In 1978, Turner et al. showed that macroorchidism was also associated with some XLMR families segregating for the cytogenetic marker.

Finally, the pedigree originally published by Martin and Bell (1943) was reevaluated by Richards and Webb (1982) and found to show both macroorchidism and the cytogenetic marker on the X chromosome. In recognition of the first published pedigree, XLMR associated with the X chromosome cytogenetic marker was named the Martin-Bell syndrome. It is also referred to as the fragile X syndrome because of its association with a unique cytogenetic marker, the fra(X) site.

A Brief Description of the Fra(X) Site as a Diagnostic Marker

The fra(X) site is one of many fragile sites observed in human chromosomes when cells are cultured under certain conditions. The sites appear as an unstained gap or break at a defined point on a chromosome and are inherited in a mendelian fashion. The fra(X) site, located at Xq27.3, is expressed only under conditions of pyrimidine deficiency.

In general, the presence of the fra(X) site seems to be an excellent marker for fra(X)-related MR in males and a relatively good one for fra(X)-related MR in females (Jacobs and Sherman 1985). Although the proportion of fra(X)-positive cells rarely exceeds 50%, there is considerable variation in the expression of the fra(X) site among affected individuals. Much of this variation is due to technical factors within the laboratory. However, other factors may influence fra(X) expression and account for this variability. First, the frequency of fra(X)-positive cells seems to be somewhat characteristic of an individual. Genetic factors have been shown to play a small role in determining the proportion of positive cells in families; however, variation caused by technical factors is far more significant (Fisch et al. 1991). Second, age at testing affects the frequency of fra(X)-positive cells in carrier females. Briefly, the frequency of positive cells in intellectually normal female carriers seems to decrease with age. Third, the level of I.Q. seems to be inversely correlated with the frequency of fra(X)-positive cells (Sherman et al. 1984; Chudley et al. 1983). However, Cronister et al. (1991) found no correlation among females with greater than 2% fragility. In general, it can be said that mentally impaired heterozygotes are more likely to demonstrate the fra(X) site than are normally functioning heterozygotes.

Epidemiology

The goal of an epidemiologic study is to obtain an accurate estimate of the prevalence of the fra(X) syndrome and, hence, the gene frequency. Unfortunately, it is impossible to estimate the prevalence directly because identification of all carriers with the fra(X) mutation is not possible. Thus, different approaches have been taken to estimate indirectly the contribution of the fra(X) syndrome to XLMR. Some have estimated the proportion of XLMR that is due to the fra(X) syndrome by screening mentally retarded populations for the fra(X) syndrome. Others have screened populations with particular characteristics such as autism, macroorchidism, or a specific level of MR to determine the contribution of the fra(X) syndrome to morbidity.

Prevalence Studies

The Prevalence of Nonspecific X-linked Mental Retardation

Nonspecific XLMR accounts for a significant proportion of retarded males in the population. The measurement of this proportion or a direct measurement of the population frequency of XLMR is impossible because the feature that distinguishes XLMR from nonspecific MR, the pattern of inheritance, is not always revealed in small families. Therefore, XLMR cannot be completely separated from the heterogeneous group of nonspecific MR. One indirect way to measure the frequency of XLMR is to identify families with two or more affected sibs, as multiple affected sibs are an indication of a genetic cause. Then, the number of affected brother pairs is compared to the number of affected sister pairs and the excess of brother pairs is assumed to be due to X-linked genes. Most studies have shown a 2:1 ratio of male:female affected sib pairs (Wright et al. 1959; Priest et al. 1961; Wortis et al. 1966; Davison 1973). Using this same strategy in a population-based study in New South Wales, Australia, Turner and Turner (1974) found that the prevalence of carrier females of X-linked moderate MR (IQ between 30 and 55) was 0.74/1000. If it is assumed that XLMR is due to an X-linked recessive lethal gene, these data suggest that the frequency of males with moderate MR due to X-linked genes is 0.55/1000. (For specific calculations, see Turner and Turner 1974.) The authors concluded that approximately 20% of the moderate retardation in males was due to X-linked genes.

Herbst and Miller (1980) did a similar study in British Columbia, Canada, during a 20-year period and included all types of nonspecific MR. They found that the prevalence of carrier females was 2.44/1000, which suggests that the prevalence of affected males due to X-linked genes is about 1.83/1000. Two reasons for the higher prevalence in the British Columbia study may be considered: individuals ascertained included those with all levels of MR who were either dead or alive at the time of study, whereas those ascertained in the New South Wales study included only moderately retarded individuals who were living at the time of the study. Given a prevalence of XLMR between 0.55/1000 and 1.83/1000 in males, the number of X-linked genes involved in the etiology of MR may be estimated under the following assumptions: (1) the average mutation rate is between 3 and 9×10^{-5} per locus and (2) the reproductive ability in affected males is zero and in carrier females is 100%. Under these assumptions, it is estimated that 7–19 X-linked genes may cause nonspecific MR. Morton et al. (1977), using a different approach, estimated that approximately 18 X-linked genes cause nonspecific XLMR, a result similar to those in the above two studies.

The Prevalence of the Fra(X) Syndrome

Once the fra(X) syndrome could be distinguished from the heterogeneous group of nonspecific XLMR, it was possible to estimate the disease frequency of this particular type of XLMR. To date, however, complete ascertainment of all carriers with the fra(X) site in a defined geographic area has not been attempted in large part because the requisite cytogenetic testing is extremely labor intensive. In addition, only a proportion of gene carriers express the fra(X) site; approximately 44% of female carriers and 20% of male carriers show no obvious MR and are fra(X) negative. Thus, a more accurate marker and one that is more efficient must be available before extensive population screening is feasible. Because of these complications, other strategies have been used to obtain estimates of the prevalence of the fra(X) syndrome.

The earliest estimate of prevalence was extrapolated from data obtained from the affected brothers study of Herbst and Miller (1980). Based on literature at that time (Turner et al. 1980b; Howard-Peebles and Stoddard 1980; Jacobs et al. 1979, 1980), Herbst and Miller assumed that approximately 50% of XLMR was due to the fra(X) mutation; thus, they estimated the prevalence of the fra(X) syndrome in males to be one-half of 1.83/1000, or 0.92/1000 male births.

A more direct approach was taken by Fishburn et al. (1983). They reexamined the moderately retarded brother pairs ascertained in the study of Turner and Turner (1974) for the fra(X) site and macroorchidism. They estimated the prevalence of the fra(X) syndrome to be 0.19/1000 male births, the prevalence of XLMR and macroorchidism and no fra(X) to be 0.09/1000, and the prevalence of other forms of XLMR to be 0.28/1000. Thus, approximately one-third of moderate XLMR was due to the fra(X) syndrome.

Table 2.1 shows the estimates of prevalence of fra(X)-related MR obtained from four studies that attempted to ascertain all individuals with the fra(X) syndrome in a defined population. In each, mentally retarded individuals were identified and screened for the presence of the fra(X) site and prevalence figures were then estimated on the basis of vital statistics. The two Scandinavian studies were based on registries, whereas the other two studies were based on screening of school-aged children.

In 1977, Gustavson et al. studied an unselected series of children with an IQ of less than 50 in a northern Swedish county born between 1959 and 1970 and found the prevalence of moderate to severe MR to be 3.5/1000. In this same population, Blomquist et al. (1981) found the prevalence of mild retardation (IQ between 50 and 69) to be 3.8/1000. Later, this population was screened for the fra(X) mutation, and 7.3% of severe to moderately retarded males and 4.5% of mildly retarded males were fra(X) positive (Blomquist et al. 1982, 1983). Extrapolating to the total population, Gustavson et al. (1986) estimated that the prevalence of fra(X)-related MR in males was 0.6/1000 in this Swedish county.

Kähkönen et al. (1987) studied the fra(X) mutation in the province of Kuopio in Finland by screening MR individuals identified through a registry and through achievement tests in normal schools. They found that 8.7% of severely retarded males and no severely retarded females had the fra(X) syndrome and that none of the mildly retarded males and 5.4% of the mildly retarded females had the fra(X) mutation. Overall, they estimated the prevalence to be 0.8/1000 and 0.4/1000 in males and females, respectively.

Turner et al. (1986) surveyed one area of Sydney, Australia, to evaluate the potential public health applications of cytogenetic screening for the fra(X) syndrome among mentally impaired individuals. They found a prevalence of 0.4/1000 in males and 0.2/1000 in females.

Webb et al. (1986) surveyed schools for the educationally subnormal including children between the ages of 11 and 16 in the County of Coventry in the United Kingdom. The prevalence of the fra(X) mutation was 0.7/1000 in males and almost the same in females, 0.6/1000.

Sutherland (1982, 1985) examined a series of unselected neonates for the

Table 2.1
Prevalence of Fragile (X) Syndrome Obtained from Population-Based Studies

Country Studied	Population Size	No. Studied	Prevalence	% of Fra(X) Individuals		Reference
				Severely Mentally Retarded	Mildly Mentally Retarded	
Males						
Sweden	40,871[a]	89	0.6/1000	7.3	4.5	Gustavson et al. 1986
Finland	6,594	61	0.8/1000	8.7	0	Kähkönen et al. 1987
Australia	58,094	472	0.4/1000	2.6	1.0	Turner et al. 1986
United Kingdom	28,611	219	0.7/1000	4.4	3.2	Webb et al. 1986
Females						
Finland	6,288	50	0.4/1000	0	5.4	Kähkönen et al. 1987
Australia	54,641	203	0.2/1000	1.0	2.9	Turner et al. 1986
United Kingdom	26,945	128	0.6/1000	3.2	5.2	Webb et al. 1986

[a]Includes both males and females.

fra(X) syndrome and did not find fra(X) expression in 1810 males nor 1648 females. If it is assumed that the prevalence of fra(X) is approximately 0.6/1000 male births, or 1/1667, and approximately 0.4/1000 female births, or 1/2500, it is not surprising that fra(X) individuals were not identified in this relatively small sample.

Based on the above studies, prevalence estimates of the fra(X) syndrome in a predominantly Caucasian population range from 0.4/1000 to 0.8/1000 in males and from 0.2/1000 to 0.6/1000 in females. These numbers are underestimates because they are based on screening of individuals with overt MR and do not include those with borderline or nearly normal intelligence. Nevertheless, these values make it clear that the fra(X) syndrome is the most common inherited cause of mental retardation and, after trisomy 21, the most common identified cause of mental retardation.

The Frequency of the Fra(X) Syndrome in Selected Populations

Tables 2.2 and 2.3 summarize studies that have estimated the proportion of fra(X) cases among males and females, respectively, in populations selected using various criteria. These studies are usually based on surveys of institutions, sheltered workshops, or special schools. Comparison of estimates among studies is difficult, and figures must be interpreted with caution for two reasons. First, the selection is not always well defined in each study and cannot always be followed precisely. Furthermore, it is likely that institutions and workshops differ in the proportion of individuals with severe and mild MR in the various populations. Second, surveys of institutionalized populations are difficult to interpret because each society has a different policy of institutionalization of mentally impaired individuals. Thus, these data cannot be used to estimate the prevalence of the fra(X) syndrome, but they can be used to measure the contribution of the fra(X) syndrome to morbidity. A representative study from each section of the tables is discussed to provide a better description of each selected population.

Unselected Retarded Individuals

In these studies, all individuals with MR were studied cytogenetically irrespective of clinical features or etiology. The wide range of frequencies is due, in part, to the variation in the size of the population studied. The studies done in Hawaii are reviewed as they are community based. Proops et al. (1983) studied 81 mentally retarded school-aged children and found 0/54 males and 4/27 (14.8%) females with the fra(X) syndrome, giving an overall rate of 4.9%. Later, Jacobs et al. (1986a) reported a study of three further populations in Hawaii: individuals in community placement, those in day care facilities, and those in special education schools. The frequencies were similar in all three

Table 2.2
Frequencies of Fragile (X) Syndrome in Male Populations

Selection Criteria	Population Base	Area Studied	Population Size	% of Fra(X) Cases	Reference
Unselected retarded males					
	Institution	Germany	242	6.2	Froster-Iskenius et al. 1983
	Institution	Finland	150	4.0	Kähkönen et al. 1983
	Institution	Taiwan	219	3.6	Li et al. 1988
	Institution	United States	65	9.2	Carpenter et al. 1982
	Institution[a]	United States	267	2.6	Hagerman et al. 1988
	Institution	United Kingdom	512	5.9	English et al. 1989
	Institution	Australia	444	1.6	Sutherland 1982
	Institution	Italy	91	4.4	Sanfilippo et al. 1986
	Sheltered workshop	Australia	127	11.0	Turner et al. 1986
	Sheltered workshop	Australia	84	0	Sutherland 1985
	Community	Hawaii	376	1.9	Jacobs et al. 1986a
	Special schools	Hawaii	54	0	Proops et al. 1983
	Special schools	Australia	328	3.4	Sutherland 1985
	Referred mentally retarded[b]	Australia	1012	3.1	Voullaire et al. 1989
Major congenital anomalies/dysmorphic					
Normal	Institution	Belgium	354	16.1	Fryns et al. 1984
	Institution	Finland	68	8.8	Kähkönen et al. 1983
	Institution	United States	44	13.6	Paika et al. 1984
	Institution	Canada	818	4.0	Kirkilionis et al. 1983
	Institution	United Kingdom	100	7.0	Primrose et al. 1986
	Referred mentally retarded[b]	Australia	892	3.0	Voullaire et al. 1989

			Country	N	%	Reference
Abnormal		Institution[c]	Finland	82	0	Kähkönen et al. 1983
		Referred mentally retarded[b]	Australia	120	3.3	Voullaire et al. 1989
Intellectual impairment						
Severe	(IQ < 50)	Institution	United Kingdom	22	0	Kinnell and Banu 1983
		Institution	Belgium	3	0	Dereymaeker et al. 1988
		Institution	Belgium	36	5.0	Fryns et al. 1986
		Institution	Japan	53	1.9	Aoi et al. 1989
		Institution	Japan	243	5.3	Arinami et al. 1986
Mild/Dull		Institution	United Kingdom	42	0	Kinnell and Banu 1983
	(IQ ≥ 50)	Special Schools	United Kingdom	155	6.5	Thake et al. 1987
		Special Schools	United Kingdom	96	0	Lamont et al. 1986
Testes size						
Macroorchidism		Institution	United States	23	43.5	Shapiro et al. 1983
		Institution	United States	18	38.9	Howard-Peebles and Finley 1983
		Institution	United States	5	80.0	Brown et al. 1981
		Institution[a]	United States	36	16.7	Hagerman et al. 1988
		Institution	Canada	167	11.0	Kirkilionis et al. 1983
		Institution	Denmark	52	3.8	Nielsen et al. 1982
Microorchidism		Institution	Canada	421	1.3	Kirkilionis et al. 1983
Normal testes size		Institution	Canada	230	1.8	Kirkilionis et al. 1983
Autism			United States	183	13.1	Brown et al. 1986b
			Canada	16	6.3	Chudley[d]
			United States	37	0	Goldfine et al. 1985
			Sweden	20	20.0	Gillberg et al. 1987
			United States	25	0	Leckman[d]

(continued)

77

Table 2.2 (*Continued*)

Selection Criteria	Population Base	Area Studied	Population Size	% of Fra(X) Cases	Reference
		Japan	39	5.1	Matsuishi et al. 1987
		United States	40	7.5	McGillivray et al. 1984
		Denmark	20	5.0	Mikkelsen[a]
		United States	85	2.4	Payton et al. 1989
		United States	18	0	Pueschel et al. 1985
		Denmark	20	10.0	Tranebjaerg and Kure 1991
		Australia	70	1.4	Turner[a]
		South Africa	40	0	Venter et al. 1984
		Sweden	101	15.8	Wahlstrom et al. 1986
		United States	76	5.3	Watson et al. 1984
		United States	6	0	White[a]
Family history					
Positive	Institution	Germany	18	38.8	Froster-Iskenius et al. 1983
	Institution	United States	36	13.9	Carpenter et al. 1982
Negative	Institution	Germany	224	3.6	Froster-Iskenius et al. 1983
	Institution	United States	29	3.4	Carpenter et al. 1982

[a] Patients with known etiology of mental retardation (MR) were excluded.
[b] Patients with developmental disabilities referred to a cytogenetic laboratory; includes both males and females.
[c] Abnormal includes dysmorphic features, neurologic symptoms, and childhood psychoses.
[d] Data from Opitz and Sutherland 1984.

Table 2.3

Frequencies of Fragile (X) Syndrome in Female Populations

Selection Criteria	Population Base	Area Studied	Population Size	% of Fra(X) Cases	Reference
Unselected retarded females					
	Institution	Australia	80	0	Sutherland 1982
	Institution	Taiwan	122	4.1	Li et al. 1988
	Institution[a]	United States	173	2.3	Hagerman et al. 1988
	Community	Hawaii	350	0.3	Jacobs et al. 1986a
	Special schools	Hawaii	27	14.8	Proops et al. 1983
	Special schools	Australia	174	1.1	Sutherland 1985
	Sheltered workshop	Australia	119	1.0	Turner et al. 1986
	Sheltered workshop	Australia	44	0	Sutherland 1985
Major congenital anomalies/dysmorphic					
Normal	Institution	Belgium	30	3.3	Fryns et al. 1984
	Special schools[b]	Australia	72	6.9	Turner et al. 1980b
	Special schools[b]	United Kingdom	104	9.6	Thake et al. 1987
Abnormal	Special schools[b]	Australia	55	0	Turner et al. 1980b
Intellectual impairment					
Severe (IQ < 50)	Institution	Japan	190	1.1	Arinami et al. 1987
	Institution	Belgium	10	0	Dereymaeker et al. 1988
Mild/Dull (IQ ≥ 50)	Special schools	Australia	128	3.9	Turner et al. 1980b
	Special schools	United Kingdom	70	0	Lamont et al. 1986

[a]Patients with known etiology of mental retardation were excluded.
[b]Clinically normal and mildly retarded.

populations: 5/274, 2/71, and 1/71 fra(X) males, respectively, and 1/278, 0/85, and 0/43 fra(X) females, respectively. These give overall rates of 1.9% fra(X) males and 0.3% fra(X) females after multiple ascertainments are removed.

Major Congenital Anomalies and Malformations

In general, most studies find that the frequency of fra(X) cases is higher in mentally retarded populations with no obvious congenital anomalies or malformations. Voullaire et al. (1989) found that 3.1% of the patients referred for cytogenetic studies because of developmental disabilities were fra(X) positive. Before the cytogenetic study, patients were separated based on the presence of multiple congenital anomalies. The frequency of fra(X) cases among those without anomalies was 3.0% (27/892) and among those with anomalies was 3.3% (4/120). However, when the four cases with anomalies were reassessed clinically, they were found either not to be dysmorphic or to have only minor facial anomalies.

In a study of 150 mentally retarded institutionalized males, Kähkönen et al. (1983) separated males into four groups: those with dysmorphic features ($N = 18$), with neurologic symptoms ($N = 46$), with childhood psychosis ($N = 18$), and with no clinical signs ($N = 68$). They identified six fra(X) cases, and all fell into the last category, resulting in a frequency of 8.8% among otherwise normal males with MR, or an overall frequency of 4.0%.

Intellectual Impairment

The most accurate estimates of the frequency of fra(X) cases among the severely and mildly retarded are given in table 2.1 as these studies were population based. In general, the frequency of fra(X) males is higher among the severely retarded, whereas the frequency of fra(X) females is higher among the mildly retarded. Further studies have been done among institutionalized individuals and show a wide range of estimates (tables 2.2 and 2.3).

Testes Size

Most, but not all, adult fra(X) males have macroorchidism. The large testes are more readily identified in postpubertal males although they are sometimes enlarged early in life. Unfortunately, macroorchidism is not specific to fra(X)-related MR as it is sometimes seen in association with other forms of non-specific MR. However, the correlation of fra(X) and large testes is strong enough to make this feature a useful preliminary screening tool to identify males at risk for having the fra(X) syndrome. Brown et al. (1981) measured the testes size of 15 randomly selected males with nonspecific MR. They found that 5 males had volumes above the ninetieth percentile (>25 ml) and that, of these, 4 had the fra(X) syndrome. Other studies did not find as high a rate as did Brown et al., although they did find increased rates (table 2.2). Shapiro et al. (1983) found that 43.5% (10/23) of males with macroorchidism and nonspecific MR had the fra(X) syndrome. They concluded that macroorchidism along with clinical features characteristic of the fra(X) syndrome would be good criteria for screening individuals with MR.

Autism

The prevalence of autism is estimated to be about 0.45/1000 in the general population. Significant concordance for autism in monozygotic twins, 36%, compared to 0% concordance in dizygotic twins suggests a genetic etiology. Also, autism is found to be 50 times more frequent in siblings of autistic children than in the general population. Sex-linked genetic factors have been indicated because there is a high male:female ratio, approximately 3:1. Although no primary genetic cause has been found, several genetic conditions such as phenylketonuria, trisomy 21, tuberous sclerosis, and Williams syndrome are associated with autism.

The relationship between autism and the fra(X) syndrome is not clear. Although there have been many documented cases of autism associated with the fra(X) syndrome, the frequency of the fra(X) syndrome among the autistic population varies greatly between studies (table 2.2). For example, several Swedish studies have shown a relatively high frequency of fra(X) syndrome among individuals with autism. Gillberg et al. (1987) found that 4 of 20 (20%) children with Kanner-type autism had the fra(X) syndrome. Wahlstrom et al. (1986) studied 101 boys and 21 girls and found that 16 of the autistic boys and none of the girls had the fra(X) syndrome (15.8%). In a large study conducted in the United States, Brown et al. (1986b) found a rate of 13.1% fra(X)-positive males among 183 autistics. When they combined this study with 12 other studies, they found that 7.7% of the 614 autistic males were fra(X) positive. Watson et al. (1984) pointed out that the frequency of fra(X) syndrome in autistic males is similar to that seen among the mentally retarded, which suggests that the finding of fra(X) among autistic patients may be related to MR rather than to autism per se. However, the frequency of autistic features in fra(X) is higher than that in other causes of MR, suggesting a close association between the fra(X) syndrome and autism (see chapter 1).

Family History of MR

Another way to identify possible fra(X) cases among those with nonspecific MR is to screen those who have other family members with mental retardation (table 2.2). Carpenter et al. (1982) found that 5 of 36 institutionalized males with a positive family history (13.9%) had the fra(X) mutation, whereas only 1 of 29 with a negative family history had the fra(X) syndrome (3.4%). Froster-Iskenius et al. (1983) found that 7 of 18 (38.8%) institutionalized males with a

Table 2.4

Estimate of Proportion of X-Linked Mental Retardation (XLMR) Families with Fragile (X) Syndrome

XLMR Families Studied	Positive for Fra(X) Syndrome	Reference
13	5	Bundey et al. (1985)
6	3	Herbst et al. (1981)
6	3	Jacobs et al. (1979)
3	2	Jennings et al. (1980)
10	6	Lopez Pajares et al. (1983)
52	16	Primrose et al. (1986)
8	1	Proops et al. (1983)
26	5	Thake et al. (1987)
23	7	Turner et al. (1980b)
147	**48**	

Table 2.5

First Reports of Fragile (X) Families of Non-European Extraction

Nationality or Ethnic Group	Reference
American black	Howard-Peebles and Stoddard (1980)
North African	Mattei et al. (1981)
South African	
Zulu	Venter et al. (1981)
Indian	Venter et al. (1981)
Cape colored	Venter et al. (1981)
White	Venter et al. (1981)
Mexican	Rivera et al. (1981)
Brazilian	Vianna-Morgante et al. (1982)
Chilean	Lacassie et al. (1983)
Sri Lankan	Soysa et al. (1982)
Pakistani	Bundey et al. (1985)
Indian	Ahuja et al. (1990)
Japanese	Rhoads (1984)
Filipino	Rhoads (1984)
Hawaiian/part-Hawaiian	Rhoads (1984)
Dutch Indonesian	Rhoads (1984)

positive family history had the fra(X) syndrome. Table 2.4 shows several studies that have screened families with XLMR for the fra(X) syndrome. If all studies are added together, they indicate that approximately 33% of XLMR is due to the fra(X) syndrome, an estimate similar to that suggested by Turner et al. (1980b).

Fra(X) Syndrome in Different Ethnic Groups

At one time, it was thought that XLMR was most prevalent in families of northern European origin. The distribution of the fra(X) syndrome shows that this finding may have been an ascertainment bias as the fra(X) syndrome has been identified in almost every ethnic group in which it has been studied. Although it is not comprehensive, table 2.5 presents a list of non-European groups in which the fra(X) syndrome has been identified. Most studies completed to date have not been adequate to determine whether there is a significant difference in the prevalence of the fra(X) syndrome among ethnic groups. In a study of the racially mixed population of Hawaii, Jacobs et al. (1986a) found no differences in the prevalence of the fra(X) syndrome in Caucasian, Hawaiian, Oriental, and Filipino families, although this sample was relatively small.

Genetic Epidemiology

Genetic epidemiology is the study of the familial distribution of a disorder with the goal of understanding the possible genetic basis. This task seemed simple for the fra(X) syndrome: fra(X)-related mental retardation was known to be transmitted as an X-linked trait and to co-segregate with the marker on the X chromosome, the fra(X) site. However, there were several observations that were exceptions to the simple rules of X-linked inheritance, and these were noted even before the fra(X) syndrome was fully delineated. Martin and Bell (1943) reported two apparently normal brothers who both had affected grandsons. Losowsky (1961) reported a family with a normal male who had an affected brother and affected grandsons and great grandsons. In 1963, Dunn et al. posed several genetic epidemiologic questions based on the inheritance pattern observed in a large XLMR pedigree: (1) Through whom did the defect enter the pedigree? (2) Why is there a deficiency of affected males? (3) Do the males and females of low-normal intelligence have the disease in a mild form? (4) Can we be sure that this defect is inherited by sex-linked recessive rather than dominant sex-limited transmission? In 1978, Wolff et al. were some of the first to speculate on how males could carry a mutation on the X chromosome and not express it. They suggested that the unaffected male carrier noted in their pedigree may be a mosaic with normal cells and mutant cells that carry the X-linked defect. They proposed three mechanisms for the mosaicism: (1) a half-chromatid mutation in the maternal gamete, (2) an early embryonic mutation, or (3) a mutation in the primordial germ cell.

Although we have been able to quantify some of the parameters of inheritance in the fra(X) syndrome and to suggest several models to explain some of the unique features, we still do not understand the cause of the syndrome. The following sections describe the unique features of the inheritance of the fra(X) syndrome and how they affect genetic counseling. Before describing the transmission of the fra(X) syndrome, it is important to examine the original segregation studies and discuss the limitations of those results. In the early 1980s, a large collaborative study was established to collect data on over 200 fra(X) families (Sherman et al. 1984, 1985). For the segregation study, family members diagnosed with the fra(X) syndrome of probands cytogenetically were said to be affected if they were mentally impaired in any way. Results from cytogenetic tests were available on only a few family members; therefore, these were not used in the description of affection. This limited phenotypic measurement of the fra(X) syndrome was sufficient for males because most have overt MR. However, it was not accurate for females because they have milder MR and their level of intellectual functioning was usually judged subjectively by a family member or the investigator. Thus, recurrence risks for fra(X)-related MR for females are less reliable than those for males. With these limitations in mind, the following sections describe the unique features of the fra(X) syndrome.

Expression of the Mutation in Males: Transmitting or Nonexpressing Males

One of the unique features of the fra(X) syndrome is the high proportion of males who carry the X-linked mutation but are clinically unaffected. These "transmitting" or "nonpenetrant" males are intellectually normal, show no expression of the fra(X) site, and transmit the mutation to all their daughters (table 2.6). From segregation studies, it has been estimated that 20% of all male carriers are nonpenetrant males, and recently this estimate has been confirmed using deoxyribonucleic acid (DNA) studies (Brown et al. 1991). However, current reports indicate the necessity to reevaluate these so-called "nonexpressing" males as several normally functioning males with a significant frequency of fra(X)-positive cells have been identified (Voelckel et al. 1988; Brown et al. 1986a; Veenema et al. 1987; P. A. Jacobs, personal communication). Because most intellectually normal males are not cytogenetically investigated, the frequency of unaffected, fra(X)-expressing males remains unknown. Furthermore, Voelckel et al. (1989) reported a family that did not have mental retardation but did have high expression of the fra(X) site segregating in several family members. It may be that there is a second fragile site located at Xq27.2, which

Table 2.6
Estimate of Penetrance of Mental Retardation (MR) and
Fragile (X) Expression

Mutation	MR	Fra(X) Expression	Penetrance
		Males	
+	+	+	.79
+	+	−	.01
+	−	+	.03[a]
+	−	−	.17
		Females	
+	+	+	.27
+	+	−	.03
+	−	+	.26
+	−	−	.44

Source: Data from Sherman et al. (1984).
[a] Approximation based on literature data. See text.

explains some of these unexpected findings, as suggested by Sutherland and Baker (1990). In any case, it is clear that we do not yet understand the significance of the fra(X) site.

There are two general hypotheses to explain the phenotype of normal carrier males. One hypothesis suggests that all male carriers of the fra(X) mutation show some expression of the gene, although it may be only subtle dysmorphic features or only minor deficits in some areas of learning (Loesch et al. 1987). Clearly, many other genetic and environmental factors play a role in the overall level of MR in fra(X) gene carriers. Alternatively, it may be that there is a proportion of carrier males who show no expression because they carry a different form of the mutation (Laird 1987; Nussbaum et al. 1986; Pembrey et al. 1985) or because they carry a modifying autosomal gene (Steinbach 1986; Israel 1987). Irrespective of the model, it is evident that a significant proportion of the males who carry the mutation are intellectually normal and transmit the mutation to all of their daughters.

Expression of the Mutation in Females: High Rate of Expression in Heterozygotes

About one-third of obligate carrier females are mentally impaired, although less severely than males (Turner et al. 1980a, Sherman et al. 1985). Furthermore, over one-half of carrier females show either mild mental retardation and/or fra(X) expression (table 2.6). If we base this estimate only on daughters of obligate carrier females, the penetrance is estimated to be about 74% (Sherman et al. 1988b). This proportion would be even larger if those with mild learning disabilities were included (Kemper et al. 1986; Miezejeski et al. 1986; Loesch and Hay 1988; Cronister et al. 1991). This high rate of heterozygote expression is unprecedented for other XLMR syndromes.

Expression of the Mutation: Dependent on the Phenotype of the Parent

Sex of the Carrier Parent

The expression of the mutation is dependent on the sex of the carrier parent. This is most obvious in the daughters of transmitting males. All are obligate carriers; thus, approximately one-third are expected to be mentally retarded; however, almost all daughters of transmitting males are intellectually normal (fig. 2.1). In the collaborative study (Sherman et al. 1985), only 3 of the 46 daughters of transmitting males (7%) had slight intellectual handicaps, but the assessment of all 3 was not rigorous. Thus, it may be that fra(X)-related MR is not seen in daughters of transmitting males. Cytogenetic expression in these daughters is almost always negative or, if positive, observed at a very low frequency. Thus, the sex of the carrier parent influences the expression of the mutation in offspring.

Intellectual Functioning of the Carrier Mother

The expression of the mutation is also dependent on the presence of fra(X)-related mental impairment (IQ estimated to be <85) in carrier mothers (fig. 2.2). For mentally impaired mothers, penetrance is virtually complete among carrier sons; for intellectually normal mothers, however, penetrance is only 76%. The same trend is seen in daughters: the mutation is 55% penetrant in carrier daughters of mentally impaired mothers and 32% penetrant in carrier daughters of intellectually normal mothers. This may be a consequence of background genes or environment or may be inherent to the mutation.

If it is true that the mutation is completely penetrant in sons of mentally impaired mothers, then it should follow that mothers of transmitting males are always intellectually normal. This is difficult to test because three generations are needed to identify a transmitting male and thus their mothers are usually not alive at the time of study. However, for several large published pedigrees (see pedigrees from Sherman et al. 1985), no overt MR has been documented in the direct ancestors of transmitting males. This can be tested when DNA markers become available to identify gene carriers accurately.

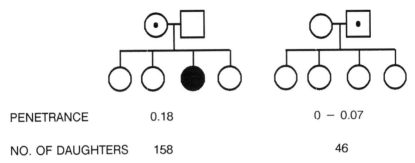

PENETRANCE   0.18   0 – 0.07

NO. OF DAUGHTERS   158   46

Figure 2.1 The penetrance of mental retardation in carrier daughters of intellectually normal female and male carriers. [Data from Sherman et al. (1985)]

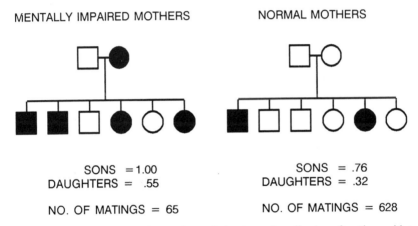

MENTALLY IMPAIRED MOTHERS   NORMAL MOTHERS

SONS   = 1.00   SONS   = .76
DAUGHTERS = .55   DAUGHTERS = .32

NO. OF MATINGS = 65   NO. OF MATINGS = 628

Figure 2.2 The penetrance of mental retardation in carrier offspring of matings with a mentally impaired mother compared to those with a mentally normal mother. [Data from Sherman et al. (1985)]

First Degree Relatives of Carrier Males: "The Sherman Paradox"

In 1986, Dr. John Opitz used the term the *Sherman paradox* to describe the characteristics of the expression of the fra(X) mutation in relatives of transmitting males. The mothers and daughters of transmitting males are rarely, if ever, mentally retarded and brothers of transmitting males are much less likely to be mentally retarded than are the brothers of affected males. A statistical test of this observation was done by comparing the penetrance of the brothers of transmitting males with the penetrance of the grandsons of transmitting males (fig. 2.3). A significant difference was found. The penetrance of fra(X)-related

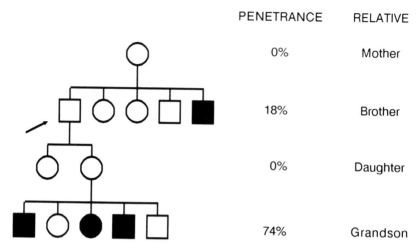

Figure 2.3 The penetrance of mental retardation in relatives of a transmitting male (*arrow*). [Data from Sherman et al. (1985)]

MR was only 18% in brothers compared to 74% in grandsons. The paradox is this: the mothers of these two sibship types are phenotypically similar, that is, they are both obligate carriers and intellectually normal. Under any simple genetic model, the expression of the mutation in their sons would be expected to be the same, but this is not the case.

Lack of New Mutations among Affected Individuals

For an X-linked recessive lethal disease such as Duchenne muscular dystrophy, we expect one-third of the isolated affected males to be due to new mutations. This assumes equilibrium between selection and mutation and equal mutation rates between egg and sperm. Under these same assumptions, approximately 37% of isolated fra(X) males would be due to new mutations (Sherman et al. 1984). In our first study, however, we found the estimate of new mutations among isolated affected males to be zero, suggesting that mutations do not occur in eggs and, consequently, that all mothers of affected males are obligate carriers. From this, we estimated the mutation rate in sperm to be 7.2×10^{-4} (Sherman et al. 1984), one of the highest mutation rates found in humans. Although a dearth of isolated cases among affected individuals was confirmed in later studies (Jacobs et al. 1986b; Sherman et al. 1988a), the complex inheritance pattern of the fra(X) syndrome may mean that our explanation of a lack of mutation in eggs is too simplistic. For example, if the mechanism for the fra(X) mutation involves a multistep process, new mutations would be expected among the clinically normal individuals, with subsequent steps being necessary to produce individuals with clinical signs.

The Application of Segregation Analysis to Genetic Counseling

From the above considerations, it is clear that the transmission of the fra(X) syndrome defies the principles of classic genetics. This greatly complicates genetic counseling, as there is no genetic model on which to base recurrence risks. At present, risks used in genetic counseling are based on the results of segregation studies (Sherman et al. 1985; Mulley and Sutherland 1987; Navajas et al. 1987; Weaver and Sherman 1987; Sherman et al. 1988b; Bridge and Lillicrap 1989). Table 2.7 provides recurrence risks for situations where the sex and intellectual level of the carrier parent are known; however, these risks have two limitations. First, they are based only on fra(X)-related MR and do not include expression of the fra(X) site in the assessment of the carrier parent. Fra(X) expression may be indicative of a different form of the mutation; thus, expression of the mutation in offspring may be different for an intellectually normal, fra(X)-negative mother than for an intellectually normal, fra(X)-positive mother. This information would be vital to genetic counseling. Second, current risk estimates for fra(X)-related MR in females are unreliable as studies on which they are based did not accurately assess affection. (See chapter 8 for a complete discussion of genetic counseling.)

Table 2.8 shows the recurrence risks in families with an isolated case. These families are the most difficult to counsel as the fra(X) mutation is most likely due to a different mechanism than that controlling other known X-linked disorders. Most of the proposed genetic models suggest that there are no mutations

Table 2.7
Recurrence Risks in Families with a Known Carrier Parent Who Is Either Normal or Mentally Impaired (MI)

Offspring	Carrier Mother		Carrier Father	
	Normal	MI	Normal	MI
Carrier son				
Mentally retarded	0.38	0.50	0	0
Normal	0.12	0	0	0
Carrier daughter				
Mentally retarded	0.16	0.28	~0	?
Normal	0.34	0.22	~1	?

Source: Data from Sherman et al. (1985).

Table 2.8

Recurrence Risks of MR in Relatives of an Isolated Case
of the Fragile (X) Syndrome

Isolated	Siblings		First Cousins	
Case	Male	Female	Male	Female
Male	0.23–0.38	0.09–0.16	0.06–0.08	0.03–0.04
Female	0.16–0.38	0.07–0.16	0.03–0.08	0.02–0.03

Source: Data from Sherman et al. (1988a).

among the affected males or females; thus, the recurrence risks are high in families with isolated cases. If these models are not true and new mutations can occur among affected individuals, then recurrence risks are relatively low. At this point, a range for the recurrence risks can be given in a genetic counseling situation.

Summary

In spite of many years of intensive research, the genetics of the fra(X) syndrome remain a puzzle. In medical genetics, this syndrome is one of the most important and challenging disorders to understand because it is the most common inherited form of mental retardation and the biology of the unique mutation has far-reaching implications. Currently, research efforts are directed toward characterizing the mutation, determining the reason for its high prevalence in the population, and identifying factors that affect its expression. With the collaboration of many scientific and medical disciplines and with the enthusiasm and cooperation of concerned families, the unraveling of this perplexing disorder continues to progress.

References

Ahuja, Y. R., S. Rani, M. Sujatha, and P. Hanmantha Rao. 1990. Prevalence of fragile-X syndrome amongst mentally retarded patients at Hyderabad, India. *Am. J. Med. Genet.* In press.

Aoi, T., H. Takashima, T. Takada, and T. Okada. 1989. Fragile X chromosome in institutionalized male adults with mental retardation. *Keio J. Med.* 38:36–39.

Arinami, T., I. Kondo, and S. Nakajima. 1986. Frequency of the fragile X syndrome in Japanese mentally retarded males. *Hum. Genet.* 73:309–312.

Arinami, T., I. Kondo, S. Nakajima, and H. Hamaguchi. 1987. Frequency of the fragile

X syndrome in institutionalized mentally retarded females in Japan. *Hum. Genet.* 76:344–347.

Blomquist, H. K., K. H. Gustavson, and G. Holmgren. 1981. Mild mental retardation in children in a northern Swedish county. *J. Ment. Defic. Res.* 25:169–186.

Blomquist, H. K., K. H. Gustavson, G. Holmgren, I. Nordenson, and A. Sweins. 1982. Fragile site X chromosomes and X-linked mental retardation in severely retarded boys in a northern Swedish county. A prevalence study. *Clin. Genet.* 21:209–214.

Blomquist, H. K., K. H. Gustavson, G. Holmgren, I. Nordenson, and U. Palsson-Strae. 1983. Fragile X syndrome in mildly mentally retarded children in a northern Swedish county. A prevalence study. *Clin. Genet.* 24:393–398.

Bridge, P. J., and D. P. Lillicrap. 1989. Molecular diagnosis of the fragile X [fra(X)] syndrome: Calculation of risks based on flanking DNA markers in small phase-unknown families. *Am. J. Med. Genet.* 33:92–99.

Brown, W. T., P. M. Mezzacappa, and E. C. Jenkins. 1981. Screening for fragile X syndrome by testicular size measurement. *Lancet* 2:1055.

Brown, W. T., A. C. Gross, C. B. Chan, and E. C. Jenkins. 1986a. DNA linkage studies in the fragile X syndrome suggest genetic heterogeneity. *Am. J. Med. Genet.* 23:643–644.

Brown, W. T., E. C. Jenkins, I. L. Cohen, G. S. Fisch, E. G. Wolf-Schein, A. Gross, L. Waterhouse, D. Fein, A. Mason-Brothers, E. Ritvo, W. B. Ruttenberg, W. Bentley, and S. Castells. 1986b. Fragile X and autism: A multicenter survey. *Am. J. Med. Genet.* 23:341–352.

Brown, W. T., A. C. Gross, C. B. Chan, and E. C. Jenkins. 1986a. DNA linkage studies in the fragile X syndrome suggest genetic heterogeneity. *Am. J. Med. Genet.* 23:643–664.

Bundey, S., T. P. Webb, A. Thake, and J. Todd. 1985. A community study of severe mental retardation in the West Midlands and the importance of the fragile X chromosome in its aetiology. *J. Med. Genet.* 22:258–266.

Cantú, J. M., H. E. Scaglia, M. Medina, M. Gonzalez-Diddi, T. Morato, M. E. Moreno, G. Perez-Palacios, and G. Needa. 1976. Inherited congenital normofunctional testicular hyperplasia and mental deficiency. *Hum. Genet.* 33:23–33.

Carpenter, N. J., L. G. Leichtman, and B. Say. 1982. Fragile X-linked mental retardation. *Am. J. Dis. Child.* 136:392–398.

Chudley, A. E., J. Knoll, J. W. Gerrard, L. Shepel, E. McGahey, and J. Anderson. 1983. Fragile (X) X-linked mental retardation. I. Relationship between age and intelligence and the frequency of expression of fragile (X)(q28). *Am. J. Med. Genet.* 14:699–712.

Cronister, A., R. Schreiner, M. Wittenberger, K. Amiri, K. Harris, and R. J. Hagerman. 1991. The heterozygous fragile X female: Historical, physical, cognitive and cytogenetic features. *Am. J. Med. Genet.* 38:269–274.

Davison, B. C. C. 1973. Genetic studies in mental subnormality. I. Familial idiopathic severe subnormality: The question of a contribution by X-linked genes. *Br. J. Psychiatry Special Publ.* 8:1–60.

Dereymaeker, A. M., J. P. Fryns, J. Haegeman, J. Deroover, and H. Van den Berghe. 1988. A genetic-diagnostic survey in an institutionalized population of 158 mentally retarded patients. The Viaene experience. *Clin. Genet.* 34:126–134.

Dunn, H. G., H. Renpenning, J. W. Gerrard, J. R. Miller, T. Tabata, and S. Federoff. 1963. Mental retardation as a sex-linked defect. *Am. J. Ment. Defic.* 67:827–848.

English, C. J., E. V. Davison, M. S. Bhate, and L. Barrett. 1989. Chromosome studies of males in an institution for the mentally handicapped. *J. Med. Genet.* 26:379–381.

Escalante, J. A., and O. Frota-Pessoa. 1973. Retardamento mental. In W. Becak et al. (eds.), *Genetica medica.* São Paulo: Sarvier, pp. 300–308.

Escalante, J. A., H. Grunspun, and O. Frota-Pessoa. 1971. Severe sex-linked mental retardation. *J. Genet. Hum.* 19:137–140.

Fisch, G. S., W. Silverman, and E. C. Jenkins. 1991. Genetic (and other) factors which contribute to variability in cytogenetic expression in fragile X males. *Am. J. Med. Genet.* 38:404–407.

Fishburn, J., G. Turner, A. Daniel, and R. Brookwell. 1983. The diagnosis and frequency of X-linked conditions in a cohort of moderately retarded males with affected brothers. *Am. J. Med. Genet.* 14:713–724.

Froster-Iskenius, U., G. Felsch, C. Schirren, and E. Schwinger. 1983. Screening for fra(X)(q) in a population of mentally retarded males. *Hum. Genet.* 63:153–157.

Fryns, J. P., A. Kleczkowska, E. Kubien, and H. Van den Berghe. 1984. Cytogenetic findings in moderate and severe mental retardation. A study of an institutionalized population of 1991 patients. *Acta Paediatr. Scand. (Suppl.)* 313:4–23.

Fryns, J. P., A. Kleczkowska, A. Dereymaeker, M. Hoefnagels, G. Heremans, J. Marien, and H. Van den Berghe. 1986. A genetic-diagnostic survey in an institutionalized population of 173 severely mentally retarded patients. *Clin. Genet.* 30:315–323.

Gillberg, C., S. Steffenburg, and G. Jakobsson. 1987. Neurobiological findings in 20 relatively gifted children with Kanner-type autism or Asperger syndrome. *Dev. Med. Child Neurol.* 29:641–649.

Giraud, F., S. Ayme, J. F. Mattei, and M. G. Mattei. 1976. Constitutional chromosome breakage. *Hum. Genet.* 34:125–136.

Goldfine, P. E., P. M. McPherson, G. A. Heath, V. A. Hardesty, L. J. Beauregard, and B. Gordon. 1985. Association of fragile X syndrome with autism. *Am. J. Psychiatry* 142:108–110.

Gustavson, K. H., G. Holmgren, R. Jonsell, and H. K. Blomquist. 1977. Severe mental retardation in children in a northern Swedish county. *J. Ment. Defic. Res.* 21:161–180.

Gustavson, K. H., H. K. Blomquist, and G. Holmgren. 1986. Prevalence of the fragile-X syndrome in mentally retarded boys in a Swedish county. *Am. J. Med. Genet.* 23:581–587.

Hagerman, R., R. Berry, A. W. Jackson, J. Campbell, A. C. M. Smith, and L. McGavran. 1988. Institutional screening for the fragile X syndrome. *Am. J. Dis. Child.* 142:1216–1221.

Harvey, J., C. Judge, and S. Weiner. 1977. Familial X-linked mental retardation with an X chromosome abnormality. *J. Med. Genet.* 14:46–50.

Herbst, D. S., and J. R. Miller. 1980. Nonspecific X-linked mental retardation. II. The frequency in British Columbia. *Am. J. Med. Genet.* 7:461–469.

Herbst, D. S., H. G. Dunn, F. J. Dill, D. K. Kalousek, and L. W. Krywaniuk. 1981. Further delineation of X-linked mental retardation. *Hum. Genet.* 58:366–372.

Howard-Peebles, P. N., and W. H. Finley. 1983. Screening of mentally retarded males for macro-orchidism and the fragile-X chromosome. *Am. J. Med. Genet.* 15:631–635.

Howard-Peebles, P. N., and G. R. Stoddard. 1980. Race distribution in X-linked mental retardation with macro-orchidism and fragile site in Xq. *Am. J. Hum. Genet.* 32:629–630.

Israel, M. 1987. Autosomal suppressor gene for fragile-X: An hypothesis. *Am. J. Med. Genet.* 26:19–31.

Jacobs, P. A., M. Mayer, and E. Rudak. 1979. More on marker X chromosomes mental retardation and macro-orchidism. *N. Engl. J. Med.* 300:737–738.

Jacobs, P. A., T. W. Glover, M. Mayer, P. Fox, J. W. Gerrard, H. G. Dunn, and D. S. Herbst. 1980. X-linked mental retardation: A study of 7 families. *Am. J. Med. Genet.* 7:471–489.

Jacobs, P. A., and S. L. Sherman. 1985. The fragile(X): A marker for the Martin-Bell syndrome. *Dis. Markers* 3:9–25.

Jacobs, P. A., M. Mayer, and M. A. Abruzzo. 1986a. Studies of the fragile(X) syndrome in mentally retarded populations in Hawaii. *Am. J. Med. Genet.* 23:567–572.

Jacobs, P. A., S. L. Sherman, G. Turner, and T. Webb. 1986b. The fragile(X) syndrome: The mutation problem. *Am. J. Med. Genet.* 23:611–617.

Jennings, M., J. G. Hall, and H. Hoehn. 1980. Significance of phenotypic and chromosomal abnormalities in X-linked mental retardation (Martin-Bell or Renpenning syndrome). *Am. J. Med. Genet.* 7:417–432.

Johnson, G. E. 1896–7. Contribution to the psychology and pedagogy of feeble minded children. *J. Psycho-asthenics* 2:26–32.

Kähkönen, M., J. Leisti, M. Wilska, and S. Varonen. 1983. Marker X-associated mental retardation. A study of 150 retarded males. *Clin. Genet.* 23:397–404.

Kähkönen, M., T. Alitalo, E. Airaksinen, R. Matilainen, K. Launiala, S. Autio, and J. Leisti. 1987. Prevalence of the fragile X syndrome in four birth cohorts of children of school age. *Hum. Genet.* 77:85–87.

Kemper, M. B., R. J. Hagerman, R. S. Ahmad, and R. Mariner. 1986. Cognitive profiles and the spectrum of clinical manifestations in heterozygous fra(X) females. *Am. J. Med. Genet.* 23:139–156.

Kinnell, H. G., and S. P. Banu. 1983. Institutional prevalence of fragile X syndrome. *Lancet* 2:1427.

Kirkilionis, A., F. Sergovich, and J. Pozsony. 1983. Use of testicular volume as a cytogenetic screening criterion. *Am. J. Hum. Genet.* 35:138A.

Lacassie, Y., R. Moreno, F. de la Barra, T. M. Bianca Curotto, T. M. Angélica Alliende, P. E. Anríquez, G. Barahena, and S. Muzzo. 1983. Síndrome del X-frágil: Discusión del primer caso confirmado citogenéticamente en Chile. *Rev. Chil. Pediatr.* 54:410–416.

Laird, C. D. 1987. Proposed mechanism of inheritance and expression of the human fragile-X syndrome of mental retardation. *Genetics* 117:587–599.

Lamont, M. A., N. R. Dennis, and M. Seabright. 1986. Chromosome abnormalities in pupils attending ESN/M schools. *Arch. Dis. Child.* 61:223–226.

Lehrke, R. G. 1974. X-linked mental retardation and verbal disability. *Birth Defects* 10:1–100.

Li, S. Y., C. C. Tsai, M. Y. Chou, and J. K. Lin. 1988. A cytogenetic study of mentally retarded school children in Taiwan with special reference to the fragile X chromosome. *Hum. Genet.* 79:292–296.

Loesch, D. Z., and D. A. Hay. 1988. Clinical features and reproductive patterns in fragile X female heterozygotes. *J. Med. Genet.* 25:407–414.

Loesch, D. Z., D. A. Hay, G. R. Sutherland, J. Halliday, C. Judge, and G. C. Webb. 1987. Phenotypic variation in male-transmitted fragile X: Genetic inferences. *Am. J. Med. Genet.* 27:401–417.

Lopez Pajares, I., A. Delicado, A. Gallego, and I. Pascual Castroviejo. 1983. Familial X-linked mental retardation and fragile X chromosomes in 6 Spanish families. *Clin. Genet.* 23:236. Losowsky, M. S. 1961. Hereditary mental defect showing the pattern of sex influence. *J. Ment. Defic. Res.* 5:60–62.

Lubs, H. A. 1969. A marker X chromosome. *Am. J. Hum. Genet.* 21:231–244.

Martin, J. P., and J. Bell. 1943. A pedigree of mental defect showing sex-linkage. *J. Neurol. Psychiatry* 6:154–157.

Matsuishi, T., Y. Shiotsuki, K. Yoshimura, H. Shoji, F. Imuta, and F. Yamashita. 1987. High prevalence of infantile autism in Kurume City, Japan. *J. Child. Neurol.* 2:268–271.

Mattei, J. F., M. G. Mattei, C. Aumeras, M. Auger, and F. Giraud. 1981. X-linked mental retardation with fragile X: A study of 15 families. *Hum. Genet.* 59:281–289.

McGillivray, B. C., F. J. Dill, J. Sandercock, D. S. Herbst, and B. Tischler. 1984. Infantile autism—an occasional feature of X-linked mental retardation. *Am. J. Hum. Genet.* 36:3s.

Miezejeski, C. M., E. C. Jenkins, A. L. Hill, K. Wisniewski, J. H. French, and W. T. Brown. 1986. A profile of cognitive deficit in females from fragile X families. *Neuropsychologia* 24:405–409.

Morton, N. E., D. C. Rao, H. Lang-Brown, C. J. Maclean, R. D. Bart, and R. Lew. 1977. Colchester revisited: A genetic study of mental defect. *J. Med. Genet.* 14:1–9.

Mulley, J. C., and G. R. Sutherland. 1987. Letter to the editor: Fragile X transmission and the determination of carrier probabilities for genetic counseling. *Am. J. Med. Genet.* 26:987–990.

Navajas, L., C. Rosenberg, and A. M. Vianna-Morgante. 1987. Genetic counseling in Martin-Bell syndrome. *Rev. Bras. Genet.* 10:333–340.

Nielsen, K. B., N. Tommerup, H. V. Dyggve, and C. Schou. 1982. Macroorchidism and fragile X in mentally retarded males. *Hum. Genet.* 61:113–117.

Nussbaum, R. L., S. D. Airhart, and D. H. Ledbetter. 1986. Recombination and amplification of pyrimidine-rich sequences may be responsible for initiation and progression of the Xq27 fragile site: An hypothesis. *Am. J. Med. Genet.* 23:715–722.

Opitz, J. M. 1986. On the gates of hell and a most unusual gene. Editorial comment. *Am. J. Med. Genet.* 23:1–10.

Opitz, J. M., and G. R. Sutherland. 1984. Conference report: International Workshop on the Fragile X and X-linked Mental Retardation. *Am. J. Med. Genet.* 17:5–94.

Paika, I. J., F. Lai, N. M. McAllister, and W. A. Miller. 1984. The fragile-X marker survey: Preliminary report on the screening of suspected fragile-X syndrome patients at the Fernald state school. *Am. J. Hum. Genet.* 36:108s.

Payton, J. B., M. W. Steele, S. L. Wenger, and N. J. Minshaw. 1989. The fragile X marker and autism in perspective. *J. Am. Acad. Child Adolesc. Psychiatry* 28:417–421.

Pembrey, M. E., R. M. Winter, and K. E. Davies. 1985. A premutation that generates a defect at crossing over explains the inheritance of fragile X-mental retardation. *Am. J. Med. Genet.* 21:709–717.

Penrose, L. S. 1938. A clinical and genetic study of 1,280 cases of mental defect. *Ment. Res. Council Spec. Rep. Ser.* 229.

Priest, J. H., H. C. Thuline, G. D. LaVeck, and D. B. Jarvis. 1961. An approach to genetic factors in mental retardation. *Am. J. Ment. Defic.* 66:42–50.

Primrose, D. A., R. El-Matmati, E. Boyd, C. Gosden, and M. Newton. 1986. Prevalence of the fragile X syndrome in an institution for the mentally handicapped. *Br. J. Psychiatry* 148:655–657.

Proops, R., M. Mayer, and P. A. Jacobs. 1983. A study of mental retardation in children in the island of Hawaii. *Clin. Genet.* 23:81–96.

Pueschel, S. M., R. Herman, and G. Groden. 1985. Brief report: Screening children with autism for fragile-X syndrome and phenylketonuria. *J. Autism Dev. Disord.* 15:335–338.

Renpenning, H., J. W. Gerrard, W. A. Zaleski, and T. Tabata. 1962. Familial sex-linked mental retardation. *Can. Med. Assoc. J.* 87:954–956.

Rhoads, F. A. 1984. Fragile-X syndrome in Hawaii: A summary of clinical experience. *Am. J. Med. Genet.* 17:209–214.

Richards, B. W., and T. Webb. 1982. The Martin-Bell-Renpenning syndrome. *J. Med. Genet.* 19:79.

Rivera, H., A. Hernandez, L. Plascencia, J. Sanchez-Corona, D. Garcia-Cruz, and J. M. Cantú. 1981. Some observations on the mental deficiency normo-functional testicular hyperplasia and fra(X)(q28) chromosome syndrome. *Ann. Genet. (Paris)* 24:220–222.

Ruvalcaba, R. H. A., S. A. Myhre, E. C. Roosen-Runge, and J. B. Beckwith. 1977. X-linked mental deficiency megalotestes syndrome. *JAMA* 238:1646–1650.

Sanfilippo, S., R. M. Ragusa, S. Musumeci, and G. Neri. 1986. Fragile X mental retardation: Prevalence in a group of institutionalized patients in Italy and description of a novel EEG pattern. *Am. J. Med. Genet.* 23:589–595.

Shapiro, L. R., G. M. Summa, P. L. Wilmot, and E. Gloth. 1983. Screening and detection of the fragile X syndrome. *Am. J. Hum. Genet.* 35:117A.

Sherman, S. L., N. E. Morton, P. A. Jacobs, and G. Turner. 1984. The marker (X) syndrome: A cytogenetic and genetic analysis. *Ann. Hum. Genet.* 48:21–37.

Sherman, S. L., P. A. Jacobs, N. E. Morton, U. Froster-Iskenius, P. N. Howard-Peebles, K. B. Nielsen, M. W. Partington, G. R. Sutherland, G. Turner, and M. Watson. 1985. Further segregation analysis of the fragile X syndrome with special reference to transmitting males. *Hum. Genet.* 69:289–299.

Sherman, S. L., A. Rogatko, and G. Turner. 1988a. Recurrence risks for relatives in families with an isolated case of the fragile X syndrome. *Am. J. Med. Genet.* 31:753–765.

Sherman, S. L., G. Turner, H. Robinson, and S. Laing. 1988b. Investigation of the segregation of the fragile X mutation in daughters of obligate carrier women. *Am. J. Med. Genet.* 30:633–639.

Snyder, R. D., and A. Robinson. 1969. Recessive sex-linked mental retardation in the absence of other recognizable abnormalities. *Clin. Pediatr.* 8:669–674.

Soysa, P., M. Senanayahe, M. Mikkelsen, and H. Poulsen. 1982. Martin-Bell syndrome fra(X) (q28) in a Sri Lankan family. *J. Ment. Defic. Res.* 26:251–257.

Steinbach, P. 1986. Mental impairment in Martin-Bell syndrome is probably determined by interaction of several genes: Simple explanation of phenotypic differences between unaffected and affected males with the same X chromosome. *Hum. Genet.* 72:248–252.

Sutherland, G. R. 1977. Fragile sites on human chromosomes: Demonstration of their dependence on the type of tissue culture medium. *Science* 197:265–266.

———. 1982. Heritable fragile sites on human chromosomes. VIII. Preliminary population cytogenetics data on the folic-acid-sensitive fragile sites. *Am. J. Hum. Genet.* 34:452–458.

———. 1985. Heritable fragile sites on human chromosomes. XII. Population cytogenetics. *Ann. Hum. Genet.* 49:153–161.

Sutherland, G. R., and E. Baker. 1990. The common fragile site in band q27 of the human X chromosome is not coincident with the fragile X. *Clin. Genet.* 37:167–172.

Thake, A., J. Todd, T. Webb, and S. Bundey. 1987. Children with the fragile X chromosome at schools for the mildly mentally retarded. *Dev. Med. Child Neurol.* 29:711–719.

Tranebjaerg, L., and P. Kure. 1991. Prevalence of fra(X) and other specific diagnoses in autistics in a Danish county. *Am. J. Med. Genet.* 38:212–214.

Turner, G., and B. Turner. 1974. X-linked mental retardation. *J. Med. Genet.* 11:109–113.

Turner, G., B. Turner, and E. Collins. 1971. X-linked mental retardation without physical abnormality: Renpenning's syndrome. *Dev. Med. Child Neurol.* 13:71–78.

Turner, G., C. Eastman, J. Casey, A. McLeary, P. Procopis, and B. Turner. 1975. X-linked mental retardation associated with macro-orchidism. *J. Med. Genet.* 12:367–371.

Turner, G., R. Till, and A. Daniel. 1978. Marker X chromosomes, mental retardation and macro-orchidism. *N. Engl. J. Med.* 299:1472.

Turner, G., R. Brookwell, A. Daniel, M. Selikowitz, and M. Zilibowitz. 1980a. Heterozygous expression of X-linked mental retardation and X-chromosome marker fra(X)(q27). *N. Engl. J. Med.* 303:662–664.

Turner, G., A. Daniel, and M. Frost. 1980b. X-linked mental retardation, macroorchidism, and the Xq27 fragile site. *J. Pediatr.* 96:837–841.

Turner, G., H. Robinson, S. Laing, and S. Purvis-Smith. 1986. Preventive screening for the fragile X syndrome. *N. Engl. J. Med.* 315:607–609.

Veenema, H., N. J. Carpenter, E. Baker, M. H. Hofker, A. Millington-Ward, and P. L. Pearson. 1987. The fragile X syndrome in a large family. III. Investigation on linkage of flanking DNA markers with the fragile X site Xq27. *J. Med. Genet.* 24:101–106.

Venter, P. A., G. S. Gericke, B. Dawson, and J. Op't Hof. 1981. A marker X chromosome associated with nonspecific male mental retardation. *S. Afr. Med. J.* 21:807–811.

Venter, P. A., J. Op't Hof, D. J. Coetzee, C. Van der Walt, and A. E. Retief. 1984. No marker (X) syndrome in autistic children. *Hum. Genet.* 67:107–111.

Vianna-Morgante, A. M., I. Armando, and O. Frota-Pessoa. 1982. Escalante syndrome and the marker X chromosome. *Am. J. Med. Genet.* 12:237–240.

Voelckel, M. A., M. G. Mattei, C. N'Guyen, N. Philip, F. Berg, and J. F. Mattei. 1988. Dissociation between mental retardation and fragile site expression in a family with fragile X-linked mental retardation. *Hum. Genet.* 80:375–378.

Voelckel, M. A., N. Philip, C. Piquet, M. C. Pellissier, I. Oberlé, F. Berg, M. G. Mattei, and J. F. Mattei. 1989. Study of a family with a fragile site of the X chromosome at Xq27–28 without mental retardation. *Hum. Genet.* 81:353–357.

Voullaire, L. E., G. C. Webb, and M. Leversha. 1989. Fragile X testing in a diagnostic cytogenetics laboratory. *J. Med. Genet.* 26:439–442.

Wahlstrom, J., C. Gillberg, K. H. Gustavson, and G. Holmgren. 1986. Infantile autism and the fragile X: A Swedish multicenter study. *Am. J. Med. Genet.* 23:403–408.

Watson, M. S., J. F. Leckman, B. Annex, W. R. Breg, D. Boles, F. R. Volkmar, D. J. Cohen, and C. Carter. 1984. Fragile X in a survey of 75 autistic males. Letter to the editor. *N. Engl. J. Med.* 310:1462.

Weaver, D. D., and S. L. Sherman. 1987. A counseling guide to the Martin-Bell syndrome. Letter to the editor. *Am. J. Med. Genet.* 26:39–44.

Webb, T. P., S. Bundey, A. Thake, and J. Todd. 1986. The frequency of the fragile X chromosome among school children in Coventry. *J. Med. Genet.* 23:396–399.

Wolff, G., H. Hameister, and H. H. Ropers. 1978. X-linked mental retardation: Transmission of the trait of an apparently unaffected male. *Am. J. Med. Genet.* 2:217–224.

Wortis, H., M. Pollack, and J. Wortis. 1966. Families with two or more mentally retarded or mentally disturbed siblings: The preponderance of males. *Am. J. Ment. Defic.* 70:745–752.

Wright, S. W., G. Tarjan, and L. Eyer. 1959. Investigation of families with two or more mentally retarded siblings. *Am. J. Dis. Child.* 97:445–463.

CHAPTER 3

Cytogenetics

Peter Jacky, Ph.D.

Historical Perspective

If you were to ask a clinical cytogeneticist today to pick a human chromosome abnormality that is both important in terms of its overall contribution to human genetic disease and yet poorly understood in terms of its "behavior" as a chromosomal abnormality, the cytogeneticist would very likely choose the fragile X chromosome. There are very few human chromosomal abnormalities for which we have any concern about the behavior of the anomalous chromosome. Usually human chromosomal abnormalities are either present or absent, and we ascribe a constellation of physical or mental abnormalities to a chromosomal abnormality if it is present or look for an alternative explanation if it is absent. Most clinical human chromosomal abnormality is a function of numerical abnormality, either wholly or partially, and we usually have little concern about the actual cytogenetic behavior of the extra, or deleted, chromosome material in an individual. This is certainly not true of the fra(X) chromosome. Since the original description of a fragile site lesion on the X chromosome and its association with a common heritable form of mental retardation (Lubs 1969), a tremendous effort has been devoted to understanding the behavior of this chromosomal abnormality, both in terms of its behavior in the laboratory and our ability to use it as a reliable diagnostic chromosome marker for the syndrome and in terms of its behavior in individuals and within families.

Unlike most other human chromosomal abnormalities, the fragile site lesion is present in only a portion of dividing cells examined from an affected individual. This is probably largely explained by the fact that expression of the fragile site lesion on the X chromosome is a function of the tissue culture conditions that are imposed on cells during chromosome preparation in the laboratory. When the correct cellular metabolic requirements for fragile site expression are achieved, the fragile site lesion on the chromosome is evident and, when they are not, it is absent. There is little, if any, evidence that the fragile site per se exists in vivo in individuals. Furthermore, although the fra(X) site seems to be quite a reliable cytogenetic marker for diagnosis of the syndrome in individuals, we have no understanding of the relationship between the expression of the chromosomal lesion and the underlying mutation responsible for the manifestation of the mental retardation syndrome.

The behavior of the fra(X) can also be distinctly different in affected and unaffected individuals. The fra(X) site is relatively easy to elicit in males and females who demonstrate varying degrees of intellectual impairment but difficult to elicit in unaffected female or male carriers, regardless of how stringently tissue culture requirements are applied. This may be fundamentally explained by X chromosome inactivation mechanisms that are normally invoked in all females to suppress genetically one of the X chromosomes. However, unlike most other X-linked genetic disorders or X chromosome abnormalities in which the X inactivation mechanism allows most carrier females to go largely unaffected, the fra(X) carrier female is at substantial risk of realizing some clinical effect from the mutation.

Herbert Lubs's (1969) original observation and description of the fra(X), or *marker X,* was in many respects both insightful and lucky. He was using tissue culture medium (TC 199) appropriate for eliciting the fragile site in a family in which two males with the syndrome and an apparently unaffected mother all showed the marker at relatively high frequencies. Lubs described much of the morphologic variation in the fra(X) site that would lead to our appreciation of the variability evident in expression of fragile site lesions in clinical cytogenetics today and would later be important in the broader definition of both rare heritable and relatively common fragile sites on other human chromosomes.

Large families with mental retardation segregating as an X-linked trait were well documented in human genetics at the time (Martin and Bell 1943; Renpenning et al. 1962; Dunn et al. 1963), and, given Lubs's report, many clinical geneticists retrieved such families and requested that chromosome studies be initiated. Lubs's observation, however, went largely unconfirmed, and most geneticists filed away his report as a serendipitous finding. Almost 10 years would pass before the fra(X) site would reemerge as perhaps one of the most significant discoveries in human cytogenetics.

The reemergence was set in motion by a report by Grant Sutherland in Australia in 1977. He showed that the expression of the fragile site on the X chromosome and other apparently rare and heritable fragile sites on other human chromosomes was a function of the type of tissue culture medium used in the cell culture for chromosome preparation. Sutherland also demonstrated that the fra(X) and other heritable fragile sites were generally expressed in only a portion of cells analyzed but at significantly higher frequencies in tissue culture medium TC 199 as opposed to, for instance, RPMI 1640 or Ham's F10. Because TC 199 was considered one of the old standard media in cell culture and it contained a huge variety of components, many of which were probably not essential to good lymphocyte growth, many laboratories had switched to better-defined, simpler media for culturing lymphocytes. This understanding about the tissue culture requirements for fragile site expression made sense to a very few cytogeneticists still routinely using TC 199 and observing fra(X) sites and other constitutional chromosomal breaks (Giraud et al. 1976; Harvey et al. 1977). It did encourage cytogeneticists to reinitiate studies of X-linked mental retardation families, this time with TC 199. Subsequently, several of the large sex-linked mental retardation families described in the literature were found to be fra(X) positive (Dunn et al. 1963, restudied by Jacobs et al. 1980; Ruvalcaba et al. 1977, restudied by Jennings et al. 1980; Bowen et al. 1978, restudied by Martin et al. 1980).

Sutherland's discovery also encouraged investigators to reexamine their clinical files for case reports of nonspecific familial X-linked mental retardation and to study the chromosomes of these families using the appropriate culturing conditions. Soudek et al. (1984) found that 10 of 22 families restudied exhibited the fra(X) chromosome. Turner et al. (1980b) found the fra(X) chromosome to be segregating in 7 of 23 families, and Jacobs et al. (1980) found the fra(X) in 6 of 7 families. The one family that did not exhibit the marker in the study by Jacobs et al. was the family originally reported by Renpenning et al. (1962). In the initial families studied or surveyed, fra(X)-linked mental retardation was turning out to be very common and, perhaps more importantly, it was heritable, frequently with numerous individuals affected within the same family or kindred.

In 1979, Sutherland followed through on his initial observation about the specific culture medium requirements for fragile site expression and produced perhaps the landmark paper in our present understanding and definition of heritable sites on human chromosomes and tissue culture factors that influence their expression. What Sutherland (1979a) showed then was that it was the relative deficiency of the vitamin folic acid and a DNA pyrimidine base thymidine, which were responsible for the effectiveness of TC 199 in eliciting expression, when compared to other more modern tissue culture media. Medium containing normal levels of folic acid and/or thymidine suppressed the expression of the fra(X), and one could take fragile site-expressing medium containing no folic acid or thymidine and, in a dose-response fashion, add either of these components and gradually suppress the frequency of expression. A thymidine analog 5-bromodeoxyuridine would similarly suppress fragile site expression, or one could effectively induce folate/thymidine depletion with the folate antagonist methotrexate and elicit expression of the site.

In an accompanying paper, Sutherland (1979b) also put forward the current working definition of heritable fragile sites on human chromosomes: (1) that they are nonrandom achromatic lesions bridging one or both chromatids of a chromosome arm; (2) that they are usually present in only a portion of cells analyzed but, when expressed, are present at exactly the same chromosome position in all cells from an individual or kindred; (3) that fragile sites are indeed fragile as evidenced by deletion of the chromosome fragment distal to the fragile site or by the formation of tri-radial type figures; and (4) that the fragile site tendency in a chromosome is heritable and segregates in a mendelian co-dominant fashion through families.

From his cell culture observations, Sutherland also hypothesized about the fundamental mechanism underlying the expression of folate/thymidine-sensitive fragile sites, and surmised that it was through the metabolic integration of folate metabolism with pyrimidine biosynthesis and a relative shortage of thymidylate available for de novo DNA synthesis that folic acid/thymidine depletion elicited fragile site expression. Independently, Glover (1981) and Tommerup et al. (1981) confirmed his suspicion by showing that the fragile site could be elicited in medium containing normal levels of folic acid with the thymidylate synthetase antagonist 5-fluorodeoxyuridine.

There was still, however, much that was troublesome about heritable fragile sites in general and about the fra(X) in particular. The expression of the lesion in only a portion of cells analyzed, difficulty in eliciting the site in obligate carrier females or in tissues other than peripheral blood lymphocytes, and increasing evidence that fra(X) Martin-Bell syndrome was a relatively common human genetic abnormality that had clinically escaped us all led to renewed enthusiasm to solve some of these problems in the human cytogenetics community. In the hope of improving frequencies of expression, alternative cell culture methods were developed. Other thymidylate synthetase inhibitors such as fluorodeoxyycytidine and trifluorothymidine (Jacky and Sutherland 1983) or substances that somehow affected folate metabolism (Howard-Peebles et al. 1980) were used. Other chromosome structure-affecting compounds (Jacky and Dill 1983) were added to existing methods. Jacky and Dill (1980) first demonstrated the fra(X) in cultured skin fibroblasts, and confirmation by Tommerup et al. (1981), Fonatsch (1981), Mattei et al. (1981), and Steinbach et al. (1983) indicated that the syndrome would probably be amenable to prenatal diagnosis. Rapid developments in the cytogenetic area were being paralleled by clinical delineation of the fra(X) syndrome and its segregation through families (discussed in chapters 1 and 2). Combined with methodologic improvements, these developments moved the fra(X) rapidly to the forefront of clinical cytogenetics, as evidenced by ad hoc workshops at international meetings (Hecht et al. 1982) and the eventual gathering at the First International Fragile X Workshop in Bethesda in 1983 (Opitz and Sutherland 1984).

Heritable Fragile Sites

Fragile sites, in a much broader sense, have been observed on human chromosomes for many years. They were generally considered preparational artifacts or common human chromosome variants of little or no clinical significance. There was certainly no equation between the expression of such a chromosomal lesion and the tissue culture conditions to which an individual's cells had been exposed.

Sutherland's report in 1977 of such a relationship between fragile sites at 2q13, 10q23, 20p11, and Xq27 and the medium TC 199 drew attention to this correlation and opened an important period in the definition of some 107 fragile sites on human chromosomes and of various culture conditions that are required for their expression (Hecht 1988a; Hecht et al. 1990).

Fragile sites have categorically been broken down into several separate groups largely based on their tissue culture requirements for eliciting expression and their frequency in the population. The relatively rare heritable fragile sites are divided into two fairly discrete groups. Folate-sensitive fragile sites require folic acid/thymidine depletion for expression (Sutherland 1979a). Bromodeoxyuridine/distamycin A-inducible fragile sites seem relatively insensitive to tissue culture medium composition and often occur in individuals at relatively low spontaneous frequencies (Magenis et al. 1970) but show dramatic increases in frequency of expression when bromodeoxyuridine (BrdU) (Scheres and Hustinx 1980; Sutherland et al. 1980; Croci 1983), bromodeoxycytidine (BrdC) (Sutherland et al. 1984), or distamycin A (DistA) (Schmid et al. 1980) is added to the culture medium for a certain period before chromosome harvest. This latter group is also induced by the adenine/thymidine-(AT)-specific DNA base binding substances Netropsin and Hoechst 33258 (Sutherland et al. 1984). There is also some evidence that these fragile sites are induced by interferon (Thestrup-Pederson et al. 1980; Hecht et al. 1981; Shabati et al. 1983). In terms of induction, the two categories of rare heritable fragile sites seem to behave in almost opposite fashions. There are some 19 known rare heritable folate-sensitive fragile sites, including a site at 19p13, and 5 BrdU/DistA sites, summarized in figure 3.1.

A third category of fragile sites is a group that is generally also folate sensitive but relatively common and in fact may reflect a normal aspect of human chromosome structure and/or base DNA composition of specific regions of human chromosomes. These fragile sites have variously been called constitutive (Daniel et al. 1984a; Yunis and Soreng 1984) or constitutional and, because they are so common, have become a functional index for the cytogeneticist in recognizing that the folate/thymidine depletion conditions required for fra(X) expression have been achieved. Many constitutive sites are also induced with the DNA polymerase inhibitor aphidicolin (Glover et al.

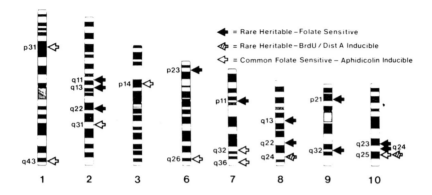

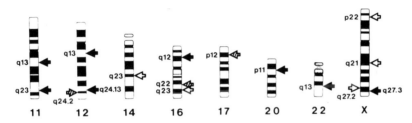

Figure 3.1 The rare and the most common constitutive fragile sites on human chromosomes, distinguished on the basis of their required method of induction.

1984) so that their expression is apparently tightly integrated with DNA replication and subsequent condensation. The most commonly seen folate-sensitive constitutive sites are marked on the idiogram in figure 3.1, and some examples of simultaneous expression of some constitutive sites and the fra(X) are shown in figure 3.2.

The categorical breakdown of fragile sites is continuing to evolve. For instance, the constitutive category now also includes a small group of BrdU-inducible sites and a small group of unique fragile sites that are induced by 5-azacytidine and largely confined to heterochromatic chromosome regions, i.e., 1q12, 9q12, and Yq12 (Sutherland et al. 1985b; Hecht et al. 1990). There are also apparently constitutive 5-azacytidine sites at 1q42 and 19q13. Also, a number of fragile sites with distinctly different requirements for induction seem to coincide in chromosomal location. Whether this represents double ascertainment of certain fragile sites through methodologic quirks or in fact distinctly different closely linked fragile site sequences remains uncertain. It may be that certain fragile sites detected at the cytogenetic level contain all of the required

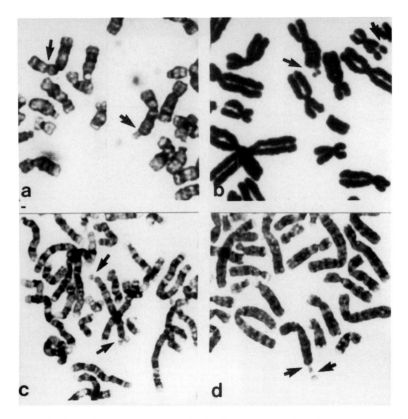

Figure 3.2 Examples of common constitutive fragile sites and the fra(X), expressed in the same metaphase. *a:* fra(3)(p14), fra(X)(q27.3). *b:* fra(16)(q23), fra(X)(q27.3). *c:* fra(X)(p22), tri-radial fra(X)(q27.3). *d:* fra(X)(q27.2), fra(X)(q27.3).

molecular base sequences for induction by distinctly different methods.

Of the rare heritable fragile sites, the sites at 2q13, 10q23, 10q25, 16q22, 20p11, and Xq27.3 are the best documented. All have been shown to be inherited in a simple mendelian fashion (reviewed by Sutherland and Hecht 1985). Most of the autosomal fragile sites have been demonstrated in phenotypically normal individuals, and none has been clearly associated with any specific clinical disorder (Schmid and Vischer 1969; Buhler et al. 1970; Magenis et al. 1970; Reeves and Lawler 1970; Fraccaro et al. 1972; Ferguson-Smith 1973; Oliver et al. 1978; Sorensen et al. 1979). An exception to this may be an association that exists between some fragile sites and specific hematologic malignancies or solid tumors (Hecht 1988b; LeBeau 1988; Hecht and

Sandberg 1988). The lack of clinical significance of rare autosomal fragile sites is at least partially explained by their presence nearly always in the hetero-zygous condition. The only rare fragile site ever observed homozygous in individuals is the relatively common BrdU site at 10q25 in two phenotypically normal siblings (Sutherland 1981).

The estimated frequency of occurrence of heritable fragile sites in the popu-lation differs substantially for the two categories of rare heritable fragile sites. The rare folate-sensitive autosomal sites occur in substantially less than 1% of the normal population (Hecht and Kaiser-McCaw 1979; Sutherland 1982a; Sutherland and Hecht 1985), but frequencies may be higher in selected groups. Petit et al. (1986) ascertained the folate-sensitive autosomal sites in 3.2% of a mentally retarded population surveyed. The rare BrdU/DistA-inducible herita-ble autosomal fragile sites are generally more common than are folate-sensitive heritable sites, although the fragile sites at 16q22 and 17p12 have been poorly ascertained, probably because of the required induction method (Sanfilippo et al. 1983). The BrdU site at 10q25 occurs in 1 of 40 individuals in the Australian population and can be considered a chromosomal polymorphism (Sutherland 1982b). The folate-sensitive aphidicolon-inducible fragile sites are extremely common and probably reflect a normal aspect of human chromosome structure and/or specific DNA base composition at particular chromosomal sites (Yunis and Soreng 1984). These sites are not infrequently expressed on both chromo-some homologs in a single metaphase cell.

An alphabetical gene symbol designation for each fragile site was initiated and adopted at the Eighth International Workshop on Human Gene Mapping (Berger et al. 1985; Sutherland and Mattei 1987; Sutherland and Ledbetter 1988). The designation was based on order of consideration of individual fragile sites by the committee and not on their sequential distribution along a chromosome and can be somewhat confusing. For example, fra(X)(q27.3) is FRAXA, whereas fra(X)(p22.31) is FRAXB, fra(X)(q22.1) is FRAXC, and FRAXD is the folic acid/aphidicolon-sensitive constitutive site at Xq27.2 just proximal to the Xq27.3 mental retardation site (Hecht et al. 1990).

Fra(X) Morphology and Variability in Expression

The fragile site on the X chromosome, like other heritable fragile sites, appears as an achromatic discontinuity traversing one or often both chromatids of the metaphase chromosome arm. Fragile sites cytologically appear very much like secondary constrictions that have been associated with nucleolar activity in classic plant and animal cytogenetics. Fragile sites at lesions in chromosome arms are frequently more easily discriminated in conventionally or homogeneously stained chromosome preparations (Sutherland and Hecht 1985) and are often more evident in less condensed chromosome preparations (Barbi and Steinbach 1982; Jacky and Dill 1983).

Figure 3.3 illustrates some of the variability in morphology of the fra(X) in homogeneously stained chromosome preparations. There is little difficulty in discriminating the fragile site lesion in the top row of figures (fig. 3.3*a–d*). The fra(X) can sometimes be more difficult to discriminate simply because of the overall quality of a metaphase spread (fig. 3.3*e,g,h*). The fragile site lesion is evident on more condensed chromosomes (fig. 3.3*i,j*), although seeing the fragile site is more difficult as chromosomes compact and, generally, overall frequencies of expression for a patient will be lower if analysis is confined to such metaphase spreads (Barbi and Steinbach 1982; Jacky and Dill 1983). Occasionally, rather bizarre variations in expression become apparent, as in the "bleeding-away" of the distal fragment (fig. 3.3*k,l*). Expression of the fragile site on a single chromatid and actual separation of the chromosome fragment distal to the fragile site are occasionally seen.

Fragile sites always occur in the same position on their respective chromosomes. The fra(X) mental retardation site has been positioned in the distal portion of sub-band Xq27.3 based on high resolution G- and R-banding chromosome studies (Turleau et al. 1979; Brookwell and Turner 1983; Krawczun et al. 1985) (fig. 3.4). On more extended chromosome preparations, a distinct, small, dark cap, the most distal portion of band q27, will be evident on the Xq28 distal fragment (fig. 3.2*c*). Banded chromosome preparations often show the fragile site less clearly, and less of the morphologic variation in the fragile site is evident than in homogeneously stained preparations (fig. 3.4). However, chromosome banding should always be used to confirm the presence of the Xq27.3 site in a patient, even when laboratories find scoring homogeneously stained chromosomes more desirable in detecting the lesion. This is important given descriptions of constitutive sites at 6q26, 7q36, and Xq27.2 that are induced under fra(X) culture conditions and morphologically appear nearly identical to the fra(X) in homogeneously stained material (Howard-Peebles 1981; Soudek and McGregor 1981). Chromosome banding is also essential for a routine constitutional chromosome analysis, which should be done on all patients referred for fra(X) analysis (Jacky et al. 1991).

R- and G-banding studies have also shown that the banding pattern of the chromosome arm adjacent to the fragile site is consistent with the banding pattern of the normal X (Harvey et al. 1977; Sutherland 1979a; Turleau et al. 1979; Howard-Peebles and Stoddard 1979). There is a striking similarity in appearance between the distal fragment on the terminal end of the fra(X) chromosome and the short arm satellites on D and G group chromosomes (e.g., see figure 3.1; chromosomes 14 and 22 have "satellited" pieces of chromatin connected by stalks to the main body of the chromosome); for this reason there

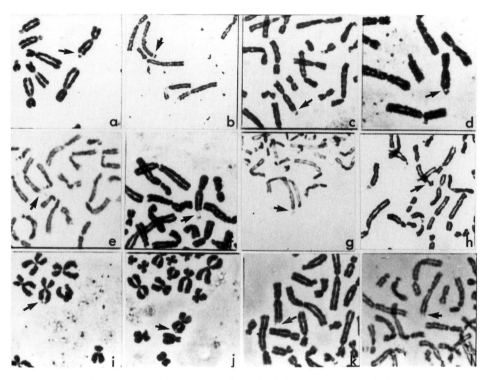

Figure 3.3 Examples of homogeneously stained (1% aceto-orcein) fra(X) chromosomes.

was initially some concern that the distal fragment was in fact a translocated satellite from one of these chromosomes. However, studies by Turleau et al. (1979) showed the Xq27–28 fragile site to be C-band negative, or lacking any translocated centrometric heterochromatin, and studies using silver staining, which is specific for satellited nucleolar regions (AgNOR banding), did not reveal any nucleolar organizer activity at the Xq27.3 fragile site (Howard-Peebles and Howell 1979; Sutherland and Leonard 1979; Turleau et al. 1979). The fact that satellite stalks from acrocentric chromosomes known to be involved in translocation are still stainable with this technique suggested that it was unlikely that the fra(X) includes material translocated from one of the D or G group chromosomes.

Although rare, perhaps the most dramatic appearances of the fra(X), or of other heritable fragile sites for that matter, is the appearance of apparent re-duplication of the Xq28 fragment distal to the fragile site (see figures 3.2c and 3.3h). This tri-radial configuration of fragile site-bearing chromosomes was

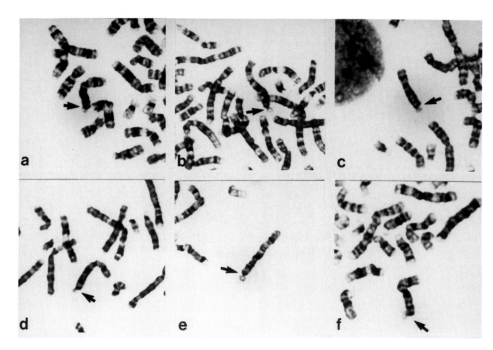

Figure 3.4 Trypsin/Wright's stain G-banded examples of the fra(X)(q27.3). Note the apparent expression of the fragile site on a single chromatid (*c* and *d*) and the precise location of the fragile site in distal band q27, such that a portion of distal band q27 either "bridges" the fragile site lesion or "caps" the distal q28 fragment (*b, c, e,* and *f*).

initially interpreted as selective endoreduplication or autonomous replication of the distal fragment (LeJeune et al. 1966, 1968; Noel et al. 1977) but perhaps was better explained by Ferguson-Smith (1973) as breakage of the fragile site lesion on one chromatid and subsequent segregation and replication of the chromatid carrying the entire distal chromosome fragment. This behavior has been interpreted as evidence of the fact that fragile sites are indeed fragile. The tri-radial appearance has been described for other fragile site chromosomes (Fraccaro et al. 1972; Sutherland 1979b; Glover et al. 1984) and is a more dramatic figure when the fragile site is more proximal on the chromosome arm and the distal fragment is larger (fig. 3.5). This breakage and unequal distribution of the distal fragment may occur repeatedly, giving rise to quadri-radial (see figure 3.5*g*) or even penta-radial type figures (Fraccaro et al. 1972).

The recent description of a common constitutive folate/thymidine depletion-induced fragile site at Xq27.2 not associated with familial retardation (Sutherland and Baker 1990) (see figure 3.2*d*) suggests that a proportion of fra(X) tri-

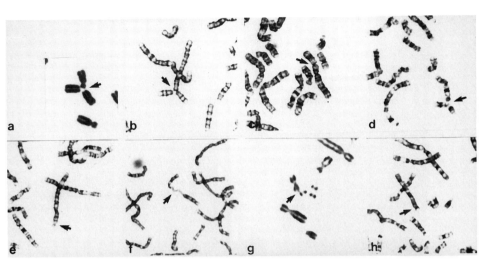

Figure 3.5 Examples of rare and common fragile sites on human chromosomes in response to folate/thymidylate depletion. *a*, tri-radial fra(2)(q13); *b*, tri-radial fra(2)(q31); *c*, fra(3)(p14); *d*, tri-radial fra(10)(q23); *e*, fra(6)(q26); *f*, 9qh "uncoiler" phenomenon; *g*, quadri-radial fra(16)(q23); *h*, fra(X)(q27.2).

radial figures may in fact be tandem expression of the Xq27.2 and Xq27.3 fragile sites. The constitutive fragile site at Xq27.2 may also be responsible for reports of apparent fra(X) sites in normal male individuals (Daker et al. 1981; Ledbetter et al. 1986; Sutherland and Baker 1990). In any case the tri-radial figure is well-documented for other heritable fragile sites and, even though rarely observed, is important in the basic fragility definition of fragile sites on human chromosomes (Sutherland 1979b).

Cell Culture Requirements in Eliciting Fra(X)

Folate/Thymidylate Deprivation and Folate Metabolism

In a more conventional sense, cytogenetic detection of the fragile site at Xq27.3 requires that, before chromosome analysis, cells be cultured under conditions that either restrict the availability of folic acid entering or being processed through the folate pathway (Sutherland 1979a) or more specifically interfere with the production of thymidylate and its availability for DNA replication (Glover 1981; Tommerup et al. 1981). Practically speaking, this is achieved by using culture medium either low in (TC 199) or entirely lacking (MEM-FA) folic acid, in which proliferating cells over time deplete folate reserves and effectively induce restricted conditions, or by using medium containing normal levels of folate but incorporating a folate or a thymidylate antagonist for a significant period before chromosome harvest to induce restricted conditions. Neither culture system should, of course, contain exogenous thymidine, which would metabolically permit bypassing of depletion or antagonist methods.

Sutherland (1979a) originally postulated that the metabolic mode of action of folate deprivation on fragile site expression was through pyrimidine biosynthesis, specifically in the conversion of dUMP to dTMP mediated by the coenzyme 5,10-meTHF: uridine monophosphate (dUMP) + 5,10-methylene tetrahydrofolate (5,10-meTHF) → thymidine monophosphate (dTMP) + dihydrofolate (DHF) (fig. 3.6). If this reaction is inhibited even mildly, the resulting deficiency in dTMP, thymidylate, would restrict DNA synthesis and potentially lead to lesions in the chromosomes. That this reaction may be the area of metabolism involved in fragile site expression is supported by the expression-enhancing effects of the folate antagonists methotrexate (Sutherland 1979a; Fonatsch 1981; Mattei et al. 1981), trimethoprim and pyrimethamine (LeJeune et al. 1982; Calva-Mercado et al. 1983), and Bactrim®, a mixture of trimethoprim and sulphamethoxazole (Jacky and Sutherland communication in Sutherland and Hecht 1985). These compounds all competitively inhibit dihydrofolate reductase (DHFR), blocking the conversion of DHF to tetrahydrofolic acid (THF) or in the initial reduction reaction converting dietary folic acid into DHF (Erbe 1975, 1979). Conversion of DHF to THF is tightly integrated with the production of coenzyme 5,10-meTHF (fig. 3.6), which is the methyl donor in converting dUMP to dTMP through thymidylate synthetase (TS).

Thymidylate biosynthesis itself can be attacked more specifically in eliciting the fragile site. Fluoropyrimidines such as 5-fluorodeoxyuridine (FUdR), 5-fluorodeoxycytidine (FCdR), and trifluorothymidine are powerful, highly specific, and irreversible inhibitors of thymidylate synthetase (Glover 1981; Tommerup et al. 1981; Jacky and Sutherland 1983) (fig. 3.6). FUdR is metabolized by thymidine kinase to FdUMP, which is the competitive agent. Methotrexate, in addition to its competitive inhibition of dihydrofolate reductase, can be converted intracellularly to diglutamyl methotrexate, which also inhibits thymidylate synthetase (Erbe and Wang 1984).

As would be predicted from the use of the specific metabolic antagonists, the concentration of folic acid in tissue culture media or in medium serum supplements, or the folate status of patients themselves for that matter, generally has much less bearing on the effectiveness of the culture system in eliciting fra(X) expression. FUdR is an effective inducer in the presence of folic acid but not in the presence of thymidine (Glover 1981; Brookwell et al. 1982; Gardiner et al.

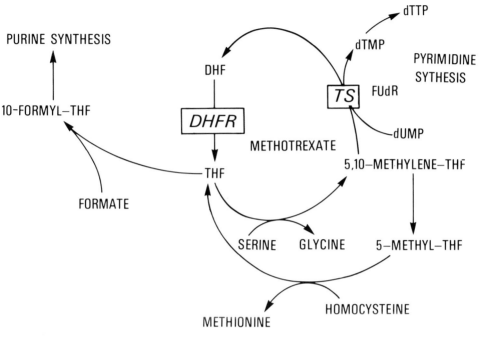

Figure 3.6 The folate metabolism pathway. *DHF*, dihydrofolate; *THF*, tetrahydrofolate; *dUMP*, uridylate; *dTMP*, thymidylate; *DHFR*, dihydrofolate reductase; *TS*, thy-
mydilate synthetase; *FUdR*, fluorodeoxyuridine. [Abstracted from Erbe (1975)]

1984), and therefore tissue culture media lacking thymidine (e.g., RPMI 1640)
are frequently preferred as background media in antagonist culture systems.

Methionine

In addition to its central position in thymidylate biosynthesis, folate metabolism is an active participant in purine synthesis and in the metabolic conversion
of several amino acids (Erbe and Wang 1984) (fig. 3.6). Howard-Peebles et al.
(1980) and Howard-Peebles and Pryor (1981) reported that the amino acid
methionine was apparently essential for fra(X) expression even under folate
depletion conditions. Methionine is synthesized from homocysteine by methionine synthase in the presence of vitamin B_{12} and the reduction of 5-meTHF to
THF (fig. 3.6). 6-meTHF is the main tissue and serum storage form of folate
(Erbe and Wang 1984). The basis for the methionine requirement for fragile site
expression is not well understood.

Glover and Howard-Peebles (1983) later showed that the methionine requirement in folate depletion was apparently overridden if FUdR was the fragile site-inducing agent. Erbe (personal communication) and Sutherland and Hecht (1985) also suggested that methionine is so essential to active cell proliferation in culture that any reduction in methionine may lead to poor cell growth and failure to deplete folate and thymidine effectively in the culture medium. Reliable detection of the fragile site generally requires a healthy, actively proliferating cell population (Kennerknecht et al. 1991).

Excess Thymidine

Sutherland et al. (1985a) recently showed that very high concentrations of thymidine will effectively elicit the fragile site. This "thymidine block" method inhibits DNA replication and has been effectively applied in cell synchronization procedures for high resolution chromosome banding (Viegas-Pequignot and Dutrillaux 1978). Excess thymidine leads to an elevated pool of deoxyribothymidine 5'-triphosphate (dTTP), which inhibits ribonucleotide reductase in the reduction of cytidine diphosphate to deoxycytidine diphosphate (Reichard et al. 1961). The expression of fra(X) elicited by excess thymidine can be inhibited with the addition of deoxycytidine (Sutherland et al. 1985a). The excess thymidine method is remarkable in that it basically provides evidence for the involvement of an alternative pathway for fragile site expression. Any molecular mechanism to explain fragile site expression (e.g., through specific nucleotide pool depletion or specific DNA base sequences that may be particularly sensitive to nucleotide pool imbalances) must now include both thymidylate and deoxycytidine.

Serum, pH, and Culture Period

Serum is a cell growth-promoting component added to most defined media for cell culture purposes. Its overall concentration in a medium is usually a function of the type of cells being grown, with concentrations roughly varying from 2–15% for cells, like lymphocytes, grown in suspension culture to concentrations of 25–30% for more finicky cells like amniocytes grown in monolayer culture. Serum is an expensive culture medium component and is obtained most frequently as either fetal bovine serum (FBS) or fetal calf serum and more rarely as pooled human serum or autologous patient serum. Serum contains a variety of substances including folates and other vitamins, most amino acids associated with the folate pathway, and ribonucleosides and deoxyribonucleosides (Erbe and Wang 1984). The concentration of these components can vary substantially from one lot of serum to another. So that the effects of this undefined component in medium on fra(X) expression are minimized, serum concentrations are kept relatively low (i.e., 2–5%) (Howard-Peebles and Pryor 1979; Sutherland 1979a; Howard-Peebles 1983). Concerns about adding exogenous folate from serum are more important in culture systems employing simple folate/thymidine depletion, as opposed to antagonist systems. Erbe and Wang (1984) and Erbe (personal communication) cautioned that the folates present in serum are biologically much more potent than folic acid as a vitamin constituent in a defined medium, and they encouraged the use of dialyzed serum to minimize this effect. Other investigators found little or no effect of higher serum concentrations on fra(X) frequencies and preferred higher concentrations (e.g., 15% FBS) for better mitotic yield (Webb et al. 1982).

Sutherland (1979a) showed a significant positive correlation between increasing pH over a range of 7–8 and frequencies of expression of the fra(X) and some other folate-sensitive fragile sites cultured in MEM-FA. This observation was confirmed for TC 199 as well (Gustavson et al. 1981; Howard-Peebles and Pryor 1981) but is apparently not so important in medium M (Jacobs et al. 1980). The optimal pH for fra(X) expression seems to be around 7.6; a pH much above this begins to retard cell growth seriously. So that this elevated pH is maintained for the duration of cell culture, medium is strongly buffered with 20–25 mM N-2-hydroxyethylpiperazine-N′-2-ethanesulfonic acid (HEPES). It is unclear precisely why pH is an important factor in fra(X) expression in lymphocytes, and again this concern seems to be limited to folate/thymidine depletion systems and not antagonist systems. Branda and Nelson (1982) showed that cellular uptake of folates inversely correlates with pH and that, at lower pH, intracellular levels of folate are substantially higher.

The time that cells spend in depleted conditions or exposed to a metabolic antagonist is also a significant factor in the expression of fragile sites. Sutherland (1979a) found that, in adding either folic acid or thymidine to lymphocyte culture to suppress fragile site expression, both compounds were most effective in inhibiting expression if they were added at least 24 hours before chromosome harvest. The inhibitory effects substantially decreased when either factor was added closer to harvest, and the findings seemed to indicate that the influences of culture media on fragile site expression are most effective before or early in the replicative phase of the cell cycle preceding chromosome harvest. This timing effect is consistent with the postulated mode of action of folate deprivation, namely, reduced pyrimidine biosynthesis. Low folate levels would lead to substantially reduced levels of thymidylate available for DNA synthesis. The original observation is consistent with the single round of replication required for fragile site expression induced with metabolic antagonists (Cantú and Jacobs 1984).

From a more practical standpoint, a number of reports have shown that extending the culture of lymphocytes from 72 to 96 hours will generally improve frequencies of fra(X) expression (Jacobs et al. 1980; Jennings et al. 1980;

Howard-Peebles and Pryor 1981; Mattei et al. 1981). Again, these findings largely pertain to folate/thymidine depletion systems where an extended period in culture perhaps more effectively depletes medium and serum components that suppress fragile site expression (e.g., folic acid and thymidine). Fragile site frequencies generally begin to decline after 96 hours, most likely as a result of overall culture deterioration and poor cell proliferation (Beek et al. 1980, 1983; Jacky et al. 1983). Fragile sites may in fact select against cells that express them because of breakage of the fragile site and loss of the distal chromosome fragment at anaphase. This is at least evidenced with a peak in the expression of interphase micronuclei containing lagging chromosome fragments at 120 hours under conditions of folate/thymidine depletion (Beek et al. 1983).

Culture duration is much less problematic in eliciting fragile sites with metabolic inhibitors. Generally, these compounds are required only in the last 24 hours before chromosome harvest (Glover 1981; Trommerup et al. 1981) and are effectively used with 72-hour culture duration. Simple folate/thymidine depletion culture conditions are considered diagnostically unsatisfactory at a culture duration of 48 hours and probably optimal at 96 hours.

Exogenous Folates, Folate Therapy, and Multivitamins

Several other controllable patient and culture preparation parameters seem to be able to influence a fra(X) result. Storage of peripheral blood either intentionally or through delay in transportation reduces frequencies of expression (Jacobs et al. 1980; Fonatsch 1981; Mattei et al. 1981; Brookwell et al. 1982; Fonatsch and Schwinger 1983). Brookwell et al. (1982) found that this effect could be overcome using the FUdR method of induction, as opposed to folate/thymidine depletion. Fonatsch and Schwinger (1983) and Soudek (1985) reported conflicting results, finding no benefit in improving frequencies of expression for older blood specimens with methotrexate, aminopterin, or FUdR induction. Jacky and Sutherland (1983), in a more controlled protocol, stored blood from four fra(X) male patients for up to seven days at 4°C and found no consistent decrease in overall frequencies of expression, nor did they find consistent differences in frequencies of expression between folate/thymidine depletion and the use of thymidylate synthetase antagonists.

Taken collectively, the reports on blood storage and transit delay are somewhat contradictory, and more systematic studies are required. Plausible explanations for reduced frequencies of expression related to blood storage are poor cell proliferation, possible efflux or leaching of folic acid and thymidine from dead or dying cells (Tommerup 1989b), and a decline in overall metaphase quality for scoring (Mattei et al. 1981), all of which may negatively influence a fra(X) result.

A number of authors have reported reduced frequencies of fra(X) expression in patients being therapeutically treated with folic acid (Lejeune et al. 1982; Brown et al. 1984, 1986; Erbe 1984; Neilsen and Tommerup 1984; Gustavson et al. 1985; Froster-Iskenius et al. 1986). Although the efficacy of such treatment remains uncertain, the cytogenetic findings have increased practical concerns about the effects of individual physiologic levels of folic acid on fra(X) studies and the effects of dietary supplements of folic acid taken regularly in multivitamins (Nielsen et al. 1983a; Froster-Iskenius et al. 1987). Reduced frequencies of fra(X) expression in patients receiving folate therapy have been largely confined to folate/thymidine depletion methods and not antagonist methods. FUdR generally elicits the fragile site at frequencies comparable to or only moderately decreased from frequencies elicited before treatment, whereas frequencies may drop dramatically when folate/thymidine depletion systems are used (Brown et al. 1984; Nielsen and Tommerup 1984). Brown et al. (1984) reported pretreatment frequencies in two fra(X) brothers of 32% and 49% with FUdR which dropped to 14% and 24%, respectively, on day 18 with daily folic acid doses of 500 and 1000 mg, respectively, in the two individuals. Frequencies in TC 199 for the same treatment period dropped to 4% in each male. These data were also interesting in the precipitous drop that can take place in serum folate levels once treatment is discontinued. Both males showed a greater than 25-fold decrease in serum folate levels five days after cessation of treatment, after which serum levels declined less rapidly. Serum levels were still essentially twice pretreatment levels three and one-half weeks after therapy was discontinued.

Froster-Iskenius et al. (1987) reported false-negative results in fra(X) patients taking oral dietary vitamin supplements studied initially only with folate/thymidylate depletion. The patients were clearly positive when vitamin supplements were withheld and cells were cultured according to the FUdR protocol. The results from both patients on folate therapy and dietary supplements of folic acid indicate that patient serum and red cell folate levels can have a significant effect on fra(X) cytogenetic results. A five- to six-week clearance of any folic acid supplementation may be prudent before fra(X) chromosome studies, and these results also point to the benefits derived in setting up blood from questionable fra(X) patients under multiple culture conditions employing both depletion and antagonist systems (Erbe and Wang 1984; Froster-Iskenius et al. 1987).

Concern about any bacterial contamination leading to the addition of exogenous folate to fra(X) cultures should disqualify cultures from fra(X) analysis in spite of good cell growth and chromosome slide preparations (Sutherland and Hecht 1985). Many enteric species of bacteria secrete folates as metabolic biproducts, and they will effectively destroy intended folate-depleted culture conditions.

The cell density of lymphocyte cultures influences fra(X) frequencies, particularly with the FUdR antagonist system (Cantu et al. 1985; Krawczun et al. 1986, 1988). Krawczun et al. (1986) recommended that whole blood be inoculated at a concentration of no more than 10^5 cells/ml (i.e, 5–7 drops of whole blood per 5 ml of culture). These studies suggested that either chemical decay of FUdR over time or complete utilization of metabolic antagonists at higher cell densities may allow cells to resume normal thymidylate metabolism and suppress fragile site expression.

Methods for Fra(X) Chromosome Preparation and Analysis

Standards of practice in the actual preparation, analysis, and scoring of fra(X) studies vary considerably. Heritable fragile sites are expressed in only a variable fraction of cells analyzed; thus, concerns exist about which cell culture methods will maximize frequencies of expression, how many positive cells are essential for a positive diagnosis, and how many cells must be analyzed reasonably to exclude the diagnosis.

Peripheral Blood Lymphocytes

Culture Methods

Numerous alternative methods for eliciting the fra(X) in lymphocytes have been published and those currently considered most reliable are listed in table 3.1. Generally, simple folate/thymidine deprivation by using TC 199 (Sutherland 1977), MEM-FA (Sutherland 1979a; Jacky and Sutherland 1983), or other commercially available folic acid/thymidine-deficient media [RPMI-FA (Irvine), Medium M (GIBCO)] is not by itself sufficiently reliable. The risk of a false-negative result is minimized with multiple culture systems, with at least one employing a folate or thymidylate antagonist. Practically speaking, this means that many laboratories routinely use two separate methods, frequently the older TC 199 or an equivalent standard and an antagonist method or simply two different antagonist methods. This is generally now considered to be an appropriate standard of practice (Jacky et al. 1991) and, perhaps more importantly, it not uncommonly assures satisfactory results in a sufficient number of analyzable cells. Both types of systems often compromise the mitotic index of a culture; poor cell proliferation in culture may negatively influence a fra(X) outcome (Kennerknecht et al. 1991). For this and other reasons noted previously, multiple culture systems are appropriate.

Although simple folate/thymidine depletion methods may lack a degree of reliability, they collectively have certain advantages over the antagonist methods. They are simple, are imposed at culture initiation, and require no further

Table 3.1
Culture Methods for Eliciting the Xq27.3 Fragile Site

1. **Folate/Thymidine Depletion:** TC 199 (Sutherland 1977) or MEM-FA (Sutherland 1979a; Jacky and Sutherland 1983), or RPMI 1640-FA (Irvine), or RPMI-FA 1640-FA (Irvine), Medium M (GIBCO), with 2–5% FBS.
2. **Dihydrofolate Reductase Inhibitors:** 10^{-5}, -10^{-7} methotrexate (Sutherland 1979a; Mattei et al. 1981), 16 mg/L aminopterin (Fonatsch 1981), or 13–26 mg/L trimethoprim (Lejeune et al. 1982; Calva-Mercado et al. 1983), or 300–600 mg/L Bactrim (Roche) (roughly equivalent to 50–100 mg/L trimethoprim) (Jacky and Sutherland in Sutherland and Hecht 1985).
3. **Thymidylate Synthetase Inhibitors:** RPMI 1640, or Ham's F10 + 0.005–0.1 mg/L, FUdR (Glover 1981; Tommerup et al. 1981), or FCdR (Jacky and Sutherland 1983).
4. **Ribonucleotide Reductase Inhibitors:** 300–1200 mg/L excess thymidine (Sutherland et al. 1985a).

attention for the duration of culture. Frequently, such media can be used as a routine lymphocyte medium in the laboratory. Dr. Sutherland's laboratory in Australia and my own laboratory have been using MEM-FA as a routine lymphocyte culture medium for several years. This routine use has some inherent advantages; it assures a fresh stock of appropriate fra(X) medium on hand at all times, folate/thymidine depletion medium produces generally more extended chromosome preparations for higher band resolution analysis, and the medium is somewhat more economical, with reduced levels of fetal bovine serum. For an elevated pH, media are buffered with 25 mM HEPES, and the pH is slightly raised to 7.6 with concentrated $NaHCO_3$.

Concentrations of the various metabolic antagonists used for eliciting the fra(X) vary among laboratories. Folic acid is generally present in the antagonist background medium at 1–10 mg/L. RPMI 1640 is frequently a medium of choice because it specifically lacks thymidine, as opposed to Ham's F10 (0.7 mg/L thymidine) or CMRL 1969 (10 mg/L thymidine). McCoy's 5A medium is also a satisfactory lymphocyte medium for use with antagonist systems (Tommerup 1989b).

Simple folate restriction conditions are imposed at culture initiation, whereas specific folate/thymidylate antagonists are added 24 hours before chromosome harvest. Variations reported in the two general methods include earlier addition of antagonists (Wilhelm et al. 1988) and combining of folate/thymidine depletion with antagonist induction. However, the latter methods often are so stringent and the mitotic index of such cultures is so depressed that analysis is neither practical nor necessarily a good idea (Kennerknecht et al. 1991).

Chromosome Preparation and Staining

Hypotonic and fixation treatments of fra(X) cultures at chromosome harvest follow routine laboratory procedures. However, this is an area that has not been studied extensively. Buhler et al. (1970) showed improved frequencies of expression of the fragile site at 2q13 when treated with a hypotonic solution of sodium citrate (1%) rather than the presently more commonly used KCl (0.075 *M*). Jacky and Dill (1980) found higher frequencies of expression of the fra(X) in fibroblasts when sodium citrate was used for the hypotonic treatment compared with KCl, and their observation was supported by similar findings by Gardner et al. (1982). In is unclear what difference a hypotonic treatment should make in improving frequencies of fragile site expression. The marked difference between the appearance of chromosomes after treatment in KCl and sodium citrate suggests that sodium citrate interacts more vigorously with chromatin. In general, the chromosomes appear less contracted and the integrity of the chromatin appears more relaxed, which may permit better visualization of the fragile site lesion. With KCl, the peripheries of the chromosomes appear more distinct, which seems to indicate that KCl interacts less directly with the chromatin material than does sodium citrate.

The mechanism underlying improved frequency of expression with sodium citrate may involve the chelation of divalent cations by the citrate moiety. In discussing the nature and origin of achromatic lesions in chromosomes, Chaudhuri (1972) suggested that, in addition to disturbances caused in the DNA itself, altered concentrations of divalent cations can produce decondensation irregularities. Golomb and Bahr (1974) showed that the chelation of divalent cations, particularly Ca^{+2}, can interface with the normal condensation process. Hypotonics will not in themselves elicit fragile sites. They may, however, be significant in making already induced fragile site lesions more evident in the metaphase chromosome spread.

Many laboratories prefer to analyze fra(X) studies on routinely banded chromosome preparations and, with sufficient experience, this should be considered diagnostically satisfactory. However, fragile site lesions on chromosomes are often more evident on homogeneously stained chromosome preparations compared to banded chromosomes. This is at least partly due to chromatin swelling that occurs in the enzymatic or heat pretreatments of preparations before banding, which can effectively obliterate the fragile site lesion. Homogeneous staining is achieved with 1–2% aceto-orcein, Giemsa, or Wright's stain. Aceto-orcein (1–2%), because of its high specificity for the nucleic acid component of chromatin, may be the best choice (Jacky and Dill 1980; Zankl and Eberle 1982) but is now infrequently used in human cytogenetics laboratories.

Confirmation of the Xq27.3 fragile site should use banded chromosome preparation to distinguish definitely the fra(X) from constitutive fragile sites on the distal long arms of chromosomes 6 and 7, as well as the recently described folate-sensitive constitutive site at Xq27.2, which is clearly distinct from the Xq27.3 fra(X) syndrome site (Sutherland and Baker 1990). Chromosome banding is also essential for a standard constitutional chromosome analysis, which should be performed for all patients referred for suspicion of fra(X)-linked mental retardation (Jacky et al. 1991).

Scoring and Analysis

The degree of chromosome condensation (as discussed earlier) can affect the frequency of expression of the fra(X) determined for individuals, and scoring should generally be directed at more extended chromosome spreads (Barbi and Steinbach 1982; Jacky and Dill 1983). In practice, because of the large number of cells required in the analysis and the extra time required to discriminate the X chromosome in more extended preparations, a compromise is usually achieved that eliminates from analysis both the very condensed metaphase and the very extended prometaphase cell.

Two questions frequently raised for fra(X) studies are how many cells should be scored in a routine analysis and at what point is a patient, either male or female, considered positive. This problem in practice has been treated as a question of chromosomal mosaicism in the number of cells scored based on levels of exclusion of the chromosomal abnormality similar to those adopted in ruling out mosaicism (Hook 1977; DeArce 1983). Examples of the number of cells required for exclusion levels of 1–60% with confidence intervals of 95% and 99% are listed in table 3.2. For males, exclusion at the 3% level with 95% confidence is considered appropriate and requires the scoring of 100 cells. For females, because detection is frequently more difficult and frequencies of expression are often lower than in males, exclusion at the 2% level with 95% confidence is considered appropriate and requires the scoring of 150 cells. Generally, frequencies of less than 3–4% should be regarded as of questionable significance, and such studies should be repeated to confirm the diagnosis. Low levels of expression should be interpreted in the context of both the patient phenotype and the family history.

Constitutional Chromosomal Damage

An important concern of cytogeneticists conducting fra(X) studies is whether the fragile site induction system is working. This concern has in the past been partly addressed by running parallel control cultures from positive fra(X) individuals to improve confidence that restrictive conditions have been achieved. Such controls had several drawbacks: (1) the work required in a fra(X) chromosome study was increased; (2) difficulty was encountered in obtaining suitable controls; and (3) there was known heterogeneity of fra(X) expression among

Table 3.2

Frequency of Fragile (X) Excluded with 95% and 99% Confidence Limits for Number of Cells Scored

No. of Cells Scored	Frequency (%) at Confidence Levels of:	
	95%	99%
5	. . .	. . .
10	26	37
15	19	27
20	14	21
25	12	17
30	10	15
35	9	13
40	8	11
45	7	10
50	6	9
55	6	9
60	5	8
65	5	7
70	5	7
75	4	6
80	4	6
85	4	6
90	4	5
95	4	5
100	3	5
150	2	4
200	2	3
250	2	2
300	1	2
350	1	2
400	1	2

Source: Adapted from Hook 1977.

individuals and among different cell populations (Brown et al. 1987). More recently, an alternative internal culture control was adopted whereby constitutional or constitutive folate-sensitive fragile sites are scored along with the fra(X) site on the same slide preparations (Soudek and McGregor 1981; Steinbach et al. 1982; Daniel et al. 1984; Jacky et al. 1991). As discussed earlier, constitutive folate-sensitive fragile sites are common in the population and are distributed extensively throughout the human chromosome complement (Glover et al. 1984; Yunis and Soreng 1984). The most commonly recognized constitutive sites and those most likely occurring in the population at the highest frequencies are the sites at 1p31, 2q31, 3p14, 6q26, 7q32, 16q23, Xp22, and Xq27.2 (Daniel et al. 1984; Glover et al. 1984; Hecht 1986; Sutherland and Baker 1990) (see figs. 3.1 and 3.5). The 9qh region also frequently seems to "uncoil" or become more extended under conditions of folate/thymidylate deprivation (Schmid and Vischer 1969) (see fig. 3.5*f*). Restrictive culture conditions are considered to have been effective if the constitutive fragile sites are present in approximately 2–5% of cells analyzed (Steinbach et al. 1982). Although it is acknowledged that not all individuals demonstrate constitutive sites under appropriate restrictive conditions (Wilmot and Shapiro 1986; Jenkins et al. 1988b), this internal culture control is considered perhaps the best that can currently be achieved in monitoring the actual culture conditions to which cells are exposed. It has been suggested that each laboratory establish its own baseline values for constitutive fragile sites relative to the induction systems used (Jenkins et al. 1990).

Reporting of Fra(X) Results

The correct cytogenetic nomenclature for indicating the presence of the chromosome abnormality is 46,fra(X)(q27.3),Y in males and 46,X,fra(X)(q27.3) in females. The result is not expressed as mosaicism, and it is generally recommended that the fra(X) chromosome report include the frequency of expression and the number of cells examined (Jacky et al. 1991). Frequencies of expression may be of some clinical significance, and they are in any case important information in family studies and other diagnostic testing. The report might also list the specific tissue culture methods used and comment on the presence or absence of constitutive fragile sites, with explanation of their significance.

Guidelines

Cytogenetic quality assurance measures being developed by the Association of Cytogenetic Technologists, the College of American Pathologists, and regional genetic group proficiency testing programs in cytogenetics have attempted to establish specific criteria for the preparation, scoring, and interpretation of specimens submitted for fra(X) chromosome analysis. However, until recently, there was no widespread consensus as to the methods and the number of cells that should be analyzed in fra(X) studies and, perhaps more importantly, the limitations in detection of the fra(X) by current cytogenetic techniques because, in many instances, appropriate systematic studies have not been done. In 1989, an ad hoc committee convened at the Fourth International Workshop on the Fragile X Syndrome and X-Linked Mental Retardation to establish minimal cytogenetic standards for the preparation and analysis of the fra(X) chromosome in lymphocytes (Jacky et al. 1991). The intention of the committee was to develop practical standards for the routine cytogenetic detec-

Table 3.3

Guidelines for Fragile X Chromosome Preparation and Analysis in Lymphocytes

---

At least two or three fragile X induction systems should be used for whole-blood cultures; the folate/thymidine deficient system (i.e., TC 199) should not be used alone

At least 100 cells should be scored for males and 150 for females

The presence of the Xq27.3 fragile site should be confirmed with chromosome banding

When a frequency of less than 4% is obtained, a repeat specimen should be requested. If no higher frequency of expression is obtained, the results should be interpreted with caution and on a case-by-case basis

Proper cytogenetic ISCN nomenclature should be used, i.e.

46,fra(X)(q27.3),Y

46,X,fra(X)(q27.3)

Fragile X studies for suspected X-linked mental retardation should include a standard constitutional chromosome analysis

---

Source: Adapted from Jacky et al. 1991.

tion of the fra(X). The guidelines are listed in table 3.3 and describe reasonable criteria for effective tissue culture methods for eliciting the Xq27.3 fragile site in vitro and for the analysis of such chromosome preparations.

Given limited cytogenetic resources, such scoring guidelines require a degree of flexibility and some interpretation in their application on a routine basis. The fra(X) should perhaps be more aggressively sought where it is more likely to be found, as for instance based on family history or clinical grounds. On the other hand, chromosome studies of additional intellectually retarded males and females in a family in which the problem has been diagnosed may not require the full cell count. Many laboratories currently routinely apply the fra(X) protocol to all bloods received from males or females with a diagnosis of developmental delay or mental handicap of unknown etiology.

Fibroblasts and Amniocytes for Prenatal Diagnosis

Demonstrating the fra(X) in skin fibroblasts cultured for a longer term was a necessary step in the eventual development of reliable prenatal testing for Martin-Bell syndrome. Jacky and Dill (1980) first showed that the fra(X) could be elicited in fibroblasts cultured under severe folate/thymidine depletion at frequencies comparable to their expression in lymphocytes in three individuals. The observation was generally confirmed in other investigations (Fonatsch 1981; Glover 1981; Mattei et al. 1981; Tommerup et al. 1981; Brookwell et al. 1982; Gardner et al. 1982; Steinbach et al. 1983; Barbi et al. 1984; Schmidt and Passarge 1986), although methods combining folate depletion and metabolic antagonists or simply using antagonists were considered more reliable (Mattei et al. 1981; Sutherland and Hecht 1985). Frequencies of expression in fibroblasts compared to lymphocytes are generally lower, probably because restrictive culture conditions are more difficult to achieve in situ for cells grown in monolayer and restrictive culture conditions compromise the mitotic index and produce poor quality chromosome preparations showing fewer clear fragile sites (Sutherland and Hecht 1985). Fra(X)-positive cells may be preferentially selected against in poorly proliferating cultures (Steinbach, personal communication) for reasons outlined earlier. Gardner et al. (1982) reported that increasing the L-methionine concentration under simple folate restriction conditions (TC 199) enhanced fragile site expression in fibroblasts. This method was used by McDermott et al. (1983) to demonstrate the fra(X) in a few males who did not express the fragile site in lymphocytes. A few of the other heritable sites on human chromosomes were demonstrated in fibroblasts (summarized by Sutherland and Hecht 1985). Aside from their methodologic importance for developing fra(X) prenatal diagnostic testing, fibroblasts may also be useful in determining fra(X) X-inactivation status in heterozygous females and may in fact be a more accurate reflection of the fra(X)-inactivation status of females showing a degree of intellectual impairment than are peripheral blood lymphocytes (Rocchi et al. 1990).

Perhaps the most difficult aspect of developing reliable methods for detecting the fra(X) in cells cultured in monolayer has been the transfer of the cells to restrictive culture conditions. Generally, cultures are not initiated and maintained in the background media that have been successfully used in lymphocyte culture, and the transition from the culture-initiating medium to medium appropriate for eliciting the fra(X) is difficult for actively dividing cells. This has been particularly true in amniocytes. Furthermore, specific medium components may be inherently antagonistic to fragile site expression. Jenkins et al. (1986a; 1988a) showed that Chang medium inhibits fra(X) expression even in the presence of FUdR or excess thymidine. Alternative methodologic protocols for eliciting the fra(X) in amniocytes are still being developed but, from our own experience, initiating cultures in MEM Alpha Medium (without Chang supplement) and eventually transferring to folate depletion in MEM-FA with an antagonist maintains a common background medium and makes the transition into depleted conditions considerably easier for cells. Perhaps the best induction method for amniocytes reported thus far combines FUdR (0.1 mM) with excess thymidine (600 mg/L) (Howard-Peebles 1991).

The offering of fra(X) prenatal diagnosis has generally been confined to pregnancies with a confirmed family history of fra(X) syndrome, and the collective experience is confined to a relatively few institutions that are developing an expertise in this area. The combined experience now includes approximately 500 specimens: 75% are from amniocenteses (Oberlé et al. 1985; Jenkins et al. 1988a; Purvis-Smith et al. 1988; Shapiro et al. 1988); 15% are fetal blood specimens (Webb et al. 1987; Shapiro et al. 1988), and approximately 10% are chorionic villi (Tommerup et al. 1985; Jenkins et al. 1988a; McKinley et al. 1988; Shapiro et al. 1988). In recently reviewing their own laboratory's fra(X) prenatal experience with 233 specimens, Shapiro et al. (1991) reported overall fra(X) detection rates for males and females of 11% and 13%, respectively. A combined false-negative rate of 4% emphasized the need for improved methods. Their experience also indicated that chorionic villi may be the least reliable tissue for fra(X) prenatal diagnosis, although this has not been the experience of other groups (Tommerup 1989b). Concordance between fra(X) expression frequencies in amniocytes or chorionic villi and peripheral blood lymphocytes is frequently difficult to show. A good example of this was reported by Rocchi et al. (1985) for male monozygotic twin fetuses who were discordant for fra(X) expression in amniocytes (0.4%, 17.5%) but concordant in lymphocytes (32%, 34%). There are also several reports of discordant results on prenatal specimens split between collaborating laboratories.

Perhaps one of the most difficult aspects of fra(X) prenatal diagnosis is predicting the possible clinical status of a fetus based on a positive fra(X) result. This is particularly difficult with respect to the expressing heterozygous female fetus, and it will be only with improved methods and better understanding of phenotype/fra(X) frequency correlations or other diagnostic criteria that such predictions will be more easily made. Approximately half of all fra(X) prenatal diagnoses have required DNA molecular studies in addition to the cytogenetic evaluation (see chapter 4).

Fra(X) Expression in Males and Their Female Relatives

Overview

Most of our understanding of fra(X) expression in individuals and within, and between, families has been confined to the analysis of peripheral blood lymphocytes. Reliable fra(X) expression in other tissues is often more difficult to achieve or less practical in making individual and family comparisons. Much of our current understanding of the differences in fra(X) expression in males and females emerged relatively early in the fra(X) literature (Giraud et al. 1976; Sutherland 1979c; Jacobs et al. 1980; Fryns 1984; Soudek et al. 1984). Many of these studies were initiated to reexamine clinical case files of previously reported families with familial X-linked mental retardation for the presence of the fragile site. Although the analysis of peripheral blood lymphocytes provided a reliable and satisfactory method for determining whether a mentally retarded male was carrying the fra(X), it generally proved much less satisfactory in determining female carrier status. Virtually all affected males from fra(X) families demonstrated the fra(X) chromosome. Frequency of expression was reported over a wide range, 2–50%, and the fragile site was rarely if ever demonstrated in any normal related males from such families.

It seems, however, that reliable determination of female carrier status by showing the fra(X) chromosome was not possible. Less than half of the older age obligate carrier females demonstrated the fra(X) in the early studies cited above. Interestingly, about half of the potential carrier females in these families demonstrated fra(X), consistent with mendelian transmission. Demonstration of fra(X) in the daughters of obligate carriers, compared to the difficulty in eliciting expression in obligate carrier mothers, immediately suggested an age dependency in fra(X) expression in females. In his study of 30 carrier females, Sutherland (1979c) concluded that the frequency of fra(X) expression in carriers rapidly declines in females over the age of 25 years and that the marker is frequently not observed in older obligate carrier females (30 years or older).

One interesting aspect of these earlier-reported families is that occasionally the pedigrees contained females of low normal intelligence who also demonstrated the fra(X) (Giraud et al. 1976; Sutherland 1979c; Jacobs et al. 1980). Only a few of these females were studied in detail, but the limited evidence suggested that there may be a positive correlation between the frequency of expression and the degree of intellectual deficit; the lower the intelligence of the heterozygous female, the greater is the frequency of expression of the fra(X) chromosome (Jacobs et al. 1980). This seems to be true only in females with >2% expression (Cronister et al. 1991, chapters 1 and 2). With the exception of perhaps making the methodologic detection of the fragile site generally more reliable, the development and use of metabolic antagonists for eliciting expression have contributed little in changing the apparent discrepancy that exists between males and females in expressing the fragile site.

Expression in Affected Males

Frequencies of expression in affected males tend to be higher than those in females who demonstrate the fra(X) and seem to be fairly constant over time for the same individual (Eberle et al. 1982; Howard-Peebles 1983; Soudek et al. 1984; Jenkins et al. 1986b) when results are reported from a single laboratory. Turner and Partington (1988) reported a small but significant decline in frequencies of expression for males after age 40, although this may in part be attributed to poor cell proliferation with advancing age. Frequencies of expression for males in the same family are generally fairly comparable. This has been interpreted to mean that a frequency may be a genetic familial trait (Brookwell et al. 1982; Soudek et al. 1984; Hecht 1986). This is also supported by concordant monozygous male twin and triplet data for frequencies of expression (Gillberg 1983; van der Hagen et al. 1983; Rocchi et al. 1985; Rosenblatt et al. 1985; Tommerup et al. 1987), even when discrepancies in degree of clinical effect exist (Tommerup et al. 1987). Chudley et al. (1983), Turner and Jacobs (1983), and Turner and Partington (1988) reported that frequencies of expression tend to correlate with degree of intellectual handicap in males, although exceptions to this are common both within families and when comparing specific individuals. Frequencies may vary considerably for the same individual studied at different institutions (Jacobs et al. 1980; Lubs et al. 1984).

Expression in Females

It is generally accepted that fra(X) expression in carrier females is much more difficult to show. An inverse correlation between age and frequency of expression has been reported (Sutherland 1979c; Jacobs et al. 1980; Turner et al. 1980a; Nielsen et al. 1983b), although this may in whole or in part be attributed to ascertainment bias (Turner and Jacobs 1983). Hecht et al. (1982) recommended serial study of females to address the questions of less reliable detection and declines in frequency of expression with advancing age.

Clearly one-third of all heterozygous female carriers are clinically affected to some degree (Turner et al. 1980a; Mikkelsen 1984; Sherman et al. 1984; Webb et al. 1984) (see chapter 1). This is an unusually high percentage for an X-linked disorder. Generally, affected females show higher frequencies of expression than do carrier females of normal intelligence when they do express the fra(X) (Howard-Peebles et al. 1980; Jacobs et al. 1980; Fishburn et al. 1983; Nielsen et al. 1983b; Knoll et al. 1984), and frequencies can occasionally equal or exceed frequencies of expression achieved in affected males in the same family (Jacky and Dill 1980; Tuckerman et al. 1985). The apparent decrease in fra(X) frequencies in females of normal intelligence with advancing age may not apply to more severely affected female individuals (Nielsen et al. 1983b).

X-Inactivation in Females

A natural explanation for the occurrence of heterozygous females with low intelligence may be that these particular individuals represent an extreme in the distribution of paternal and maternal X chromosome inactivation. In these females, the X chromosome carrying the fragile site and therefore the abnormal genes responsible for mental retardation may be active in a high proportion of cells. In an attempt to determine whether the pattern of X chromosome inactivation in such females was unusual, Uchida and Joyce (1982) first examined the late replication patterns of X chromosomes in two carrier females with normal intelligence who exhibited the marker and then compared them to patterns in two low intelligence carrier females who also exhibited the marker. They determined that both the normal X and the fra(X) were late replicating in an equal proportion of cells in the normal intelligence female carriers. [This pattern of random inactivation in normal females had also been reported by Martin et al. (1980)]. In the two dull carrier females, the normal X was preferentially inactivated about three times more frequently than was the fra(X). An increased frequency of active early-replicating fra(X) chromosomes in affected females was subsequently confirmed in several other studies (Howell and McDermott 1982; Uchida et al. 1983; Knoll et al. 1984; Webb and Jacobs 1990). Tuckerman et al. (1985) reported a similar finding in monozygotic twin females with markedly different intelligence. However, several studies have shown an excess of early-replicating active fra(X) chromosomes in both affected and normal heterozygotes (Lubs 1969; Nielsen et al. 1983b; Fryns et al. 1984; Fryns and Vvan den Berghe 1988).

One possible explanation for these contradictory results is that the late replication method per se may influence the result. Both thymidine and its analog BrdU, used to label the late-replicating X, are known to suppress fragile site expression, although more mildly when incorporated during the last five to six hours of culture (Sutherland et al. 1980). The paler-staining late-replicating X in these methods also makes visualization of the fragile site more difficult. Wilhelm et al. (1988) observed that late BrdU incorporation per se negatively influences fra(X) frequencies in heterozygous females but has no demonstrable effect on fra(X) frequencies in hemizygous males. This suggested to the investigators that BrdU incorporation, if it were to suppress fragile site expression, did not act on active X chromosomes in either females or males. The suppressive effect of BrdU on fra(X) frequencies in females only acted on late-replicating X chromosomes, perhaps in the way of a fragile site repair process, and a more accurate comparison of fragile site frequencies in females should only involve comparing frequencies of expression on active X chromosomes in X replication studies. From their own data and the analysis of data from Knoll et al. (1984), Wilhelm et al. (1988) concluded that in heterozygotes with intellectual impairment a high proportion of active X chromosomes expressed the fragile site, whereas in heterozygotes with normal or nearly normal intelligence a low proportion of active X chromosomes expressed the fragile site.

Rocchi et al. (1990) recently showed that a more accurate assessment of a fra(X) inactivation status in female heterozygotes may be achieved in cultured skin fibroblasts, which were under some circumstances concordant with degree of intellectual deficit when lymphocytes were not. The precise cause of low intelligence in carrier females thus remains somewhat controversial, but further studies with a better understanding of the effect of the methods on fragile site expression will probably clarify the relation among fra(X) expression in heterozygotes, X chromosome inactivation, and the manifestation in some female patients of a degree of intellectual impairment.

Fragile Sites as an Abnormality of Chromosomal Structure

Most hypotheses that have been put forward to explain the expression of a fragile site lesion on the X chromosome have done it with the view that if the fragile site, in a chromosome structural sense, can be understood, then perhaps we will begin some understanding of the fundamental molecular mutation underlying the mental retardation syndrome. The relationship is no doubt complex. It has developed first with some fundamental understanding of the tissue culture requirements and possible biochemical mechanisms underlying fragile site expression and then within the context of understanding fragile site behavior among different individuals, or sexes, or within families.

Fragile site expression at the level of chromosome structure seems to be a problem related to chromosome condensation, that is, a response to altered nucleotide biosynthesis occurring earlier in the cell cycle. Superimposed on this can be the apparent increasing penetrance of the fra(X) mutation as it is passed down through families (i.e., from non-fragile site expressing, unaffected transmitting males through their unaffected daughters, who generally express at very low frequencies or not at all, to their affected sons and daughters, in whom fra(X) expression is generally not difficult to demonstrate and the clinical phenotype is profoundly evident) (Sherman et al. 1984, 1985). The behavior of the fra(X) mutation among individuals and within families is discussed more extensively in chapters 2 and 7, and this discussion will be largely confined to the fragile site as a chromosome structural abnormality.

Chromosome Condensation and DNA Replication

Cytogenetic expression of a fragile site is most obviously a problem of chromosome condensation. Whether it is a problem of localized chromosome decondensation or delayed chromosome condensation because of earlier cellular events is not precisely known. Substances that have been shown generally to influence chromosome condensation by themselves have little or no effect on fragile site expression (Jacky and Dill 1983). Expression is also apparently a transient phenomenon in the cycling of chromatin and a chromosome in a cell, and this (at least in part) probably explains it being evident only in a proportion of asynchronous cells being examined from an individual at any one time. Theoretically, all fra(X) mutation-bearing X chromosomes in an individual have the potential for expressing the lesion. If fragile site expression were a fixed phenomenon once elicited in a chromosome, there would probably be quite severe consequences in terms of cell viability and the fragile site would be more evident cytogenetically with such phenomena as tri-radial formation from breakage of the fragile site on a single chromatid or perhaps breakage of both chromatids and release of the distal fragment and the generation of micronuclei

(Beek et al. 1983). These phenomena are in fact rarely observed and probably are more an accident than a predictable outcome for a chromosome expressing a fragile site lesion.

Fragile site expression is therefore somewhat a matter of a sequence of cellular events that is transiently evident with the microscope as a chromosomal lesion. It is not surprising that a host of parameters may influence the final determination of the frequency of expression.

Measured chromosome condensation per se has only a modest influence on frequencies of fragile site expression (Jacky and Dill 1983) and seems much less important than DNA replicative disturbances occurring earlier in the cell cycle. Sutherland (1979a), for instance, showed that even the very late addition of folate or thymidine two hours before chromosome harvest inhibited fragile site expression. In studying the effects of FUdR-induced achromatic chromosome lesions, Taylor et al. (1962) observed that such lesions could be repaired with thymidine added a single hour before chromosome harvest. These observations, along with others (Chaudhuri 1972), generally indicate that the primary commitment to fragile site expression probably occurs in the preceding replicative phases of the cell cycle. In other words, the abnormal chromosome condensation evident as a fragile site lesion at metaphase reflects S-phase replication or G_2-phase repair replication problems for that region of the chromosome that develop earlier in the cell cycle. DNA in the process of replication or arrested in replication will not condense (Johnson and Rao 1970; Beek et al. 1980; Taylor and Hagerman 1983), and so the fragile site lesion seems to be a very specific region in which replicative delay has prevented the normal mitotic condensation process.

DNA replication studies have provided more direct evidence that fragile site expression is the result of delayed replication and failed chromosome condensation. Most of the known rare heritable fragile sites occur in regions that are normally late replicating (i.e., replication occurs within the last five hours of DNA synthesis) (Kondra and Ray 1978). Abnormally late replicative behavior has been reported specifically in connection with the expression of the 2q13 fragile site (Buhler et al. 1970), and a 9q12 fragile site in the 9qh heterochromatic region has also been shown to be abnormally late replicating (Schmid and Vischer 1969). Since incomplete condensation has been shown to parallel late replication (Zakharov and Egolina 1968), it is reasonable to conclude that delayed condensation is responsible for expression.

What then are the replicative disturbances that precede faulty chromatin condensation, and how might they be produced within the context of what is understood about the metabolic requirements for fragile site expression?

Fragile Site DNA Sequences

A single round of replication is all that is required to elicit the fragile site lesion in both chromatids of the chromosome. This fairly straightforward observation implies that a fragile site DNA sequence must not be biased in the DNA strand distribution of a particular nucleotide or nucleotides that are influenced by the metabolic requirements for fragile site expression. Furthermore, whatever the fundamental mechanism underlying expression, these apparently hypersensitive points on chromosomes probably involve a substantial number of DNA base pairs to be viewed at the microscopic level [the roughly 25-Å DNA fiber will undergo an approximate 5,000-fold compaction into the metaphase chromosome (Stubblefield 1973)]. The fact that they are so sensitive to specific nucleotide concentrations has also been interpreted to mean that the DNA base sequence must also be somewhat repetitive (Sutherland 1979a; Glover 1981; Li and Zhou 1985; Li et al. 1986; Vandamme et al. 1988). A compositionally repetitive region of DNA would be particularly sensitive to altered cellular concentrations of specific DNA nucleotides and, under depleted conditions for fragile site expression, would have particular difficulty in either completing normal replication or completing repair replication just before chromosome condensation.

The initial observation of Sutherland (1979a) of the requirement for thymidine depletion suggested that the fragile site sequence might be particularly rich in adenine and thymidine residues and consequently particularly sensitive to thymidylate depletion. The AT-rich sequence hypothesis has been elaborated by other investigators to explain alternative mechanisms of fragile site induction (Glover 1981; Li et al. 1986; Vandamme et al. 1988) or amplification of a fundamentally AT-rich fragile site DNA sequence that not only can be seen at the microscopic level, but also might explain the increasing penetrance of the mutation as it segregates through families (Nussbaum et al. 1986). Fragile site AT richness is also supported by the 9qh "uncoiler" phenomenon that is evident when cells are cultured under folate/thymidine restriction (see fig. 3.5*f*); the 9q heterochromatic region is known to contain highly repetitive AT-rich satellite DNA sequences. The fra(X) site sequence also seems to be more recombigenic, with an increased sensitivity to sister chromatid exchange (Tommerup 1986, 1989a; Glover and Stein 1987), and this would support a repetitive sequence and/or perhaps a replicatively damaged area that would be more sensitive to recombination events.

Hastie and Allshire (1989) proposed alternatively that it may be thymidine/guanine (TG) strand repetitive sequences that constitute fragile site sequences. They proposed an interesting model based on the interstitial distribution of residual chromosome telomeric sequences that are highly repetitive TG sequences and that have been distributed throughout the human genome by chromosome rearrangement during evolution. The evidence supporting such a model is largely circumstantial. For instance, lower organism highly repetitive telomeric sequences will hybridize to human chromosomes, and the human fragile site at 2q13 corresponds to the fusion point of two acrocentric chromosomes in other primates that constitute human chromosome 2. The model is interesting and may help to explain the somewhat nonrandom distribution of fragile sites throughout the human genome.

One of the most interesting hypotheses of how altered nucleotide pools and, more specifically, thymidylate depletion might lead to replicative delay in a specific fragile site DNA sequence involves the misincorporation of ordinarily ribonucleic acid (RNA)-directed uracil residues into DNA, when the thymidine pool is very limited (Krumdieck and Howard-Peebles 1983; Vandamme et al. 1988). Under normal cellular conditions, eukaryotic DNA polymerase is incapable of discriminating between thymidylate (dTTP) and uridylate (dUTP). Normally the dUTP level is kept very low compared to dTTP. Any uracil residues inadvertently incorporated into DNA are removed by uracil-DNA-glycosylases, and excision-repair enzymes repair the apyrimidic site. As a direct consequence of thymidylate depletion, the intercellular concentrations of dTTP and dUTP shift substantially; dTTP becomes very low and dUTP may increase to 1,000 times its normal value (Goulian et al. 1980, 1988; Sedwick et al. 1981). This shift would substantially increase the likelihood that uracil residues would be available and incorporated into DNA during normal replication and might also substantially confound uracil-DNA-glycosylase excision-repair processes; lacking available thymidylate, uridylate would be reincorporated into DNA. This cascading sequence of misincorporation and misrepair processes may lead to a DNA sequence that is futilely trying to remove uracil residues, is unable to complete G_2 repair-replication processes, and is unable to condense as the cell progresses into mitosis.

The evidence either supporting or refuting such a model is scant and awaits further analysis. Reidy (1987) showed that deoxyuridine increased expression of folate-sensitive fragile sites, and Li and Zhou (1985) showed that addition of exogenous uridine increased fra(X) expression. However, Wang et al. (1985) showed that uracil misincorporation into total DNA is within normal limits in fra(X) cells. Furthermore, the model is difficult to reconcile with fragile site induction using excess thymidine and consequent deoxycytidine depletion (Sutherland et al. 1985a). Hoegerman (personal communication) emphasized that, in testing specific nucleotide depletion models, the overall biochemistry or metabolism of the nucleotides must be better understood and considered. For instance, nucleotides generally will not pass through cell membranes and must be added to culture systems in their nucleoside form (i.e., 2'-deoxynucleoside or 3',2'-dideoxynucleoside compounds).

Fragile Sites in the Cell Cycle

Krumdieck and Howard-Peebles (1983) proposed that disturbances in the methylation of DNA cytosine residues, combined with uracil misincorporation, may be responsible for the faulty condensation of chromatin at fragile sites. Methylated cytosine interacts with histone proteins in one of the primary stages of chromatin condensation. Inhibition of fra(X) expression by the DNA methylation inhibitor 5-azacytidine (azaC) has been reported (Mixon and Dev 1983; Daniel et al. 1984; Dev and Mixon 1984) but only at very high concentrations relative to inhibition of DNA methylation (Abruzzo et al. 1985; Glover et al. 1986; Ledbetter et al. 1986). Poot et al. (1990) recently demonstrated that the hypomethylation effect by azaC is largely confined to prolonging the S and G_2 compartments of the cell cycle and that very high concentrations will effectively arrest cells in G_2. An interesting cytologic outcome of azaC-treated cultures noted by the authors was an increase in endomitotic tetraploid cells, which they attributed to the initiation of the following cycle of replication while cells remained in a prolonged G_2. Schaap (1989) reported a similar outcome in lymphoblastoid cells without azaC treatment from fra(X) individuals and indicated that an increased incidence of endoreduplicated cells may be another useful diagnostic cytogenetic marker for these individuals. Caffeine, which is a potent inhibitor of G_2 postreplication repair, improves frequencies of fra(X) expression (Yunis and Soreng 1984) but will not by itself elicit the fra(X).

The model that is emerging for a fragile site as a chromosome structural abnormality is in its simplest sense two-stage. The first stage is the primary fragile site DNA sequence that is probably somewhat repetitive and compositionally influenced or affected by changes in nucleotide metabolism and availability during the replicative S period of the cell cycle. Once these changes are effected, the fragile sequence, on entering the G_2 secondary stage, is unable to be repaired or it is sufficiently delayed in G_2 that the normal initiation and progression of chromatin condensation cannot be achieved, and the sequence proceeds into mitosis as a chromosome gap.

Conclusions

The fra(X) chromosome is now recognized as the most common human chromosomal abnormality associated with heritable mental retardation. Although the fundamental metabolic requirements for eliciting fragile site expression are understood, there is still much to be learned about the underlying chromosomal mechanisms responsible for expression and about the relationship between the fragile site lesion and the molecular mutation responsible for the clinical disorder. Improved cytogenetic methods will probably make carrier female detection more reliable and add to our understanding of why an unusually high proportion of these individuals can show a degree of clinical effect. Much of the enthusiasm and experimentation devoted to unraveling the fra(X) enigma has driven an appreciation of heritable fragile sites on other human chromosomes and their clinical significance and will continue to add to our fundamental understanding of mammalian chromosomal structure and function.

Acknowledgments

I am grateful to Olivia Lamb, Toby Berry, Catherine Olson, and Françoise Weeks for their support and encouragement in the preparation of this manuscript and give special thanks to Marvin Yoshitomi for his work on the figures. Lucy Sheehey deserves an award for her extraordinary patience, editorial comment, and organizational skill applied in the preparation of all aspects of this paper. All of these individuals are members of the staff of the Cytogenetics Department at Kaiser-Permanente, NW. A special thank you goes to my children Luca and Clare for their patience and an unbiased perspective on the occasional late supper and a table setting partly of journals and the almighty "rough draft."

References

Abruzzo, M. A., M. Mayer, and P. A. Jacobs. 1985. The effect of methionine and 5-azacytidine on fragile X expression. *Am. J. Hum. Genet.* 37:193–198.

Barbi, G., and P. Steinbach. 1982. Increase in the incidence of the fragile site Xq27 in prometaphases. *Hum. Genet.* 61:82.

Barbi, G., P. Steinbach, A. Wiedenmann, and W. Vogel. 1984. Manifestation of the fragile site Xq27 in fibroblasts. III. A method to demonstrate R-type replication patterns and the fragile site. *Hum. Genet.* 65:76–78.

Beek, B., G. Klein, and G. Obe. 1980. The fate of chromosomal aberrations in a proliferating cell system. *Biol. Cell* 99:73–84.

Beek, B., P. B. Jacky, and G. R. Sutherland. 1983. Heritable fragile sites and micronucleus formation. *Ann. Genet.* 26:5–9.

Berger, R., C. D. Bloomfield, and G. R. Sutherland. 1985. Report of the committee on chromosome rearrangements in neoplasia and on fragile sites. Eighth International Workshop on Human Gene Mapping. *Cytogenet. Cell Genet.* 40:490–535.

Bowen, P., B. Biederman, and K. A. Swallow. 1978. The X-linked syndrome of macroorchidism and mental retardation: Further observations. *Am. J. Med. Genet.* 2:409–414.

Branda, R. F., and N. L. Nelson. 1982. Effects of pH on 5-methyltetrahydrofolic acid transport in human erythrocytes. *Biochem. Pharmacol.* 31:2300–2302.

Brookwell, R., and G. Turner. 1983. High resolution banding and the locus of the Xq fragile site. *Hum. Genet.* 63:77.

Brookwell, R., A. Daniel, G. Turner, and J. Fishburn. 1982. The fragile X(q27) form of X-linked mental retardation: FUdR as an inducing agent for fra(X)(q27) expression in lymphocytes, fibroblasts and amniocytes. *Am. J. Med. Genet.* 13:139–148.

Brown, W. T., E. C. Jenkins, E. Friedman, J. Brooks, I. L. Cohen, C. Duncan, A. L. Hill, M. N. Malik, V. Morris, E. Wolf, K. Wisniewski, and J. H. French. 1984. Folic acid therapy in the fragile X syndrome. *Am. J. Med. Genet.* 17:289–297.

Brown, W. T., I. L. Cohen, G. S. Fisch, E. G. Wolf-Schein, V. A. Jenkins, M. N. Malik, and E. C. Jenkins. 1986. High dose folic acid treatment of fragile (X) males. *Am. J. Med. Genet.* 23:263–271.

Brown, W. T., E. C. Jenkins, A. C. Gross, C. B. Chan, M. S. Krawczun, C. J. Duncan, S. L. Sklower, and G. S. Fisch. 1987. Further evidence for genetic heterogeneity in the fragile X syndrome. *Hum. Genet.* 75:311–321.

Buhler, E. M., J. Luchsinger, U. K. Buhler, K. Mehes, and G. R. Stadler. 1970. Non-condensation of one segment of a chromosome No. 2 in a male with an otherwise normal karyotype (and severe hypospadias). *Hum. Genet.* 9:97–104.

Calva-Mercado, M., C. Maunoury, M. Rethore, and J. Lejeune. 1983. Fragilité de l'X et inhibition de la dihydrofolate reductase: Comparison des effets de deux antibio-tiques: Trimethoprime et pyrimethamine. *Ann. Genet.* 26:147–149.

Cantú, E. S., and P. A. Jacobs. 1984. Fragile (X) expression: Relationship to the cell cycle. *Hum. Genet.* 67:99–102.

Cantú, E. S., R. L. Nussbaum, S. D. Airhart, and D. H. Ledbetter. 1985. Fragile (X) expression induced by FUdR is transient and inversely related to levels of thymidyl-ate synthetase activity. *Am. J. Hum. Genet.* 37:947–955.

Chaudhuri, J. P. 1972. On the origin and nature of achromatic lesions. *Chromosomes Today* 3:147–151.

Chudley, A. E., J. Knoll, J. W. Gerrard, L. Shepel, E. McGahey, and J. Anderson. 1983. Fragile (X) X-linked mental retardation. I: Relationship between age and intelligence and the frequency of expression of fragile (X)(q28). *Am. J. Med. Genet.* 14:699–712.

Croci, G. 1983. BrdU-sensitive fragile site on the long arm of chromosome 16. *Am. J. Hum. Genet.* 35:530–533.

Cronister, A., R. Schreiner, M. W. Henberge, K. Amiri, K. Harris, and R. J. Hager-man. 1991. The heterozygous fragile X female: Historical, physical, cognitive, and cytogenetic features. *Am. J. Med. Genet.* 38:269–274.

Daker, M. G., P. Chidiac, C. N. Fear, and A. C. Berry. 1981. Fragile X in a normal male: A cautionary tale. *Lancet* 1:780.

Daniel, A., L. Ekblom, and S. Phillips. 1984. Constitutive fragile sites lp31, 3p14, 6q26 and 16q23 and their use as controls for false-negative results with the fragile (X). *Am. J. Med. Genet.* 18:483–491.

DeArce, M. A. 1983. Tables for the cytogenetic study of fragile X chromosomes for diagnostic purposes. *Clin. Genet.* 24:320–323.

Dev, V. G., and C. Mixon. 1984. 5-Azacytidine decreases the frequency of fragile X expression in peripheral lymphocyte culture. *Am. J. Med. Genet.* 17:253–254.

Dunn, H. G., H. Renpenning, J. W. Gerrard, J. R. Miller, T. Tabata, and S. Federoff. 1963. Mental retardation as a sex-linked defect. *Am. J. Ment. Defic.* 67:827–848.

Eberlé, G., M. Zankl, and H. Zankl. 1982. The expression of fragile X chromosomes in members of the same family at different times of examination. *Hum. Genet.* 61:254–255.

Erbe, R. W. 1975. Inborn errors of folate metabolism. *N. Engl. J. Med.* 293:753–758, 807–811.

———. 1979. Genetic aspects of folate metabolism. *Adv. Hum. Genet.* 9:293–354.

———. 1984. Folic acid therapy in the fragile X syndrome. *Am. J. Med. Genet.* 17:299–301.

Erbe, R. W., and J.-C. C. Wang. 1984. Folate metabolism in humans. *Am. J. Med. Genet.* 17:277–287.

Ferguson-Smith, M. A. 1973. Inherited constriction fragility of chromosome 2. *Ann. Genet.* 16:29–34.

Fishburn, J., G. Turner, A. Daniel, and R. Brookwell. 1983. The diagnosis and frequency of X-linked conditions in a cohort of moderately retarded males with affected brothers. *Am. J. Med. Genet.* 14:713–724.

Fonatsch, C. 1981. A simple method to demonstrate the fragile X chromosome in fibroblasts. *Hum. Genet.* 59:186.

Fonatsch, C., and E. Schwinger. 1983. Frequency of fragile X chromosomes. Fra(X) in lymphocytes in relation to blood storage time and culture techniques. *Hum. Genet.* 64:39–41.

Fraccaro, M., J. Lindsten, L. Tiepolo, and N. Ricci. 1972. Instability of the paracentric region and selective reduplication of chromosome 2 in man. *Chromosomes Today* 3:138–146.

Froster-Iskenius, U., K. Bodeker, T. Oepen, R. Matthes, U. Piper, and E. Schwinger. 1986. Folic acid treatment in males and females with fragile-(X) syndrome. *Am. J. Med. Genet.* 23:273–289.

Froster-Iskenius, U., J. G. Hall, and C. J. R. Curry. 1987. False negative results in patients with fra(X)(q) mental retardation taking oral vitamin supplements. *N. Engl. J. Med.* 316:1093.

Fryns, J. P. 1984. The fragile X syndrome: A study of 83 families. *Clin. Genet.* 26:497–528.

Fryns, J. P., and H. Van den Berghe. 1988. Inactivation pattern of the fragile X in heterozygous carriers. *Am. J. Med. Genet.* 30:401–406.

Fryns, J. P., A. Kleczkowska., E. Kubien, P. Petit, and H. Van den Berghe. 1984. Inactivation pattern of the fragile X in heterozygous carriers. *Hum. Genet.* 65:401–405.

Gardiner, G. B., S. L. Wenger, and M. W. Steel. 1984. In vitro reversal of fragile-X expression by exogenous thymidine. *Clin. Genet.* 25:135–139.

Gardner, A. P., R. T. Howell, and A. McDermott. 1982. Fragile X chromosome: Consistent demonstration of fragile site in fibroblast cultures. *Lancet* 1:101.

Gillberg, C. 1983. Identical triplets with infantile autism and the fragile-X syndrome. *Br. J. Psychiatry* 143:256–260.

Giraud, F., S. Ayme., J. F. Mattei, and M. G. Mattei. 1976. Constitutional chromosomal breakage. *Hum. Genet.* 34:125–136.

Glover, T. W. 1981. FUdR induction of the X chromosome fragile site: Evidence for the mechanism of folic acid and thymidine inhibition. *Am. J. Genet.* 33:234–242.

Glover, T. W., and P. N. Howard-Peebles. 1983. The combined effects of FUdR addition and methionine depletion on the X-chromosome fragile site. *Am. J. Hum. Genet.* 35:117–122.

Glover, T. W., and C. K. Stein. 1987. Induction of sister chromatid exchanges in common fragile sites. *Am. J. Hum. Genet.* 41:882–890.

Glover, T. W., C. Berger, J. Coyle, and B. Echo. 1984. DNA polymerase X inhibition by aphidicolon induces gaps and breaks at common fragile sites in human chromosomes. *Hum. Genet.* 67:136–142.

Glover, T. W., J. Coyle-Morris, L. Pearce-Birge, C. Berger, and R. M. Genmill. 1986. DNA demethylation induced by 5-azacytidine does not affect fragile X expression. *Am. J. Hum. Genet.* 38:309–318.

Golomb, H. M., and G. F. Bahr. 1974. Electron microscopy of human interphase nuclei: Determination of total dry mass and DNA-packing ratio. *Chromosoma* 46:233–245.

Goulian, M., B. Bleile, and B. Y. Tseng. 1980. Methotrexate-induced misincorporation of uracil into DNA. *Proc. Natl. Acad. Sci. U.S.A.* 77:1956–1960.

Goulian, M., B. M. Bleile, L. M. Dickey, R. H. Grafstrom, H. A. Ingraham, S. A. Neynaker, M. S. Peterson, and B. Y. Tseng. 1988. Mechanism of thymineless death. *Adv. Exp. Med. Biol.* 195b:89–95.

Gustavson, K.-H., G. Holmgren, H. K. Blomquist, M. Mikkelson, I. Nordenson, H. Poulsen, and N. Tommerup. 1981. Familial X-linked mental retardation and fragile X chromosomes in two Swedish families. *Clin. Genet.* 19:101–110.

Gustavson, K.-H., K. Dahlbom, A. Flood, G. Holmgren, H. K. Blomquist, and G. Sanner. 1985. Effect of folic acid treatment in fragile X syndrome. *Clin. Genet.* 27:463–467.

Harvey, J., C. Judge, and S. Wiener. 1977. Familial X-linked mental retardation with an X chromosome abnormality. *J. Med. Genet.* 14:46–50.

Hastie, N. D., and R. C. Allshire. 1989. Human telomeres: Fusion and interstitial sites. *Trends Genet.* 5:326–331.

Hecht, F. 1986. Rare, polymorphic, and common fragile sites: A classification. *Hum. Genet.* 74:207–208.

———. 1988a. Fragile site update. *Cancer Genet. Cytogenet.* 31:125–131.

———. 1988b. Fragile sites, cancer chromosome breakpoints, and oncogenes all cluster in light G bands. *Cancer Genet. Cytogenet.* 31:17–24.

Hecht, F., and B. Kaiser-McCaw. 1979. The importance of being a fragile site. *Am. J. Hum. Genet.* 31:223–225.

Hecht, F., and A. A. Sandberg. 1988. Of fragile sites and cancer chromosome breakpoints. *Cancer Genet. Cytogenet.* 31:1–3.

Hecht, F., and G. R. Sutherland. 1984. Detection of the fragile X chromosome and other fragile sites. *Clin. Genet.* 26:301–303.

Hecht, F., B. Kaiser-McCaw, and P. B. Jacky. 1981. Interferon-inducible fragile site on chromosome 16. *Lancet* 1:108.

Hecht, F., P. B. Jacky, and G. R. Sutherland. 1982. The fragile X chromosome: Current methods. *Am. J. Med. Genet.* 11:489–495.

Hecht, F., K. H. Ramesh, and D. H. Lockwood. 1990. A guide to fragile sites on human chromosomes. *Cancer Genet. Cytogenet.* 44:37–45.

Hook, E. B. 1977. Exclusion of chromosomal mosaicism: Table of 90%, 95% and 99% confidence limits and comments on use. *Am. J. Hum. Genet.* 29:94–97.

Howard-Peebles, P. N. 1981. Chromosome banding in X-linked mental retardation. *Lancet* 1:494.

———. 1983. Conditions affecting fragile X chromosome structure in vitro. In *Cytogenetics of the mammalian X chromosome*, part B: X chromosome anomalies and their clinical manifestations. New York: Alan R. Liss, pp. 431–443.

———. 1991. Fragils X expression: Use of a double introduction system. Letter to the editor. *Am J. Med. Genet.* 38:445–446.

Howard-Peebles, P. N., and W. M. Howell. 1979. Mental retardation, marker X chromosomes and silver staining (NORS). *Cytogenet. Cell Genet.* 23:277–278.

Howard-Peebles, P. N., and J. C. Pryor. 1979. Marker X chromosomes and tissue-culture conditions. *N. Engl. J. Med.* 301:166.

———. 1981. Fragile sites on human chromosomes. I. The effect of methionine on the Xq fragile site. *Clin. Genet.* 19:228–232.

Howard-Peebles, P. N., and G. R. Stoddard. 1979. X-linked mental retardation with macroorchidism and marker X chromosomes. *Hum. Genet.* 50:247–251.

Howard-Peebles, P. N., G. R. Stoddard, and M. G. Mims. 1979. Familial X-linked mental retardation, verbal disability, and marker X chromosomes. *Am. J. Hum. Genet.* 31:214–222.

Howard-Peebles, P. N., J. C. Pryor, and G. R. Stoddard. 1980. X-linked mental retardation, the fragile site in Xq and the role of methionine. *Am. J. Hum. Genet.* 32:73A.

Howell, R. T., and A. McDermott. 1982. Replication status of the fragile X chromosome, fra(X)(q27), in three heterozygous females. *Hum. Genet.* 62:282–284.

Jacky, P. B. 1990. Fragile X and other heritable fragile sites on human chromosomes. In M. J. Barch (ed.), *ACT Cytogenetics Laboratory Manual.* New York: Raven. In press.

Jacky, P. B., and F. J. Dill. 1980. Expression in fibroblast culture of the satellited-X chromosome associated with familial sex-linked mental retardation. *Hum. Genet.* 53:267–269.

———. 1983. Fragile X chromosome and chromosome condensation. *Ann. Genet.* 26:171–173.

Jacky, P. B., and G. R. Sutherland. 1983. Thymidylate synthetase inhibition and fragile site expression in lymphocytes. *Am. J. Hum. Genet.* 35:1276–1283.

Jacky, P. B., B. Beek, and G. R. Sutherland. 1983. Fragile sites in chromosomes: Possible model for the study of spontaneous chromosome breakage. *Science* 220:69–70.

Jacky, P. B., Y. R. Ahuja, K. Anyane-Yeboa, W. R. Breg, N. J. Carpenter, U. G. Froster-Iskenius, J.-P. Fryns, T. W. Glover, K.-H. Gustavson, S. F. Hoegerman, G. Holmgren, P. N. Howard-Peebles, E. C. Jenkins, M. S. Krawczun, G. Neri, A. Pettigrew, T. Schaap, S. A. Schonberg, L. R. Shapiro, N. Spinner, P. Steinbach,

M. Vianna-Morgante, M. S. Watson, and P. L. Wilmot. 1991. Guidelines for the preparation and analysis of the fragile X chromosome in lymphocytes. *Am. J. Med. Genet.* 38:400–403.

Jacobs, P. A., T. W. Glover, M. Mayer, P. Fox, J. W. Gerrard, H. G. Dunn, and D. S. Herbst. 1980. X-linked mental retardation: A study of 7 families. *Am. J. Med. Genet.* 7:471–489.

Jenkins, E. C., W. T. Brown, M. G. Wilson, M. S. Lin, O. S. Alfi, E. R. Wassman, J. Brooks, C. J. Duncan, A. Masia, and M. S. Krawczun. 1986a. The prenatal detection of the fragile X chromosome: Review of recent experience. *Am. J. Med. Genet.* 23:297–311.

Jenkins, E. C., B. R. Kastin, M. S. Krawczun, K. P. Lele, W. P. Silverman, and W. T. Brown. 1986b. Fragile chromosome frequency is consistent temporally and within replicate cultures. *Am. J. Med. Genet.* 23:475–482.

Jenkins, E. C., W. T. Brown, M. S. Krawczun, C. J. Duncan, K. P. Lele, E. S. Cantu, S. Schonberg, M. S. Golbus, G. S. Sekhon, S. Stark, S. Kunaporn, and W. P. Silverman. 1988a. Recent experience in prenatal fra(X) detection. *Am. J. Med. Genet.* 20:329–336.

Jenkins, E. C., K. P. Lele, M. S. Krawczun, A. C. Gross, C. J. Duncan, and W. T. Brown. 1988b. Constitutive fragile sites in fra(X) individuals. *Am. J. Med. Genet.* 30:429–434.

Jenkins, E. C., C. J. Duncan, M. S. Sanz, M. Genovese, H. Gu, C. Schwartz-Richstein, K. P. Lele, M. L. Salandi, and M. S. Krawczun. 1991. Progress toward an internal control system for fra(X) induction by FUdR in whole blood cultures. *Pathobiology* 58:236–240.

Jennings, M., J. G. Hall, and H. Hoehn. 1980. Significance of phenotypic and chromosomal abnormalities in X-linked mental retardation (Martin-Bell or Renpenning syndrome). *Am. J. Med. Genet.* 7:417–432.

Johnson, R. T., and P. N. Rao. 1970. Mammalian cell fusion induction of premature chromosome condensation in interphase nuclei. *Nature* 226:717–722.

Kennerknecht, I., G. Barbi, N. Dahl, and P. Steinbach. 1991. How can the frequency of false-negative findings in prenatal diagnoses of fra(X) be reduced? Experience with first trimester chorionic villi sampling. *Am. J. Med. Genet.* 38:467–475.

Knoll, J. H., A. E. Chudley, and J. W. Gerrard. 1984. Fragile(X) X-linked mental retardation. II. Frequency and replication pattern of fragile(X)(q28) in heterozygotes. *Am J. Hum. Genet.* 36:640–645.

Knutsen, T., H. Bixenman, H. Lance, and P. Martin. Association of cytogenetic technologists task force, 1989. Chromosome analysis guidelines preliminary report. *Karyogram* 6:131–135.

Kondra, P. M., and M. Ray. 1978. Analysis of DNA replication pattern of human fibroblast chromosomes: The replication map. *Hum. Genet.* 43:139–149.

Krawczun, M. S., E. C. Jenkins, and W. T. Brown. 1985. Analysis of the fragile-X chromosome: Localization and detection of the fragile site in high resolution preparations. *Hum. Genet.* 69:209–211.

Krawczun, M. S., K. P. Lele, E. C. Jenkins, and W. T. Brown. 1986. Fragile X expression increased by low cell-culture density. *Am. J. Med. Genet.* 23:467–474.

Krawczun, M. S., K. P. Lele, E. C. Jenkins, W. T. Brown, and W. P. Silverman. 1988.

Fragile X expression in short-term whole blood cultures is affected by cell density. *Am. J. Med. Genet.* 30:435–442.

Krumdieck, C. L., and P. N. Howard-Peebles. 1983. On the nature of folic-acid-sensitive fragile sites in human chromosomes: An hypothesis. *Am. J. Med. Genet.* 16:23–28.

LeBeau, M. M. 1988. Editorial: Chromosomal fragile sites and cancer specific breakpoints. A moderating viewpoint. *Cancer Genet. Cytogenet.* 31:55–61.

Ledbetter, D. H., S. A. Ledbetter, and R. L. Nussbaum. 1986. Implications of fragile X expression in normal males for the nature of the mutation. *Nature* 324:161–163.

Lejeune, J., R. Berger, and M. O. Rethore. 1966. Sur l'endoréduplication sélective de certains segments du génome. *C. R. Acad. Sci. (Paris)* 263:1880–1882.

Lejeune, J., B. Dutrillaux, J. Lafourcade, R. Berger, D. Abonyi, and M. O. Rethore. 1968. Endoreduplication selective du bras du chromosome 2 chez une femme et sa fille. *C. R. Acad. Sci. (Paris)* 266:24–26.

Lejeune, J., N. Legrand, J. Lafourcade, M. O. Rethore, O. Raoul, and C. Manuoury. 1982. Fragilité du chromosome X et effets de la trimethoprime. *Ann. Genet.* 25:149–151.

Leversha, M. A., G. C. Webb, and S. M. Pavey. 1981. Chromosome banding required for studies on X-linked mental retardation. *Lancet* 1:49.

Li, N., and X. T. Zhou. 1985. Human chromosome hot points. IV. Uridine induced hot points break at 3p14 and 16q23.24 and increased expression of the fragile site Xq27 in folate-free medium. *Hum. Genet.* 71:363–365.

Li, N., Y. Wu, and X. Zhou. 1986. Human chromosome hot points. V. The effect of four nucleosides on chromosomes in folate-free medium. *Hum. Genet.* 74:101–103.

Lubs, H. A. 1969. A marker X chromosome. *Am. J. Hum. Genet.* 21:231–244.

Lubs, H. A., M. Watson, R. Breg, and J. E. Lujan. 1984. Restudy of the original marker X family. *Am. J. Med. Genet.* 17:133–144.

Magenis, R. E., F. Hecht, and E. W. Lovrien. 1970. Heritable fragile site on chromosome 16: Probable localization of haptoglobin locus in man. *Science* 170:85–87.

Martin, J. P., and J. Bell. 1943. A pedigree of mental defect showing sex-linkage. *J. Neurol. Psychiatry* 6:154–157.

Martin, R. H., C. C. Linn, B. J. Mathies, and R. B. Lowry. 1980. X-linked mental retardation with macroorchidism and marker X chromosomes. *Am. J. Med. Genet.* 7:433–441.

Mattei, M. G., J. F. Mattei, I. Vidal, and F. Giraud. 1981. Expression in lymphocyte and fibroblast culture of the fragile X chromosome: A new technical approach. *Hum. Genet.* 59:166–169.

McDermott, A., R. Walters, R. T. Howell, and A. Gardner. 1983. Fragile X chromosome: Clinical and cytogenetic studies on cases from 7 families. *J. Med. Genet.* 20:169–178.

McKinley, M. J., L. U. Kearney, K. H. Nicolaides, C. M. Gosden, T. P. Webb, and J. P. Fryns. 1988. Prenatal diagnosis of fragile X syndrome by placental (chorionic villi) biopsy culture. *Am. J. Med. Genet.* 30:355–368.

Mikkelsen, M. 1984. Conference report. Prenatal diagnosis. *Am. J. Med. Genet.* 17:55.

Mixon, C. and V. G. Dex. 1983. Fragile X expression is decreased by 5-azacytidine and by S-adenosylhomocysteine. *Am. J. Hum. Genet.* 35:1270–1275.

Nielsen, K. B., and N. Tommerup. 1984. Cytogenetic investigations in mentally re-tarded and normal males from 14 families with the fragile site at Xq28: Result of folic acid treatment on fra(X) expression. *Hum. Genet.* 66:225–229.

Nielsen, K. B., N. Tommerup, B. Frilis, K. Hjelt, and E. Hippe. 1983a. Folic acid metabolism in a patient with fragile X. *Clin. Genet.* 24:153–155.

Nielsen, K. B., N. Tommerup, H. Poulsen, P. Jacobsen, B. Beck, and M. Mikkelsen. 1983b. Carrier detection and X-inactivation studies in the fragile X syndrome. Cytogenetic studies in 63 obligate and potential carriers of the fragile X. *Hum. Genet.* 64:240–245.

Noel, B., B. Quack, J. Mottet, Y. Nantois, and B. Dutrillaux. 1977. Selective en-doreduplication of branched chromosome? *Exp. Cell Res.* 104:425–426.

Nussbaum, R. L., S. D. Airhart, and D. H. Ledbetter. 1986b. Recombination and amplification of pyrimidine-rich sequences may be responsible for initiation and progression of the Xq27 fragile site: An hypothesis. *Am. J. Med. Genet.* 23:715–722.

Oberlé, I., J. L. Mandel, J. Bone, M. G. Mattei, and J. F. Mattei. 1985. Polymorphic DNA markers in prenatal diagnosis of fragile X syndrome. *Lancet* 1:871.

Oliver, N., U. Francke, and K. M. Taylor. 1978. Silver staining studies of the short arm variant of human chromosome 17. *Hum. Genet.* 42:79–82.

Opitz, J. M., and G. R. Sutherland. 1984. Conference report: International Workshop on the Fragile X and X-linked Mental Retardation. *Am. J. Med. Genet.* 17:5–94.

Petit, P., J. P. Fryns, H. Van den Berghe, and F. Hecht. 1986. Population cytogenetics of autosomal fragile sites. *Clin. Genet.* 29:96–100.

Poot, M., J. Koehler, P. S. Rabinovitch, H. Hoehn, and J. H. Priest. 1990. Cell kinetic disturbances induced by treatment of human diploid fibroblasts with 5-azacytidine indicate a major role for DNA methylation in the regulation of the chromosome cycle. *Hum. Genet.* 84:258–262.

Purvis-Smith, S. T., S. Laing, G. R. Sutherland, and S. E. Baker. 1988. Prenatal diagnosis of the fragile X: The Australian experience. *Am. J. Med. Genet.* 30:337–345.

Reeves, B. R., and S. D. Lawler. 1970. Preferential breakage of sensitive regions of human chromosomes. *Humangenetik* 8:295–301.

Reichard, P., Z. N Callenakis, and E. S. Callenakis. 1961. Studies on a possible regulatory mechanism for the biosynthesis of deoxyribonucleic acid. *J. Biol. Chem.* 236:2514–2519.

Reidy, J. A. 1987. Deoxyuridine increases folate-sensitive fragile site expression in human lymphocytes. *Am. J. Med. Genet.* 26:1–5.

Renpenning, H., J. W. Gerrard, W. A. Zaleski, and T. Tabata. 1962. Familial sex-linked mental retardation. *Can. Med. Assoc. J.* 87:954–956.

Rocchi, M., V. Pecile, N. Archidiacono, G. Monni, Y. Dumey, and G. Filippi. 1985. Prenatal diagnosis of the fragile-X in male monozygotic twins: Discordant expres-sion of the fragile site in amniocytes. *Prenat. Diagn.* 5:229–231.

Rocchi, M., N. Archidiacono, A. Rinaldi, G. Filippi, G. Bartolucci, G. S. Fancello, and M. Siniscalco. 1990. Mental retardation in heterozygotes for the fragile-X mutation: Evidence in favor of an X inactivation-dependent effect. *Am. J. Hum. Genet.* 46:738–743.

Rosenblatt, D. S., E. A. Duschenes, F. V. Hellstrom, M. F. Golick, M. J. J. Vekemans, S. F. Zeesman, and E. Andermann. 1985. Folic acid blinded trial in identical twins with fragile X syndrome. *Am. J. Hum. Genet.* 37:543–552.

Ruvalcaba, R. H. A., S. A. Myhre, E. C. Roosen-Runge, and J. B. Beckwith. 1977. X-linked mental deficiency megalotestes syndrome. *JAMA* 238:1646–1650.

Sanfilippo, S., G. Neri, B. Tedeschi, N. Carlo-Stella, O. Triolo, and A. Serra. 1983. Chromosomal fragile sites: Preliminary data of a population survey. *Clin. Genet.* 24:295.

Schaap, T. 1989. Communication at the Fourth International Workshop on the Fragile X Syndrome and X-linked Mental Retardation, Harriman, NY, 1990. *Am. J. Med. Genet.* In press.

Scheres, J. M. J. C., and T. W. J. Hustinx. 1980. Heritable fragile sites and lymphocyte culture medium containing BrdU. *Am. J. Hum. Genet.* 32:628–629.

Schmid, M., C. Klett, and A. Niederhofer. 1980. Demonstration of a heritable fragile site in human chromosome 16 with distamycin A. *Cytogenet. Cell Genet.* 28:87–94.

Schmid, W., and D. Vischer. 1969. Spontaneous fragility of an abnormally wide secondary constriction region on human chromosome no. 9. *Humangenetik* 7:22–27.

Schmidt, A., and E. Passarge. 1986. Differential expression of fragile site Xq27 in cultured fibroblasts from hemizygotes and heterozygotes and its implications for prenatal diagnosis. *Am. J. Med. Genet.* 23:515–526.

Sedwick, W. D., M. Kutler, and O. E. Brown. 1981. Antifolate-induced misincorporation of deoxyuridine monophosphate into DNA: Inhibition of high molecular weight DNA synthesis in human lymphoblastoid cells. *Proc. Natl. Acad. Sci. U.S.A.* 78:917–921.

Shabati, F., D. Klar, S. Bichacho, J. Hart, and I. Hallorecht. 1983. Familial fragility on chromosome 16 (fra16q22) enhanced by both interferon and distamycin A. *Hum. Genet.* 63:341–344.

Shapiro, L. R., P. L. Wilmot, P. D. Murphy, and W. G. Breg. 1988. Experience with multiple approaches to the prenatal diagnosis of the fragile-X syndrome: Amniotic fluid, chorionic villi, fetal blood and molecular methods. *Am. J. Med. Genet.* 30:347–354.

Shapiro, L. R., P. L. Wilmot, D. A. Shapiro, I. M. Pettersen, and A. C. Casamassima. 1991. Cytogenetic diagnosis of the fragile X syndrome: Efficiency, utilization, and trends. *Am. J. Med. Genet.* 38:408–410.

Sherman, S. L., N. E. Morton, P. A. Jacobs, and G. Turner. 1984. The marker (X) syndrome: A cytogenetic and genetic analysis. *Ann. Hum. Genet.* 48:21–37.

Sherman, S. L., P. A. Jacobs, N. E. Morton, U. Froster-Iskenius, P. N. Howard-Peebles, K. B. Nielsen, M. W. Partington, G. R. Sutherland, G. Turner, and M. Watson. 1985. Further segregation analysis of the fragile X syndrome with special reference to transmitting males. *Hum. Genet.* 69:289–299.

Sorensen, K., J. Nielsen, V. Holm, and J. Haahr. 1979. Fragile site long arm chromosome 16. *Hum. Genet.* 48:131–134.

Soudek, D. 1985. Decrease of fragile X frequency in stored blood samples: Individual variability. *Clin. Genet.* 28:399–400.

Soudek, D., and T. McGregor. 1981. Sources of error in fragile X determination. *Lancet* 1:556–567.

Soudek, D., M. W. Partington, and J. S. Lawson. 1984. The fragile X syndrome. I: Familial variation in the proportion of lymphocytes with the fragile site in males. *Am. J. Hum. Genet.* 17:241–252.

Steinbach, P., G. Barbi, and T. Boller. 1982. On the frequency of telomeric chromosomal changes induced by culture conditions suitable for fragile X expression. *Hum. Genet.* 61:160–162.

Steinbach, P., G. Barbi, S. Baur, and A. Wiedenmann. 1983. Expression of the fragile site Xq27 in fibroblasts. I. Detection of fra(X)(q27) in fibroblast clones from males with X-linked mental retardation. *Hum. Genet.* 63:404–405.

Stubblefield, E. 1973. The structure of mammalian chromosomes. *Int. Rev. Cytol.* 35:1–60.

Sutherland, G. R. 1977. Fragile sites on human chromosomes: Demonstration of their dependence on the type of tissue culture medium. *Science* 197:265–266.

———. 1979a. Heritable fragile sites on human chromosomes. I. Factors affecting expression in lymphocyte culture. *Am. J. Hum. Genet.* 31:125–135.

———. 1979b. Heritable fragile sites on human chromosomes. II. Distribution, phenotypic effects and cytogenetics. *Am. J. Hum. Genet.* 31:136–148.

———. 1979c. Heritable fragile sites on human chromosomes. III. Detection of fra(X)(q27) in males with X-linked mental retardation and in their female relatives. *Am. J. Hum. Genet.* 53:23–27.

———. 1981. Heritable fragile sites on human chromosomes. VII. Children homozygous for the BrdU-requiring fra(X)(q25) are phenotypically normal. *Am. J. Hum. Genet.* 33:946–949.

———. 1982a. Heritable fragile sites on human chromosomes. VIII. Preliminary population cytogenetics data on the folic-acid-sensitive fragile sites. *Am. J. Hum. Genet.* 34:452–458.

———. 1982b. Heritable fragile sites on human chromosomes. IX. Population cytogenetics and segregation analysis of the BrdU-requiring fragile site at 10q25. *Am. J. Hum. Genet.* 34:753–756.

Sutherland, G. R., and E. Baker. 1990. The common fragile site in band q27 of the human X chromosome is not coincident with the fragile X. *Clin. Genet.* 37:167–172.

Sutherland, G. R., and F. Hecht. 1985. *Fragile sites on human chromosomes.* Oxford: Oxford University Press.

Sutherland, G. R., and D. H. Ledbetter. 1988. Report of the committee on cytogenetic markers. Human Gene Mapping 9.5 (1988): Update to the Ninth International Workshop on Human Gene Mapping. *Cytogenet. Cell Genet.* 49:221–223.

Sutherland, G. R., and P. Leonard. 1979. Heritable fragile sites on human chromosomes. IV. Silver staining. *Am. J. Hum. Genet.* 53:29–30.

Sutherland, G. R., and J. F. Mattei. 1987. Report of the committee on cytogenetic markers. Ninth International Workshop on Human Gene Mapping. *Cytogenet. Cell Genet.* 46:316–324.

Sutherland, G. R., E. Baker, and R. S. Seshadri. 1980. Heritable fragile sites on human chromosomes. V. A new class of fragile site requiring BrdU for expression. *Am. J. Hum. Genet.* 32:542–548.

Sutherland, G. R., P. B. Jacky, and E. Baker. 1984. Heritable fragile sites on human chromosomes. XI. Factors affecting expression of fragile sites at 10q25, 16q22 and 17p12. *Am. J. Hum. Genet.* 36:110–122.

Sutherland, G. R., E. Baker, and A. Fratini. 1985a. Excess thymidine induces folate sensitive fragile sites. *Am. J. Med. Genet.* 22:433–443.

Sutherland, G. R., M. I. Parslow, and E. Baker. 1985b. New classes of common fragile sites induced by 5-azacytidine and bromodeoxyuridine. *Hum. Genet.* 69:233–237.

Taylor, W., and P. Hagerman. 1983. Biochemistry of the fragile X syndrome. In R. J. Hagerman and P. M. McBogg (eds.), *The fragile X syndrome: Diagnosis, biochemistry, and intervention.* Dillon, Colo.: Spectra Publishing, pp. 115–151.

Taylor, J. H., W. F. Haut, and J. Tung. 1962. Effects of fluorodeoxyuridine on DNA replication, chromosome breakage, and reunion. *Proc. Natl. Acad. Sci. U.S.A.* 48:190–198.

Thestrup-Pederson, K., V. Esmann, J. R. Jensen, J. Hastrup, K. Thorling, A. K. Saemundsen, S. Bisballe, G. Pallesen, M. Madsen, M. Grazia-Masucci, and I. Ernberg. 1980. Espstein-Barr-virus-induced lymphoproliferative disorder converting to fatal Burkitt-like lymphoma in a boy with interferon-inducible chromosomal defect. *Lancet* 2: 997–1002.

Tommerup, N. 1986. Induction of the fragile X with simultaneous demonstration of early and late replicating regions and sister chromatid exchanges, abstract. In *Proceedings of the 7th International Congress of Human Genetics, Berlin, West Germany,* p. 221.

———. 1989a. Induction of the fragile X on BrdU-substituted chromosomes with direct visualization of sister chromatid exchanges on banded chromosomes. *Hum. Genet.* 81:377–381.

———. 1989b. Cytogenetics of the fragile site at Xq27. In K. E. Davies (ed.), *The fragile X syndrome.* New York: Oxford University Press, pp. 102–135.

Tommerup, N., H. Poulsen, and K. B. Nielsen. 1981. 5-Fluoro-2' deoxyuridine induction of the fragile site on Xq28 associated with X linked mental retardation. *J. Med. Genet.* 18:374–376.

Tommerup, N., F. Sondergaard, T. Tonnensen, M. Kristensen, B. Arveiler, and A. Schinzel. 1985. First trimester prenatal diagnosis of a male fetus with fragile X. *Lancet* 1:870.

Tommerup, N., L. Tranebjaerg, T. Tonnesen, W. Kastern, H. Hansen, and J. Dissing. 1987. Identical expression of the fragile X but discordant clinical affection in two monozygotic twins with Martin-Bell syndrome. Presented at the Third International Workshop on the Fragile X and X-linked Mental Retardation, Troina, September 13–16.

Tuckerman, E., T. Webb, and S. E. Bundey. 1985. Frequency and replication status of the fragile X, fra(X)(q27–28), in a pair of monozygotic twins of markedly differing intelligence. *J. Med. Genet.* 22:85–91.

Tuckerman, E., T. Webb, and A. Thake. 1986. Replication status of fragile X(q27.3) in 13 female heterozygotes. *J. Med. Genet.* 23:407–410.

Turleau, C., P. Czernichow, R. Gorin, P. Royer, and J. de Grouchy. 1979. Debilité mentale lieu au sexe, visage particulier, macroorchidie et zone de fragilité de l'X. *Ann. Genet.* 22:205–209.

Turner, G., and P. A. Jacobs. 1983. Marker X linked mental retardation. *Adv. Hum. Genet.* 13:83–112.

Turner, G., and M. W. Partington. 1988. Fragile X expression, age and the degree of mental handicap in the male. *Am. J. Med. Genet.* 30:423–428.

Turner, G., R. Brookwell, A. Daniel, M. DeSelikowitz, and M. Zilibowitz. 1980a. Heterozygous expression of X-linked mental retardation and X-chromosome marker fra(X)(q27). *N. Engl. J. Med.* 303:622–664.

Turner, G., A. Daniel, and M. Frost. 1980b. X-linked mental retardation, macroorchidism and the Xq27 fragile site. *J. Pediatr.* 96:837–841.

Uchida, I. A., and E. M. Joyce. 1982. Activity of the fragile X in heterozygous carriers. *Am. J. Hum. Genet.* 34:286–293.

Uchida, I. A., V. C. P. Freeman, H. Jamro, M. W. Partington, and H. C. Soltan. 1983. Additional evidence for fragile X activity in heterozygous carriers. *Am. J. Hum. Genet.* 35:861–868.

Van der Hagen, C. B., K. H. van der Orstavik, J. Blakke, and K. Berg. 1983. Monozygous male triplets with mental retardation and a fragile X chromosome. *Clin. Genet.* 23:232.

Vandamme, B., I. Liebaers, L. Hens, J. L. Bernheim, and G. Roobol. 1988. The role of fluorinated pyrimidine analogues in the induction of the in vitro expression of the fragile X chromosome. *Hum. Genet.* 79:341–346.

Viegas-Pequignot, E., and B. Dutrillaux. 1978. Une methode simple pour obtenir des prosphases et des prometaphases. *Ann. Genet.* 21:122–125.

Wang, J. C., and R. W. Erbe. 1985. Thymidylate metabolism in fragile X syndrome cells. *Somatic Cell Mol. Genet.* 11:353–357.

Wang, J. C., G. P. Beardsley, and R. W. Erbe. 1985. Antifolate-induced misincorporation of deoxyuridine monophosphate into DNA by cells from patients with the fragile X syndrome. *Am. J. Med. Genet.* 21:691–696.

Webb, G. C., J. L. Halliday, D. B. Pitt, C. G. Judge, and M. Leversha. 1982. Fragile(X)(q27) sites in a pedigree with female carriers showing mild to severe mental retardation. *J. Med. Genet.* 19:44–48.

Webb, T., and P. A. Jocobs. 1990. Fragile Xq27.3 in female heterozygotes for the Martin-Bell syndrome. *J. Med. Genet.* 27:627–631.

Webb, T. P., S. E. Bundey, A. Thake, and J. Todd. 1984. Study of the fragile X chromosome and mental retardation. *J. Med. Genet.* 21:293A.

Webb, T. P., C. H. Rodeck, K. H. Nicolaides, and C. M. Gosden. 1987. Prenatal diagnosis of the fragile X syndrome using fetal blood and amniotic fluid. *Prenat. Diagn.* 7:203–214.

Wilhelm, P. L., U. Froster-Iskenius, J. Paul, and E. Schwinger. 1988. Fra(X) frequency on the active X-chromosome and phenotype in heterozygous carriers of the fra(X) form of mental retardation. *Am. J. Med. Genet.* 30:407–415.

Wilmot, P. L., and L. R. Shapiro. 1986. The value of folate sensitive fragile sites in detecting false negative fragile X prenatal cytogenetic results in amniotic fluid cell cultures. *Am. J. Hum. Genet.* 39(Suppl.):A269.

Yunis, J. J., and A. L. Soreng. 1984. Constitutive fragile sites and cancer. *Science* 226:1199–1204.

Zakharov, A. F., and N. A. Egolina. 1968. Asynchrony of DNA replication and mitotic spiralization along hetero-chromatic portions of Chinese hamster chromosomes. *Chromosoma* 23:365–385.

Zankl, H., and G. Eberle. 1982. Methods of increasing the visibility of fragile X chromosomes. *Hum. Genet.* 60:80–81.

Editor's Note

The fragile X mental retardation (FMR-1) gene was sequenced by Dr. Stephen Warren and his collaborators (see Verkerk et al. 1991). For more information see page 172.

References Added in Proof

Oberlé, I., F. Rousseau, D. Heitz, C. Kretz, D. Devys, A. Hanauer, J. Boué, M. F. Bertheas, and J. L. Mandel. 1991. Instability of a 550-base pair DNA segment and abnormal methylation in fragile X syndrome. *Science* 252:1097–1102.

Verkerk, A. J. M. H., M. Plerettl, J. S. Sutcliffe, Y.-H. Fu, D. P. A. Kuhl, A. Pizzuti, O. Reiner, S. Richards, M. F. Victoria, F. Zhang, B. E. Eussen, G.-J. B. van Ommen, L. A. J. Blonden, G. J. Riggins, J. L. Chastain, C. B. Kunst, H. Galjaard, C. T. Caskey, D. L. Nelson, B. A. Oostra, and S. T. Warren. 1991. Identification of a gene (FMR-1) containing a CGG repeat coincident with a breakpoint cluster region exhibiting length variation in fragile X syndrome. *Cell* 65:905–914.

Yu, S., M. Pritchard, E. Kremer, M. Lynch, J. Nancarrow, E. Baker, K. Holman, J. C. Mulley, S. T. Warren, D. Schlessinger, G. R. Sutherland, and R. I. Richards. 1991. Fragile X genotype characterized by an unstable region of DNA. *Science* 252:1179–1181.

CHAPTER 4

The Molecular Biology of the Fragile X Mutation

W. Ted Brown, M.D., Ph.D.

The molecular biology of the fragile X site is an area of active investigation and research. However, the molecular nature of the mutation underlying the fra(X) site is virtually unknown. No abnormal gene or gene product related to the fra(X) mutation has yet been identified. Because knowledge about which genes might be involved is lacking, only indirect approaches are available to identify and help characterize the underlying mutation. With DNA probes that detect polymorphic variations or markers on the X chromosome, the location of the mutation has been genetically mapped. Linked DNA markers have been used to trace the inheritance of the fra(X) chromosome within families. Markers have been quite useful for clinical testing purposes. They allow carrier detection, they can identify the presence of transmitting males (both brothers and grandfathers), and they complement cytogenetic analysis for prenatal diagnosis. DNA markers are being used to help study the nature of the underlying mutation. Having closely linked DNA markers allows the application of new technologies to help isolate the fra(X) mutation. In this chapter, DNA linkage studies, clinical uses, molecular investigations, and future directions in the investigation of the fra(X) locus are reviewed.

DNA Markers and the Fra(X) Syndrome

Recent developments in the use of recombinant DNA technology have led to new methods for diagnosis of genetic diseases. The new techniques allow diagnosis by analysis of closely positioned DNA polymorphisms. This approach has been used for testing and diagnosis in fra(X) and in a number of other genetic diseases where the nature of the primary gene product or mutation is unknown. In addition to allowing carrier identification and genetic counseling, this approach can assist with the isolation and molecular characterization

146

of the basic gene mutations underlying such genetic disorders.

The development of recombinant DNA technology has depended upon two basic discoveries: endonucleases and gene cloning. In 1970, it was observed that some bacterial enzymes called restriction endonucleases degrade foreign DNA. The first such enzyme to be discovered was found in the bacteria *Haemophilus influenzae* by Smith and Wilcox (1970). This enzyme recognizes a specific sequence of six base pairs in the DNA molecule. Since their initial discovery in 1970, more than 400 different restriction enzymes have been isolated from different strains of bacteria. These enzymes generally recognize a specific sequence of four or six DNA base pairs (bp). The enzymes are named for the bacterial species from which they are isolated. The convention has been adopted that the host bacterial organism is identified by the letter of the genus name and the first two letters of the second name to form a letter abbreviation. For example, the enzyme from *Haemophilus influenzae* is known as *Hin* and that from *Escherichia coli* is known as *Eco*. A strain identification follows the genus abbreviation, for example, *EcoR*. When more than one restriction enzyme system has been identified within a given bacterial strain, these are identified separately by roman numerals, such as *EcoRI* and *HindIII*. By use of such restriction enzymes, DNA can be cut at specific and reproducible sites. Restriction enzymes cut DNA into pieces generally averaging 1,000 to 10,000 bp long. As the human genome contains about 3×10^9 bp, 300,000 to 3,000,000 pieces are produced when human DNA is digested with such an enzyme.

Restriction enzymes allowed the development of gene cloning. In this process a fragment of cut DNA can be inserted into bacterial host carriers known as vectors. Vectors include plasmids, bacteriophages, and cosmids. These vectors generally live and reproduce in the cytoplasm of bacteria. There are sites where a restriction enzyme can cut a vector and a foreign piece of DNA can be inserted. Thus, DNA from two species can be recombined. The various fragments produced by a restriction enzyme digestion of a sample of human DNA can each be individually cloned into vectors. A collection of clones (e.g., all fragments from a given chromosome) is called a library. From this library, individual clones can be selected and grown up to a very large quantity. The cloned DNA fragment can be isolated from the vector using the restriction enzyme that cuts the exact site where the DNA from the two species is joined. In this manner, a pure quantity of given gene or DNA fragment of interest can be isolated for further study. Because these vectors and their host bacteria can be grown quickly in the laboratory, large quantities of a DNA sequence can be isolated to be further studied with speed and efficiency.

To study the gene or DNA sequence of interest from a given individual, one needs a method to visualize DNA. The most widely used method for visualizing the gene of interest is the method of Southern blotting (Southern 1975). DNA from an individual is isolated from an available tissue source such as white blood cells. The DNA is cut by one of the restriction enzymes. The millions of fragments of various sizes which are produced can be separated by electrophoresis in an agarose gel. The movement of the various fragments in the gel is a function of their length. The DNA is then transferred by blotting from the agarose gel onto a supporting membrane such as nitrocellulose paper to which the DNA can be covalently bound. The position of the DNA fragments on the paper is the same as was their position in the agarose gel. For visualization of the position of a particular DNA sequence among the millions of fragments on the paper, a vector containing a cloned DNA sequence is radioactively labeled. This labeled DNA sequence is complementary to a sequence that is on the filter paper. The radioactive DNA is used to detect its complementary sequence. It hybridizes under conditions that allow the complementary sequence to be recognized. The position of the radioactive probe is visualized after exposure to X-ray film. This method allows one to detect a given sequence of DNA among the millions of sequences of DNA which are produced when a sample of human DNA is cut with a restriction enzyme.

In comparing one individual to another, it was discovered that there are random base changes or variations that occur in about 1 of every 200 to 500 bp along the genome. These variations can be detected by the use of restriction enzymes. For example, the enzyme *Hind*III recognizes the base sequence . . . AAGCTT . . . and will cut the DNA into two fragments . . . A and AGCTT. . . . However, if this sequence has a variation in some people, such as . . . TAGCTT . . . , then no cut or restriction will occur and one fragment remains. These variations are known as restriction fragment length polymorphisms (RFLPs). An example of an RFLP that is detected at a location above the fra(X) site is shown in figure 4.1. RFLPs are also referred to as DNA markers. They can be used to trace the inheritance of a gene of interest or a genetic mutation within families. When a gene of interest and an RFLP are inherited in close proximity, even if they are not at exactly the same location, the RFLP or DNA marker can be used as a disease marker to track the inheritance of the mutant gene within a family. A number of X chromosome-specific DNA fragments have been cloned using the techniques of genetic engineering and mapped at locations that are relatively close to the fra(X) locus. The inheritance of such RFLPs near the fra(X) site can be traced within families. An illustration of how this technique is applied to fra(X) is shown in fig. 4.2.

RFLPs usually exist in one of two possible variations called alleles, which are identified by numbers or letters. If a carrier mother has both type alleles of a given polymorphism (i.e., *1* and *2*), she is termed a heterozygote for that polymorphism. Otherwise, she is a homozygote. It is necessary for a mother to be a heterozygote to be informative for the inheritance of a given X-linked polymorphism. The sons and daughters of a carrier mother receive one or the

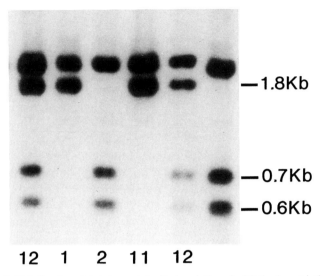

Figure 4.1 This Southern blot shows inherited variations in DNA. A restriction fragment length polymorphin is detected using the DNA probe 52A at locus DXS51. Either a 1.8-kb band (allele type 1) or both a 0.7- and a 0.6-kb (allele type 2) set of bands is seen. A female heterozygote having both alleles 1 and 2 is identified in the *left lane*.

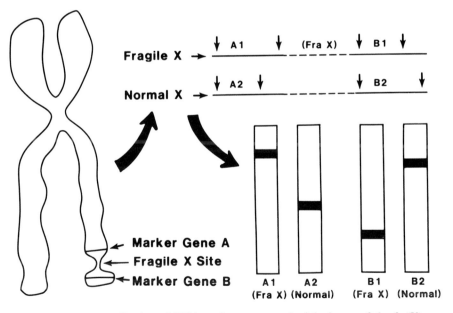

Figure 4.2 The application of DNA markers to trace the inheritance of the fra(X) chromosome. Two flanking DNA restriction fragment length polymorphins to the fra(X) locus can be used to determine who within a family has received the mutation.

149

other of her two X chromosomes. If the mother is heterozygous for a given polymorphism, her sons and daughters will receive one or the other of the two alleles and the inheritance of a given allele can be correlated with the inheritance of the fra(X) locus. If a DNA polymorphism is closely linked to the fra(X) locus and a given allele is identified in a male with fra(X), it is very likely that siblings with the same allele will also inherit the fra(X) chromosome. This can occur even though the fragile site itself may not be physically detectable or expressed, as in the case of transmitting males and some carrier females. Likewise, those siblings who inherit the opposite allele are unlikely to be carriers.

It has long been recognized that chromosomes recombine during meiosis at the formation of sexual gametes (i.e., sperm and eggs). The distance between two DNA locations on a chromosome can be measured in terms of their probability of showing a recombination at meiosis. Genetic distance is expressed in terms of centiMorgans (cM), where 10 cM is equivalent to a 10% chance of a recombination occurring. The human genome has been measured to be about 3,000 cM long. For two genetic locations to show genetic linkage, they must recombine less than 50% of the time. Otherwise, they could be on separate chromosomes and would be unlinked. To determine whether an RFLP is linked with a given disease, one determines the probabilities of inheritance. First the probability of inheriting both a disease gene and an RFLP within a family is calculated assuming that there is no genetic linkage (i.e., at each meiosis there is 50% probability of recombination). This probability is then compared with the probability of the two traits being inherited together assuming successively closer linkage distances. The odds of linkage score is determined as the probability of linkage at a given distance divided by the probability of no linkage. The logarithm of this odds score is then calculated. This is referred to as the log of the odds of linkage score or the lod score. Lod scores are logarithms and have the advantage that they can be added from one family to the next. A lod score with a value of 3 is equivalent to the log of odds of 1,000:1. A value of greater than 3 is generally accepted as proof of linkage. When the odds are less than -2, the odds are less than 1:100 for linkage. This is generally accepted as proof that no linkage exists. The actual computation of lod scores by hand is complex for a pedigree of any significant size. Computer programs that calculate linkage scores can be used on small laboratory computers. The useful range of detectable linkage between markers is defined by their separation in centiMorgans. For family DNA genetic studies, useful linkages generally range up to 30 cM. At distances of less than 10 cM, their predictive power increases because there is less than a 10% chance of a recombination and an incorrect result occurring by chance. The closer the linkage, the less the likelihood of an error and the greater the probability of a correct prediction.

The problem of isolating a gene when the nature of the gene product is unknown (i.e., when there is no known metabolic product or enzyme deficiency) is similar for many common genetic diseases. By obtaining closer and closer linked probes on either side of the locus for the genetic disease of interest, one can isolate a series of DNA segments, which can assist in identifying the mutation underlying the genetic disease. Analysis of associated polymorphisms can progressively identify DNA fragments whose inheritance more and more closely matches the disease of interest. Along with the actual physical DNA map, this information can narrow the search for the location of the gene to less than a region spanning approximately 1% recombinational distance, which is assumed to be equivalent to some 1 million base pairs. Strategies are being developed to characterize 1 million base pair stretches of human DNA and to define the mutated gene of interest. These methods should soon allow the isolation and characterization of the mutations underlying most human genetic diseases, including fra(X).

Linkage Studies of the Fra(X) Syndrome

The first RFLP that was linked to the fra(X) locus was an RFLP for clotting factor IX (F9). A large fra(X) family was studied for linkage of the fra(X) locus to F9 (Camerino et al. 1983). No recombinants were seen, and apparent tight linkage of F9 to the fra(X) locus was observed. Several other families were soon studied in which recombination was seen between F9 and the fra(X) locus (Choo et al. 1984; Davies et al. 1985; Forster-Gibson et al. 1985; Warren et al. 1985; Zoll et al. 1985). We initially studied 16 fra(X) families (Brown et al. 1985). Several large families, such as one illustrated in figure 4.3, showed a high rate of recombination, but other families, such as those shown in figures 4.4 and 4.5, had little or no recombination between F9 and fra(X). These dissimilarities in families indicated that there might be differences in rates of recombination among families. The term for such differences is genetic linkage heterogeneity. Because several of the families with no recombination had nonpenetrant (NP) or transmitting male grandfathers, it seemed likely that the presence or absence of a NP male was a distinguishing factor. We therefore divided the families into two types, either with or without an identified NP male. The analysis showed that there were significant differences among families, indicating the existence of genetic linkage heterogeneity. We concluded that there were two types of families: one type with tight linkage to F9 and one type with loose linkage.

Several other X chromosome probes were soon reported to detect polymorphic loci close to the fra(X) locus. A very useful, highly polymorphic X chromosome probe, St14, which detects locus DXS52, was discovered to exist in at least 10 different allelic types (Oberlé et al. 1985a). It was found to be linked to fra(X) on the distal side (Oberlé et al. 1986). Two other random DNA

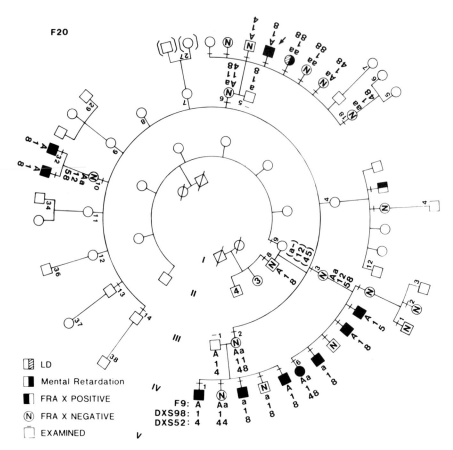

Figure 4.3 Fra(X) family F20, with frequent recombination between F9 and fra(X). The grandfather was a transmitting male; he had alleles A, 1, and 8 in common with the majority of his affected grandsons. [Reprinted with permission from Brown et al. (1987a)]

fragments were also found to be close to fra(X): one, 52A (DXS51), on the proximal side (Drayna and White 1985) and one, X13 (DXS15), also on the distal side (Davies et al. 1985).

Following our initial studies of linkage with F9, we analyzed 32 fra(X) families for the inheritance of the RFLPs associated with 52A, F9, and St14 (Brown et al. 1986). We again saw significant linkage heterogeneity for F9-fra(X). However, further studies led to the conclusion that nonpenetrance was not the correct basis for division of families into two types. We found with a larger sample of 50 families that, regardless of the presence or absence of NP

FRAGILE X PEDIGREE No. 22

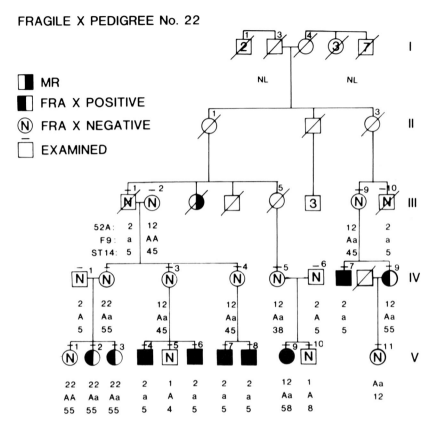

Figure 4.4 Fra(X) family 22, with tight linkage between F9 and fra(X). The grandfather (*III-1*) was a transmitting male; he had DNA markers in common with his affected grandsons and fra(X)-positive relatives of his mother and sister. [Reprinted with permission from Brown et al. (1987a)]

males, some showed tight linkage to F9 and others showed loose linkage (Brown et al. 1987a). The lod scores for two-point recombinations between the adjacent loci 52A-F9, F9-fra(X), and fra(X)-St14 for 50 families are illustrated in figure 4.6. As shown, there was significant variation in the recombination rate for F9-fra(X), much more than for fra(X)-St14 or 52A-F9. Some families showed no fra(X)-F9 recombination, whereas others showed frequent recombination. Analysis of these further families showed that many families that included a NP male also showed a high rate of F9-fra(X) recombination. Thus, the presence or absence of a NP male did not seem to be related to the observed genetic heterogeneity.

Our results indicated two classes of families with two specific recombination

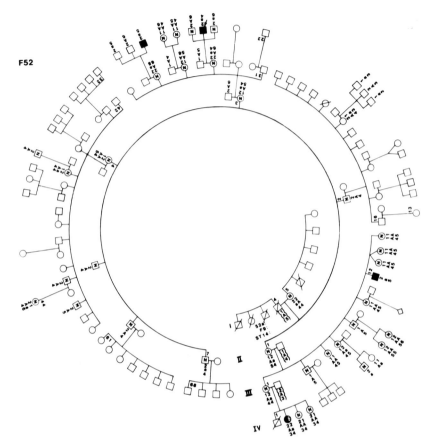

F52

Figure 4.5 Fra(X) family F52, with tight linkage between F9 and fra(X). The grand-mother (*I-5*) was a carrier; she had the same restriction fragment length polymorphins alleles as her affected grandson (*III-12*) and the majority of the affected great grand-children (*IV-1, IV-25, IV-29*). Several likely nonpenetrant males also were identified (*II-7, IV-24, IV-31*). [Reprinted with permission from Brown et al. (1987a)]

rates of 0% and 35%, with a mean of about 20%. However, it seemed possible that there actually existed two distributions of recombination rates, one close to 0 and one averaging around 35%. Risch (1988) developed a new heterogeneity test that allowed a statistical analysis of such distributions. He analyzed our data and confirmed the presence of linkage heterogeneity (Risch 1988).

DNA studies on a number of other fra(X) families were reported by various laboratories (Connor et al. 1987; Forster-Gibson et al. 1985; Goonewardena et al. 1986; Landoulsi et al. 1985; Mulligan et al. 1985; Oberlé et al. 1985b;

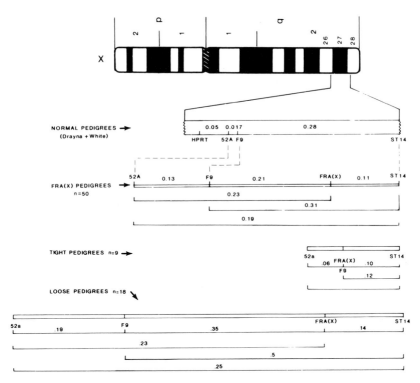

Figure 4.6 Recombination fractions around the fra(X) locus for DNA probes 52A, F9, and St14, showing linkage heterogeneity. Families could be separated into two classes: those with a high rate of recombination between fra(X) and F9, loose linkage pedigrees, and those with no recombination, tight linkage pedigrees. [Data on normal pedigrees from Drayna and White (1985); data on the fra(X) families from Brown et al. (1987a)]

Mulley et al. 1986; Oberlé et al. 1987; Thibodeau et al. 1988; Mulley et al. 1988). Giannelli et al. (1987) also reported finding F9-fra(X) linkage heterogeneity. We conducted a combined multipoint analysis of 147 fra(X) pedigrees with four flanking DNA markers including information from 14 collaborating laboratories (Brown et al. 1988b). The four probes used include F9, 52A (DXS51), St14 (DXS52), and DX13 (DXS15). Among the 147 pedigrees, 2,030 individuals were entered in the analysis, of whom 1,579 were typed for DNA markers. There were 595 fra(X)-positive males who were typed. Multipoint linkage analysis was performed using the LINKAGE program (Lathrop and Lalouel 1984). The best order and estimated recombinant distances are shown in figure 4.7. There was significant genetic heterogeneity between F9 and fra(X) in the 147 families.

Multilocus Analysis of Fragile X Syndrome Pedigrees

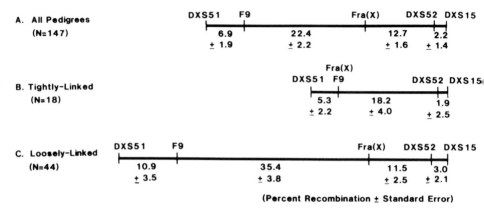

Figure 4.7 Recombination fractions for loci around fra(X) based on multipoint mapping of 147 fra(X) families based on a multicenter collaborative study. Families could be divided into two types based on linkage patterns to F9 which showed significant linkage heterogeneity. [Reprinted with permission from Brown et al. (1988b)]

The finding of linkage heterogeneity suggested several alternative explanations. One possibility was a variation in the position of the fragile site relative to the adjacent loci. However, the evidence indicated that there were altered rates of recombination between fra(X) and the proximal locus F9 but not with distal loci such as DXS52 and DX13. Another possibility was that the variation in rates of recombination may be based upon structural rearrangements of the nearby chromosomal regions. We suggested that an inhibition of recombination due to an inversion might explain our findings (Brown et al. 1985). There exist known inversions in the mammalian genome which alter recombination rates. There are at least two major inverted regions in the t complex on mouse chromosome 17, one in the proximal portion and a second in the distal portion. These inverted regions have been shown to lead to deletions and duplications after recombination (Bucan et al. 1987). If inversions are present in the human fra(X) region, they may alter recombination rates and may result in duplications or deletions that could affect nearby gene expression. Also, there may be an alteration in recombination because of variation in the number of copies of a sequence that promotes recombination. Remarkable variations in recombination rates have been found in different genetic strains of mice. For example, Steinmetz et al. (1986) showed that there are hot spots for recombination in the mouse major histocompatibility locus which are haplotype dependent. Mouse strain BIO.MOL-SGR showed a 100-fold higher rate of recombination between

K and I region marker loci than showed two other common laboratory mouse strains. Sequence data suggest that a genetic element in this region may specifically enhance recombination. A molecular understanding of the underlying sequence variation in the proximal region of the fra(X) locus is needed for a definitive explanation.

To search for new probes linked to fra(X), we localized a set of nine anonymous probes relative to F9, hypoxanthine guanine phosphoribsyltransferase (HPRT), and fra(X) in 45 fra(X) families (Brown et al. 1988a). We found probe 4D-8, which detects an *Msp*I RFLP at locus DXS98 and was known to be unlinked to HPRT (Boggs and Nussbaum 1984) and to be closely linked to fra(X). Among 40 fra(X) families, 6 were informative for the inheritance of 4D-8. They exhibited a peak lod score of 4.3 at 7% recombination between 4D-8 and fra(X). No evidence for genetic heterogeneity for 4D-8-fra(X) was seen using statistical tests, but the number of doubly informative meioses was limited. The families that showed tight F9-fra(X) linkage showed no recombinants for 4D-8-fra(X).

Other RFLPs showing linkage to fra(X) were soon identified. One of a set of random X probes, isolated by Hofker et al. (1987), cX55.7 (DXS105), was found within the region F9-fra(X) (Carpenter et al. 1987). These findings were soon confirmed (Mulley et al. 1988). An additional new probe, cX33.2 (contiguous to cX55.7) was identified by Arveiler et al. (1988). Use of this probe combined with cX55.7 created a four-allele haplotype, which increased the overall heterozygosity detected at this locus (DXS105) to nearly 70%. However, the closest proximal locus was still identified by 4D-8 (DXS98), which was found to lie between cX55.7 and fra(X), as illustrated in figure 4.8 (Carpenter et al. 1987).

From a clinical standpoint, there was a great demand for more closely linked probes to improve prenatal diagnosis and assessment of carrier status. It is most useful to have RFLPs within about 5% recombination to reduce the risk of recombination and improve the predictive certainty of DNA-based diagnostic testing. However, through 1988 none of the probes that had been identified were closer on average than about 7% (4D-8) to 12% (St14). Much effort had been expended in unsuccessful attempts to isolate closer probes. This led to the conclusion that the regions adjacent to fra(X) must be subject to unusually high rates of recombination, which might be related to the underlying nature of the mutation.

In late 1989, after much additional effort, the isolation of several closer probes was reported. The first of these was U6.2 (locus DXS304). Dahl et al. (1989a) isolated a subclone from the library of Hofker et al. (1987) which detected RFLPs with about half of enzymes tested, all of which were in disequilibrium and had heterozygosity of about 30%. This locus was soon found to be close to fra(X) on the distal side, and the best estimates placed it at about 3%

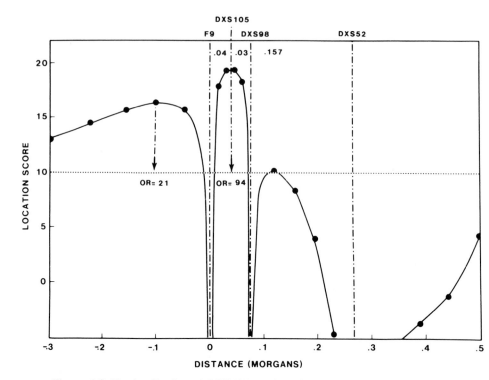

Figure 4.8 The localization of DXS105 (probe cX55.7) relative to DXS98 (probe 4D-8), F9, and DXS52 (probe St14) in 30 families using LINKMAP (Lathrop and Lalouel 1984). DXS105 was most likely more proximal and farther away from DXS52 and therefore from fra(X) than was DXS98. [Data from Carpenter et al. (1991)]

recombination (Dahl et al. 1989b; Vincent et al. 1989; Goonewardena et al. 1991). We sequenced the 1103-bp U6.2 probe and found that it contained a large 121-bp direct repeated element (Pergolizzi et al. 1991). There were also two inverted repeated elements of 19 and 20 bp. It seemed that such repeats could promote recombination in the region. They could have been involved in an insertion/deletion event that created the polymorphisms detected by U6.2.

Suthers et al. (1989) isolated probe VK21 from a somatic cell hybrid containing the distal human X chromosome region, Xq26-Xter. Several subclones were derived (VK21a and VK21c) and detected RFLPs at locus DXS296. Linkage and somatic cell hybridization studies placed the locus approximately 1 cM distal to fra(X) and just proximal to the Hunter syndrome locus [iduronate sulfatase deficiency (IDS)]. The best order was determined to be fra(X) - DXS296 - IDS - DXS304 using a combination of linkage, somatic cell hybrid, and in situ hybridization analyses.

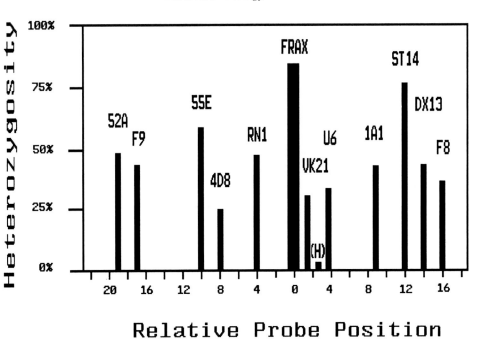

Relative Probe Position

Figure 4.9 Relative probe positions and usefulness of probes for carrier detection in fra(X). The probes are placed in their estimated best positions. The likelihood of the various probes being found to be heterozygous in a given carrier is shown at *left*.

A new probe, RN1, which detects locus DXS369 on the proximal side of fra(X), was isolated by van Oostra et al. (1990). Mapping information placed this marker in the region between DXS304 (4D8) and fra(X) at about 5% recombination. Thus, within one year, three new probes (RN1, VK21, and U6.2) and the IDS locus were mapped to within 5% recombination of fra(X). The approximate location of these new probes and the heterozygosity of each probe (the probability that a carrier mother is informative) are illustrated in figure 4.9.

Uses of DNA Probes in Clinical Testing

Families seeking genetic counseling frequently ask, "What is the probability of a sister of an affected male being a carrier?" (fig. 4.10a). The prior risk of the sister of an affected male being a carrier is 50% because she has a 50:50 chance of inheriting the fra(X) chromosome from her carrier mother. Based upon the studies of Sherman et al. (1984, 1985), if the sister is mentally unimpaired she

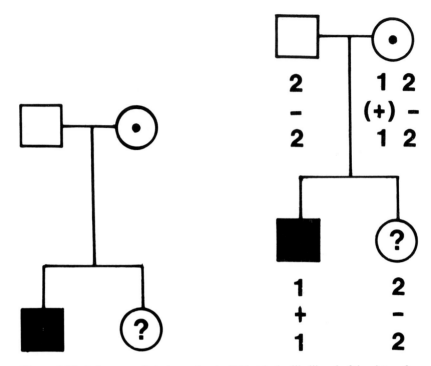

Figure 4.10 A frequent clinical question is, "What is the likelihood of the sister of an affected male being a carrier?" If adjacent alleles on either side of the fra(X) locus are different in the sister from those in the brother, her risk is greatly reduced. Depending on the loci that are informative, her risk may be as low as <1.0%.

is less likely to be a carrier and her risks are reduced to approximately 40%. If she is both mentally unimpaired and negative on cytogenetic testing, her risks are reduced to approximately 30% (see chapter 8 for a further explanation). DNA marker analysis can usually reduce the uncertainty of these risk estimates. If a carrier mother is heterozygous for the closest probes and if the sister has allele types that are different from those of her brother, the risks of the sister being a carrier are reduced from 30% to less than 1%. This situation is illustrated in figure 4.10b. If two affected sibs are available for testing, the likelihood of a recombination in both sibs is reduced and the risk calculations are even more reliable. For example, if a sister has different markers for the closest flanking markers than those of two affected brothers, the risks of her being a carrier can be reduced to less than 0.2%. We have found this method of risk analysis using LINKAGE to be of considerable use for carrier testing and genetic counseling (Brown et al. 1987c).

Another frequently asked question is whether a normal brother or a normal grandfather is a nonpenetrant carrier male. The results of the segregation analysis by Sherman et al. (1984, 1985) predict that about 1 of 6 (17%) normal sons of a carrier female will be nonpenetrant. We used DNA markers to test this prediction (Brown et al. 1991). We analyzed the normal sons from 100 families and found 51 who were doubly informative and nonrecombinant for flanking markers. Of these, 10 (19.6%) were found to be nonpenetrant males. This result closely confirmed the predictions of the Sherman studies. The true risk to the normal brothers of an affected male of being nonpenetrant are about 1 in 5 to 1 in 6. We also studied 14 families in which grandparents had all normal children including at least two daughters with fra(X)-positive sons. In 6 of these families, only two daughters had affected sons; in three daughters transmission was from the nonpenetrant grandfather. In the other 8 families, three or more daughters had affected sons and in seven the grandfather was found to be the transmitting male. Thus, DNA analysis can be applied to answer clinical questions regarding male transmission.

Molecular Approaches to Characterize the Fra(X) Mutation

A promising approach to the direct isolation of the fra(X) locus is the construction of a somatic cell hybrid containing a translocation of the human fra(X) site to a rodent chromosome. Warren et al. (1987) isolated several somatic cell hybrids that contained rearranged X chromosomes. DNA marker studies showed that the rearrangements involved the region at or near the fra(X) site. Fragility at the human X-rodent translocation junction was observed in two hybrid cells but at a lower frequency compared to the intact fra(X) chromosome. Warren et al. suggested that the fra(X) region may include a repeated sequence that is prone to recombination.

Sutherland et al. (1985) suggested that the fra(X) region involves a long, pyrimidine-rich DNA sequence, and Nussbaum et al. (1986) hypothesized that this region is prone to undergo unequal crossing over. An illustration of this possible mechanism is shown in figure 4.11. A transmitting male could have affected or unaffected grandsons depending on unequal recombinant events that might occur in his daughter's gametes, as illustrated in figure 4.12. Unequal crossing over has been shown to occur in a region of the X chromosome adjacent to fra(X). For example, studies of the genes encoding red and green visual pigment have shown inherited variations in copy number as a result of unequal recombination (Vollrath et al. 1988). The green pigment genes show one, two, or three copies, which are common alleles in the human genome. Also, studies of the murine X chromosome showed that unequal crossing over occurs at a high frequency in the pseudoautosomal region (Habers et al. 1986).

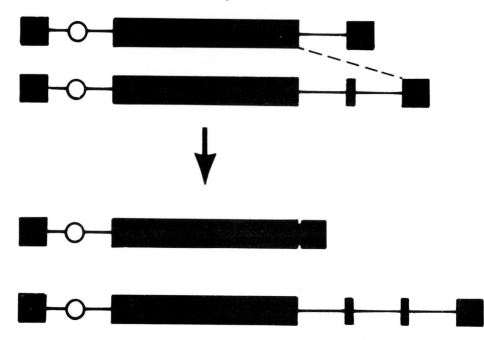

In this situation, unequal crossing over seems to be due to the presence of a sequence that is tandemly repeated and highly variable.

Most recombination presumably occurs during meiosis. However, recombination can also occur during mitosis and produce visible events such as sister chromatid exchanges (SCEs). Unequal SCEs could result in duplication or deletion of particular genes. Such a mechanism has been shown to be involved in the magnification of ribosomal RNA genes in *Drosophila* (Tartof 1974). Studies by Weinreb et al. (1988) indicated that unequal SCE has occurred at the immunoglobulin heavy chain locus in the mouse myeloma cell line MPC II. The heavy chain constant region gene has been duplicated in a tandem array on the expressed chromosome of this cell line via an unequal sister chromatid exchange. This results in the presence of a germ line and a non-germ line form of the gene, which can be detected by variations on genomic Southern blot analysis. Mutagenized derivatives of this cell line have amplified the non-germ line gene form 5- to 10-fold. Other lines also have deleted the non-germ line form. A DNA sequence in this region has the characteristics of zDNA, which may be involved in promoting recombination and may represent a hot spot for recombination. A similar type of zDNA (left-handed helix) sequence also could be involved in promoting recombination in the human fra(X) region.

Laird (1987) and Laird et al. (1987) proposed a novel hypothesis about

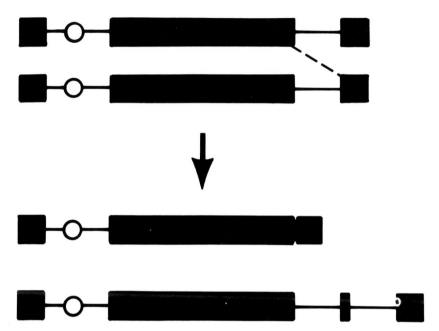

Figure 4.11 A possible mechanism of unequal crossing over. *Left*, two normal X chromosomes. *Right*, after unequal crossing over, a chromosome with an increased probability of further unequal crossing over is generated. Thus, a normal X chromosome may evolve to a transmitting nonpenetrant X chromosome to one that is likely to be found in an affected fra(X) male.

inheritance of fra(X) based upon DNA methylation. They suggested that fra(X) results from a mutation that blocks the complete reactivation of an inactivated X chromosome (see chapter 7). DNA methylation is presumed to be involved in X inactivation. The nature of the underlying sequence variation or mutation is still undefined. A large scale sequence alteration could be the basis for altered patterns of methylation. Laird also suggested that it may represent a methylation mutation and not require sequence variation. This hypothesis has many attractive features and predicts the altered ratio of affected to unaffected offspring with surprising accuracy. The theory may also explain the altered segregation ratios that may be seen among the offspring of the mothers of transmitting males (TMs) compared to the offspring of the daughters of TMs, the Sherman paradox (Turner et al. 1986) (see chapter 2).

Two recent reports (Bell et al. 1991; Vincent et al. 1991) present evidence to suggest the involvement of methylation differences in comparing fra(X) to normal X chromosomes, it is clear that DNA methylation and gene imprinting may be important factors that influence gene expression. For example, Swain et

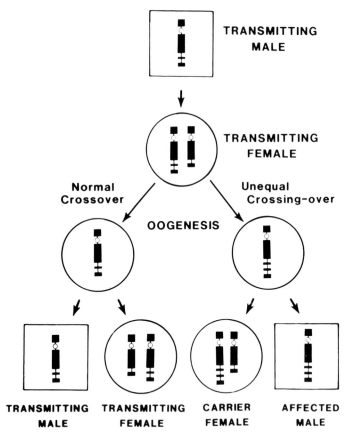

Figure 4.12 A possible mechanism of transmission of an X chromosome from a transmitting grandfather. Either affected males and carrier females or transmitting males and females may result, depending on whether unequal crossing over occurs during oogenesis.

al. (1987) reported that a gene (*myc*) introduced into a transgenetic mouse showed expression only when the offspring had inherited it from a father. This was correlated with DNA methylation patterns in that the paternally transmitted gene was less methylated than one that was maternally transmitted. Reik et al. (1987) studied genomic imprinting of transgenic loci in mice and found a locus that if derived from the father was undermethylated but if derived from the mother was highly methylated. The methylation pattern was reversed after transmission through an offspring of the opposite sex. These studies provide evidence that heritable molecular differences between maternally and paternally derived alleles are imprinted on the mouse chromosome. Direct molecular analysis of the fra(X) mutation is now beginning to show that a process of DNA methylation and resulting imprinting appear to be involved in the fra(X) mutation.

Future Directions

Rapid progress in the characterization of individual sequences adjacent to the fra(X) locus is being made, and further tightly linked probes will be useful for clinical diagnostic purposes. However, a first step toward an understanding of the nature of the underlying mutation is to develop a complete physical map of the area including fra(X). One approach is to use pulse field gel electrophoresis (PFGE) to map very large DNA fragments; they then can be analyzed and their relative orientation determined. This technique uses special restriction enzymes such as NotI, which recognize rarely occurring sequences such as 12-bp-long sequences.

Detailed PFGE physical mapping of the distal region around St14 and DXS13 has been undertaken (Patterson et al. 1987a; Bell et al. 1989). These PFGE studies have shown that St14 (DXS520) and DX13 (DXS15) detect loci that are within a DNA fragment of 470 thousand base pairs (kb). Further PFGE studies by Feil et al. (1990) physically mapped a 1.2 million base pair (Mb) region and showed that the St14 sequence actually detects a family of DXS52 loci that are dispersed within a 575–600-kb region. This region includes DXS15 and several other less-well-studied markers, including MN12 (DXS33), cpX6 (DXS130), cpX67 (134), and G1.3c (DXF22S3). PFGE studies by Patterson et al. (1989) of a new probe 1A1 (DXS374), which was genetically linked to DXS52 at about 3 cM, indicate that it lies within a 2-Mb proximal region that is not physically linked to the 1.2-Mb region containing DXS52. On the more distal side of the DXS52 region, PFGE mapping identified a 1.7-Mb region containing a cluster of genes and fragments, including the X-linked forms of color-blindness cone pigment genes (*RCP, GCP*), MD13, GdX(DXS254), G6PD, F8C, DXS115, and DXYS64. Thus, three physical regions comprising about 4 Mb on the distal side have been defined.

On the proximal side of fra(X), Nguyen et al. (1988) presented a physical map of a 1.3-Mb region surrounding F9. Patterson et al. (1987b) suggested the physical linkage of 4D-8(DXS98), cX55.7(DXS105), and cX33.2(DXS105/-DXS152) on a 400-kb fragment based on PFGE analysis of the region proximal to fra(X). In comparing fra(X) chromosomes from males in two different families, one that showed tight F9 linkage and one that showed loose linkage, Dobkin and Brown (1988) studied partial *Sfi*I PFGE products detected by cX55.7 (DXS105) using the method illustrated in figure 4.13. Results of this study indicated the presence of a large polymorphic deletion or insertion near

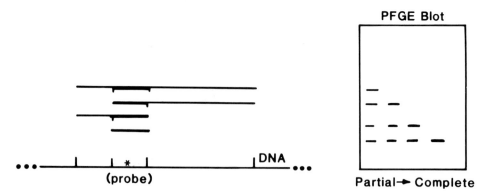

Figure 4.13 An analysis of the organization around large DNA fragments is possible using enzymatic digestions that are allowed to proceed only to partial completion. Using pulse field gel electrophoresis (PFGE), we can detect these large partials.

cX55.7 (DXS105). Additional experiments showed that these polymorphisms are observed consistently in fra(X) chromosomes from members of different families. These additional results showed that DXS105 lies within a 600-kb region that is separated from a 400-kb fragment detected by 4D-8 (DXS98) (Dobkin and Brown, unpublished results). Our results suggest that large sequence variations detectable by PFGE may be quite frequent in the proximal fra(X) region.

The cloning of the junctions between hamster and human chromosomes that seem to include the fra(X) site, as reported by Warren et al. (1987), should lead to the isolation of new probes closely linked to fra(X) and may allow characterization of DNA sequences that include the fra(X) mutation. Analysis of the mutated region in different nonpenetrant and penetrant males should reveal how the mutation arises.

As a result of initial efforts directed toward obtaining a complete sequence of the human genome, a number of developments in molecular biology techniques are being made. Many hold promise in their application to studies of the fra(X) mutation. These include the complete linking of overlapping cosmid clones, which individually are generally in the range of 10 to 50 kb, to allow the development of defined contiguous cloned sequences, *contigs*. The methods of chromosome jumping (whereby the ends of large pulse field gel fragments can be linked together) and radiation hybrid mapping are additional techniques that hold great promise. The introduction of human chromosome material into yeast artificial chromosomes (YACs) has allowed the isolation and cloning of sequences of several million base pairs. This method has already assisted in studies around the DXS52 locus (Feil et al. 1990) and promises to have application in the physical analysis of all other identified loci adjacent to fra(X). DNA transfer experiments and transgenic animals may show how the mutation affects gene expression and leads to the fra(X) syndrome. Based on these developments, it seems likely that a molecular understanding of the fra(X) mutation will soon be available.

References

Arveiler, B., I. Oberlé, A. Vincent, M. H. Hofker, P. L. Pearson, and J. L. Mandel. 1988. Genetic mapping of the Xq27–q28 region: New RFLP markers useful for diagnostic applications in fragile X and Hemophilia B families. *Am. J. Hum. Genet.* 42:380–389.

Bell, M. V., M. N. Patterson, H. R. Dorkins, and K. E. Davies. 1989. Physical mapping of DXS134 close to the DXS52 locus. *Hum. Genet.* 82:27–30.

Bell, M. V., M. C. Hirst, Y. Nakahori, R. N. MacKinnon, A. Roche, T. J. Flint, P. A. Jacobs, N. Tommerup, L. Tranebjaerg, U. Froster-Iskenius, B. Kerr, G. Turner, R. H. Lindenbau, R. Winter, M. Pembrey, S. Thibodeau, and K. E. Davies. 1991. Physical mapping across the fragile X: Hypermethylation and clinical expression of the fragile X syndrome. *Cell* 64:861–866.

Boggs, B. A., and R. L. Nussbaum. 1984. Two anonymous X-specific human sequences detecting restriction fragment length polymorphisms in region Xq26-qter. *Somatic Cell Mol. Genet.* 10:607–613.

Brown, W. T., A. C. Gross, C. B. Chan, and E. C. Jenkins. 1985. Genetic linkage heterogeneity in the fragile X syndrome. *Hum. Genet.* 71:11–18.

———. 1986. DNA linkage studies in the fragile X syndrome suggest genetic heterogeneity. *Am. J. Med. Genet.* 23:643–664.

Brown, W. T., E. C. Jenkins, A. C. Gross, C. B. Chan, M. S. Krawczun, C. J. Duncan, S. L. Sklower, and G. S. Fisch. 1987a. Further evidence for genetic heterogeneity in the fragile X syndrome. *Hum. Genet.* 75:311–321.

Brown, W. T., Y. Wu, A. C. Gross, C. B. Chan, C. S. Dobkin, and E. C. Jenkins. 1987b. RFLP for linkage analysis of fragile X syndrome. *Lancet* 1:280.

Brown, W. T., E. C. Jenkins, A. C. Gross, C. B. Chan, M. S. Krawczun, M. L. Alonso, E. S. Cantu, J. G. Davis, R. J. Hagerman, R. Laxova, M. Liebowitz, V. B. Penchaszadeh, S. Thibodeau, A. M. Wiley, M. K. Williams, J. P. Willner, and N. J. Zellers. 1987c. Clinical use of DNA markers in the fragile (X) syndrome for carrier detection and prenatal diagnosis. In A. M. Willey (ed.), *Nucleic acid probes in diagnosis of human genetic diseases.* New York: Alan R. Liss, pp. 11–34.

Brown, W. T., Y. Wu, A. C. Gross, C. B. Chan, C. S. Dobkin, and E. C. Jenkins. 1988a. Multipoint linkage of 9 anonymous probes to HPRT, factor 9, and fragile X. *Am. J. Med. Genet.* 30:551–556.

Brown, W. T., A. Gross, B. Chan, E. C. Jenkins, J. L. Mandel, I. Oberlé, B. Arveiler, G. Novelli, S. Thibodeau, R. Hagerman, K. Summers, G. Turner, B. N. White, L. Mulligan, C. Foster-Gibson, J. J. A. Holden, B. Zoll, M. Krawczak, P. Gonnewardena, K. H. Gustavson, U. Pettersson, G. Holmgren, C. Schwartz, P. N. Howard-

Peebles, P. Murphy, W. R. Breg, H. Veenema, and N. J. Carpenter. 1988b. Multi-locus analysis of the fragile X syndrome. *Hum. Genet.* 78:201–205.

Brown, W. T., A. C. Gross, P. Goonewardena, C. Ferrando, C. Dobkin, and E. C. Jenkins. 1991. Detection of fragile X non-penetrant males by DNA marker analysis. *Am. J. Med. Genet.* 38:292–297.

Bucan, M., B. G. Herrmann, A. M. Frischauf, V. L. Bautch, V. Bode, L. M. Silver, G. R. Martin, and H. Lehrach. 1987. Deletion and duplication of DNA sequences is associated with the embryonic lethal phenotype of the t9 complementation group of the mouse t complex. *Genes Dev.* 1:376–385.

Camerino, G., M. G. Mattei, J. F. Mattei, M. Jaye, and J. L. Mandel. 1983. Close linkage of fragile X linked mental retardation syndrome to haemophilia B and transmission through a normal male. *Nature* 306:701–707.

Carpenter, N. J., H. Veenema, E. Bakker, M. H. Hofker, and P. L. Pearson. 1987. A new DNA probe proximal to and closely linked to fragile X. *Am. J. Med. Genet.* 27:731–732.

Carpenter, N. J., S. N. Thibodeau, and W. T. Brown. 1991. Linkage relationships between DXS105, DXS98 and other polymorphic DNA markers flanking the fragile X locus. *Am. J. Med. Genet.* 38:349–353.

Choo, K. H., D. George, G. Filby, J. L. Halliday, M. Leversha, G. Webb, and D. M. Danks. 1984. Linkage analysis of X-linked mental retardation with and without fragile-X using factor IX gene probe. *Lancet* 1:349.

Connor, J. M., L. A. Pirritt, J. R. W. Yates, J. A. Crossley, S. J. Imrie, and J. M. Colgan. 1987. Linkage analysis using multiple Xq DNA polymorphisms in normal families, families with the fragile X syndrome and other families with X linked conditions. *J. Med. Genet.* 24:14–22.

Dahl, N., K. Hammarstrom-Heeroma, P. Goonewardena, C. Wadelius, K. H. Gustavson, G. Holmgren, G. B. van Ommen, and U. Pettersson. 1989a. Isolation of a DNA probe of potential use for diagnosis of the fragile X syndrome. *Hum. Genet.* 82:216–218.

Dahl, N., P. Goonewardena, H. Malmgren, K. H. Gustavson, G. Holmgren, E. Seemanova, G. Anneren, A. Flood, and U. Pettersson. 1989b. Linkage analysis of families with fragile-X mental retardation using a novel RFLP marker (DXS304). *Am. J. Hum. Genet.* 45:304–309.

Davies, K. E., M. G. Mattei, J. F. Mattei, H. Veenema, S. McGlade, K. Harper, N. Tommerup, K. B. Nielsen, M. Mikkelsen, P. Beighton, D. Drayna, R. White, and M. E. Pembrey, 1985. Linkage studies of X-linked mental retardation: High frequency of recombination in the telomeric region of the human X chromosome. *Hum. Genet.* 70:249–255.

Dobkin, C. S., and W. T. Brown. 1988. Pulsed-filed gradient-gel studies around the fragile site. *Am. J. Med. Genet.* 30:593–600.

Drayna, D., and R. White. 1985. The genetic linkage map of the human X chromosome. *Science* 230:753–758.

Feil, R., G. Palmieri, M. d'Urso, R. Heilig, I. Oberle, and J. L. Mandel. 1990. Physical and genetic mapping of polymorphic loci in Xq28 (DXS15, DXS52, and DXS134): Analysis of a cosmid clone and a yeast artificial chromosome. *Am. J. Hum. Genet.* 46:720–728.

Forster-Gibson, C. J., L. M. Mulligan, M. W. Partington, N. E. Simpson, J. J. A. Holden, and B. N. White. 1985. The genetic distance between the coagulation factor IX gene and the locus for the fragile-X syndrome: Clinical implications. *J. Neurogenet.* 2:231–237.

Giannelli, F., A. H. Morris, C. Garrett, M. Daker, C. Thurston, and C. A. B. Smith. 1987. Genetic heterogeneity of X-linked mental retardation with fragile X. Association of tight linkage to factor IX and incomplete penetrance in males. *Ann. Hum. Genet.* 51:107–124.

Goonewardena, P., K. H. Gustavson, G. Holgren, A. Tolun, J. Chotai, E. Johnsen, and U. Pettersson. 1986. Analysis of fragile X-mental retardation families using flanking polymorphic DNA probes. *Clin. Genet.* 30:249–254.

Goonewardena, P., W. T. Brown, A. C. Gross, C. Ferrando, C. Dobkin, V. Romano, P. Bosco, N. Ceratto, N. Dahl, and U. Pettersson. 1991. Linkage analysis of the fragile X syndrome using a new DNA marker U6.2 defining locus DXS304. *Am. J. Med. Genet.* 38:322–327.

Habers, K., P. Soriano, U. Muller, and R. Jaenisch. 1986. High frequency of unequal recombination in pseudoautosomal region shown by proviral insertion in transgenic mouse. *Nature* 324:682–685.

Hofker, M. H., A. A. Bergen, M. I. Skraastad, N. J. Carpenter, H. Veenema, J. M. Connor, E. Bakker, G. J. B. van Ommen, and P. L. Pearson. 1987. Efficient isolation of X chromosome-specific single-copy probes from a cosmic library of a human X/hamster hybrid cell line: Mapping of new probes close to the locus for X-linked mental retardation. *Am. J. Hum. Genet.* 40:312–328.

Laird, C. D. 1987. Proposed mechanism of inheritance and expression of the human fragile-X syndrome of mental retardation. *Genetics* 117:587–599.

Laird, C. D., E. Jaffe, G. Karpen, M. Lamb, and R. Nelson. 1987. Fragile sites in human chromosomes as regions of late-replicating DNA. *Trends Genet.* 3(10):274–281.

Landoulsi, A., M. C. deBlois, P. Guerin, M. O. Tethore, J. Lejeune, and G. Lucotte. 1985. Recombinaison entre le site fragile Xq27 et le gene du facteur IX de la coagulation. *Ann. Genet. (Paris)* 28(4):201–205.

Lathrop, G. M., and J. M. Lalouel. 1984. Easy calculations of lod scores and genetic risks on small computers. *Am. J. Hum. Genet.* 36:460–465.

Mulley, J. C., A. K. Geden, K. A. Thorn, L. J. Bates, and G. R. Sutherland. 1986. Linkage and genetic counseling for the fragile X using DNA probes 52A, F9, DX13, and St14. *Am. J. Med. Genet.* 27:435–449.

Mulley, J. C., G. Turner, S. Bain, and G. R. Sutherland. 1988. Linkage between the fragile X and F9, DXS52 (ST14), DXS98 (4D-8) and DXS105 (cX55.7). *Am. J. Med. Genet.* 30:567–580.

Mulligan, L. M., M. A. Phillips, C. J. Forster-Gibson, J. Beckett, M. W. Partington, N. E. Simpson, J. J. A. Holden, and B. N. White. 1985. Genetic mapping of DNA segments relative to the locus for the fragile X syndrome at Xq27.3. *Am. J. Hum. Genet.* 37:463–472.

Nguyen, C., M. G. Mattei, J. A. Rey, M.-A. Baeteman, J.-F. Mattei, and B. R. Jordan. 1988. Cytogenetic and physical mapping in the region of the X chromosome surrounding the fragile site. *Am. J. Med. Genet.* 30:601–612.

Nussbaum, R. L., S. D. Airhart, and D. H. Ledbetter. 1986. Recombination and amplification of pyrimidine-rich sequences may be responsible for initiation and progression of the Xq27 fragile site: An hypothesis. *Am. J. Med. Genet.* 23:715–722.

Oberlé, I., D. Drayna, G. Camerino, C. Kloepfer, and J. L. Mandel. 1985a. The telomeric region of the human X chromosome long arm: Presence of a highly polymorphic DNA marker and analysis of recombination frequency. *Proc. Natl. Acad. Sci. U.S.A.* 82:2824–2828.

Oberlé, I., J. L. Mandel, J. Bone, M. G. Mattei, and J. F. Mattei. 1985b. Polymorphic DNA markers in prenatal diagnosis of fragile X syndrome. *Lancet* 1:871.

Oberlé, I., R. Heilig, J. P. Moisan, C. Kloepfer, M. G. Mattei, J. F. Mattei, J. Boue, U. Froster-Iskenius, P. A. Jacobs, G. M. Lathrop, J. M. Lalouel, and J. L. Mandel. 1986. Genetic analysis of the fragile-X mental retardation syndrome with two flanking polymorphic DNA markers. *Proc. Natl. Acad. Sci. U.S.A.* 83:1016–1020.

Oberlé, I., G. Camerino, K. Wrogemann, B. Arveiler, A. Hanauer, E. Raimondi, and J. L. Mandel. 1987. Multipoint genetic mapping of the Xq26-q28 region in families with fragile X mental retardation and in normal families reveals tight linkage of markers in q26-q27. *Hum. Genet.* 77:60–65.

Patterson, M. N., S. Kenwrick, S. Thibodeau, K. Faulk, M. G. Mattei, J. F. Mattei, and K. E. Davies. 1987a. Mapping of DNA markers close to the fragile site on the human X chromosome at Xq27.3. *Nucleic Acids Res.* 15(6):2639–2651.

Patterson, M. N., C. Schwartz, M. Bell, S. Sauer, M. Hofker, B. Trask, G. van den Engh, and K. E. Davies. 1987b. Physical mapping studies on the human X chromosome in the region Xq27-Xqter. *Genomics* 1:297–306.

Patterson, M. N., M. V. Bell, J. Bloomfield, T. Flint, H. Dorkins, S. N. Thibodeau, D. Schaid, G. Bren, C. E. Schwartz, B. Wieringa, H. H. Ropers, D. F. Callen, G. Sutherland, U. Froster-Iskenius, H. Vissing, and K. E. Davies. 1989. Genetic and physical mapping of a novel region close to the fragile X site on the human X chromosome. *Genomics* 4:570–578.

Pergolizzi, R., W. T. Brown, P. Goonewardena, R. Bhan, C. Dobkin, N. Dahl, and U. Pettersson. 1991. Molecular characterization of a DNA probe, U6.2, located close to the fragile X locus. *Am. J. Med. Genet.* In press.

Reik, W., A. Collick, M. L. Norris, S. C. Barton, and M. A. Surani. 1987. Genomic imprinting determines methylation of parental alleles in transgenic mice. *Nature* 328:248–251.

Risch, N. 1988. A new statistical test for linkage heterogeneity. *Am. J. Hum. Genet.* 42:353–364.

Sherman, S. L., N. E. Morton, P. A. Jacobs, and G. Turner. 1984. The marker (X) syndrome: A cytogenetic and genetic analysis. *Ann. Hum. Genet.* 48:21–37.

Sherman, S. L., P. Jacobs, N. E. Morton, U. Froster-Iskenius, P. N. Howard-Peebles, K. B. Nielsen, M. W. Partington, G. R. Sutherland, G. Turner, and M. Watson. 1985. Further segregation analysis of the fragile X syndrome with special reference to transmitting males. *Hum. Genet.* 69:289–299.

Smith, H., and K. W. Wilcox. 1970. A restriction enzyme from *Haemophilus influenzae:* I. Purification and general properties. *J. Mol. Biol.* 51:379–391.

Southern, E. M. 1975. Detection of specific sequences among DNA fragments separated by gel electrophoresis. *J. Mol. Biol.* 98:503–517.

Steinmetz, M., D. Stephan, and K. F. Lindahl. 1986. Gene organization and recombinational hotspots in the murine major histocompatibility complex. *Cell* 44:895–904.

Sutherland, G. R., E. Baker, and A. Fratini. 1985. Excess thymidine induces folate sensitive fragile sites. *Am. J. Med. Genet.* 22:433–443.

Suthers, G. K., D. F. Callen, V. J. Hyland, H. M. Kozman, E. Baker, H. Eyre, P. S. Harper, S. H. Roberts, M. C. Hors-Cayla, K. E. Davies, M. V. Bell, and G. R. Sutherland. 1989. A new DNA marker tightly linked to the fragile X locus (FRAXA). *Science* 246:1298–1300.

Swain, J. L., T. A. Stewart, and P. Leder. 1987. Parental legacy determines methylation and expression of an autosomal transgene: A molecular mechanism for parental imprinting. *Cell* 50:719–727.

Tartof, K. 1974. Unequal meiotic sister chromatid exchange as the mechanism of ribosomal RNA gene magnification. *Proc. Natl. Acad. Sci. U.S.A.* 71:1272–1276.

Thibodeau, S. N., H. R. Dorkins, K. R. Faulk, R. Berry, A. C. M. Smith, R. Hagerman, A. King, and K. E. Davies. 1988. Linkage analysis using multiple DNA polymorphic markers in normal families and in families with fragile X syndrome. *Hum. Genet.* 79:219–227.

Turner, G., J. M. Opitz, W. T. Brown, K. E. Davies, P. A. Jacobs, E. C. Jenkins, M. Mikkelsen, M. W. Partington, and G. R. Sutherland. 1986. Conference report: Second International Workshop on the Fragile X and on X-linked Mental Retardation. *Am. J. Med. Genet.* 23:11–67.

van Oostra, B. A., P. E. Hupkes, L. F. Perdon, C. A. van Bennekom, E. Bakker, D. J. J. Halley, M. Schmidt, D. Du Sart, A. Smits, B. Wieringa, and B. A. van Oost. 1990. New polymorphic DNA marker close to the fragile site FRAXA. *Genomics* 6:129–132.

Vincent, A., N. Dahl, I. Oberlé, A. Hanauer, J. L. Mandel, H. Malmgren, and U. Pettersson. 1989. The polymorphic marker DXS304 is within 5 centimorgans of the fragile X locus. *Genomics* 5:797–801.

Vollrath, D., J. Nathans, and R. W. Davis. 1988. Tandem array of human visual pigment genes at Xq28. *Science* 240:1669–1672.

Warren, S. T., T. W. Glover, R. L. Davidson, and P. Jagadeeswaran. 1985. Linkage and recombination between fragile X-linked mental retardation and the factor IX gene. *Hum. Genet.* 69:44–46.

Warren, S. T., F. Zhang, G. R. Licameli, and J. F. Peters. 1987. The fragile X site in somatic cell hybrids: An approach for molecular cloning of fragile sites. *Science* 237:420–423.

Weinreb, A., D. R. Katzenberg, G. L. Gilmore, and B. K. Birshtein. 1988. Site of unequal sister chromatid exchange contains a potential Z-DNA-forming tract. *Proc. Natl. Acad. Sci. U.S.A.* 85:529–533.

Zoll, B., J. Arnemann, M. Krawczak, D. N. Cooper, G. Pescia, W. Wahli, P. Steinbach, and J. Schmidtke. 1985. Evidence against close linkage of the loci for fraXq of Martin-Bell syndrome and for factor IX. *Hum. Genet.* 71:122–126.

Note Added in Proof

In the spring of 1991, rapid progress was made in understanding the nature of the fragile X mutation. Oberlé et al. (1991) and Yu et al. (1991), using the approaches outlined above, independently isolated probes adjacent or overlapping fragile X that detected instability of a DNA segment. Normal transmitting males (TMs) were found to possess a 150- to 400-base pair insertion near to the GC-rich variable methylation fragment. This insertion was passed from TMs to their daughters nearly unchanged. However, among the affected offspring of these daughters, the average size of the insertion was observed to undergo a variable size increase by about 2000 bps. The size increase was heterogeneous even within a given individual. The potential technical ability to detect this insertion directly offered researchers the hope of developing a direct test of the fragile X mutation.

Verkerk et al. (1991) then used contig cloning of a YAC DNA fragment shown to span the fragile X site to identify a DNA coding gene segment that expressed a 4.8-kb message expressed in brain and lymphocytes but not in liver, lung, or kidney. It was evolutionarily highly conserved. They termed this coded gene segment FMR-1. The segment was shown by sequencing to contain a lengthy CGG repeat. This segment was 250-bp distal to the CpG island, which undergoes hypermethylation and which also was located within a coding exon segment. This CGG segment encoded a string of 30 arginine residues within a 32-amino acid stretch. It was an extremely basic region of a peptide and therefore most likely a DNA-binding nuclear type protein. Such DNA-binding proteins often are involved with gene expression. Therefore, it appears that the function of the FMR-1 gene that is mutated by insertions and also affected by hypermethylation may be to perform an important role in regulation of gene expression.

References Added in Proof

Oberlé, I., F. Rousseau, D. Heitz, C. Kretz, D. Devys, A. Hanauer, J. Boué, M. F. Bertheas, and J. L. Mandel. 1991. Instability of a 550-base pair DNA segment and abnormal methylation in fragile X syndrome. *Science* 252:1097–1102.

Verkerk, A. J. M. H., M. Plerettl, J. S. Sutcliffe, Y.-H. Fu, D. P. A. Kuhl, A. Pizzuti, O. Reiner, S. Richards, M. F. Victoria, F. Zhang, B. E. Eussen, G.-J. B. van Ommen, L. A. J. Blonden, G. J. Riggins, J. L. Chastain, C. B. Kunst, H. Galjaard, C. T. Caskey, D. L. Nelson, B. A. Oostra, and S. T. Warren. 1991. Identification of a gene (FMR-1) containing a CGG repeat coincident with a breakpoint cluster region exhibiting length variation in fragile X syndrome. *Cell* 65:905–914.

Yu, S., M. Pritchard, E. Kremer, M. Lynch, J. Nancarrow, E. Baker, K. Holman, J. C. Mulley, S. T. Warren, D. Schlessinger, G. R. Sutherland, and R. I. Richards. 1991. Fragile X genotype characterized by an unstable region of DNA. *Science* 252:1179–1181.

CHAPTER 5

Toward a Neuropsychology of Fragile X Syndrome

Bruce F. Pennington, Ph.D.,
Rebecca A. O'Connor, M.A.,
and Vicki Sudhalter, Ph.D.

The goals of this chapter are to review what is known about the neuropsychological phenotype in fragile X males and females, to point to what we would like to know, and to highlight the theoretical and methodologic issues that need to be addressed in defining the neuropsychological phenotype of this genetic syndrome. Although information about both the neurological and the psychiatric phenotypes in fra(X) is relevant to the neuropsychological phenotype, this information is covered in chapter 1 and will not be repeated here. Because fra(X) is a relatively new genetic syndrome, we may benefit from the lessons developed below that have already been learned from neuropsychological studies of other genetic syndromes. There are also issues that are specific to fra(X) because of its complex genetics and because of the unusual developmental trajectory of IQ (at least in males).

Theoretical and Methodological Issues

Our task in defining the neuropsychological phenotype in fra(X) would be much easier if there already existed a mature science of normal and abnormal neuropsychological development. Such a science would provide a catalog of both phenotypes and well-validated measures for assessing them, and our task would simply be to apply these measures to fra(X) and decide which phenotypic category, if any, best fits. Although easier, our task would also be less scientifically interesting. Instead, the relation that exists between phenotype definition of a new syndrome like fra(X) and our fledgling science of developmental neuropsychology is reciprocal and dialectic (Pennington and Smith 1988). New syndromes may compel us to carve the domain of cognition somewhat differently, with important implications for phenotype definition in other syndromes and for studies of normal behavioral development. Fra(X) syndrome is particularly exciting in this regard because it may provide insights about the intersection of neuropsychiatry and cognitive neuropsychology. For instance, fra(X) may illuminate disorders like autism, attention deficit disorder, and schizotypy, in which there are deficits both in purely cognitive functions and in social-emotional functions. Conversely, research on the neuropsychology of these related disorders and functions may provide us with theories and measures to better understand fra(X) syndrome.

Potential Analogies for the Fra(X) Phenotype

Although we do not have a mature science of developmental neuropsychology, we do at least have a preliminary taxonomy of developmental learning disorders (Pennington 1991) and a beginning understanding of the neuropsychology of different retardation syndromes. We can ask whether the neuropsychological phenotype in fra(X) females is similar to any of these better-understood developmental learning disorders and how the phenotype in fra(X) males compares and contrasts with that in other retardation syndromes. We can also ask if the phenotypes in fra(X) females and males are qualitatively similar despite varying considerably in overall level of function. Briefly, these learning disorders are developmental dyslexia, other developmental language disorders, nonverbal learning disorder, executive function disorders [e.g., attention deficit hyperactivity disorder (ADHD)], autistic spectrum disorder, and long-term memory disorder. Two better-described mental retardation syndromes are Down syndrome and Williams syndrome. In our final section, we discuss which of these analogies fit and do not fit the existing data on fra(X) females and males.

Evaluating Discriminant Validity, Specificity, Primacy, and Consistency

Finding that fra(X) males or females are impaired on the same measures as individuals with a known type of retardation syndrome or learning disorder would be interesting but would not take us very far. We also need to evaluate whether they are relatively unimpaired in other neuropsychological domains. If only areas of predicted deficit are tested, positive results are ambiguous because they may only be part of a more general pattern of impairment. This is the issue of *discriminant validity.*

This issue is well illustrated in the research done to elucidate the cognitive phenotype in Turner syndrome, another X chromosome anomaly with relevance for fra(X). Once it was discovered in the early 1960s that females with Turner syndrome had depressed performance IQs (Cohen 1962; Shaffer 1962), researchers quickly focused their attention on visuospatial tasks, neglecting the issue of discriminant validity. These overly focused studies seemed to support the hypothesis of a right hemisphere deficit (Money 1973). However, when later researchers used broader neuropsychological batteries, the deficits in Turner syndrome no longer seemed to be either exclusively right hemisphere or visuospatial (McGlone 1985; Pennington et al. 1985; Waber 1979). Despite 25 years of research on the cognitive phenotype of Turner syndrome, we still lack a clear formulation, although progress has certainly been made.

The issue of *specificity* is closely related to the issue of discriminant validity. In attempting to understand the neuropsychological phenotype in fra(X) males and females, we would like to identify specific effects of the fra(X) mutation on brain function, apart from nonspecific effects on overall developmental level. To control for this possible confound, one must utilize non-fra(X), developmentally disabled (DD) controls who are similar in overall IQ to the fra(X) subjects. Normal, younger-mental-age controls obviously do not control for the nonspecific effects of a developmental disability. In considering the phenotypic characteristics of fra(X), it is important to be able to decide which are attributable to developmental delay (nonspecific effects) and which are attributable to developmental deviance (specific effects). As we will see, very few existing studies of fra(X) have used IQ-matched, DD controls.

Not all specific effects are *primary* because some specific effects may either be secondary to primary effects (e.g., gaze avoidance may be secondary to deficits in social understanding) or be correlated effects (e.g., stereotypies in fra(X) males may be correlated rather than primary deficits). Evaluating whether observed deficits are primary, secondary, or correlated is difficult and is most definitively addressed by longitudinal studies. We should probably wait to address this issue until we are clearer about which deficits are and are not specific to fra(X).

If, in group studies of fra(X) individuals, we find a neuropsychological phenotype that has discriminant validity, specificity, and primacy, we still need to determine how *consistent* that phenotype is across individuals. Consistency is a continuous variable rather than a dichotomous one. At one extreme, there may be neuropsychological effects of a disorder that are either global or so variable across individuals as to make it meaningless to speak of *the* neuropsychological phenotype. One can imagine genetic disorders whose effects on the brain would be either global or highly variable. For example, untreated phenylketonuria (PKU) has sometimes been discussed as having a uniformly toxic effect on all of brain development, whereas neurocutaneous disorders may have a highly variable effect. If there is no consistency across affected individuals, then we will not find discriminant validity, specificity, or primacy. At the other, unlikely extreme, every affected individual will have the same phenotype. The actual situation in many genetic disorders probably falls somewhere between these two extremes; thus, we need to develop criteria for significant but less than complete consistency. These criteria must allow for the inevitable phenotypic variability across affected individuals; this variability is caused by their genetic and environmental differences. It is easy to forget that individuals with a given genetic syndrome are different in the vast majority of both their genes and their specific environmental experiences. Consequently, the genetic defect must emit a strong signal for us to detect it in the noise caused by genetic and environmental differences. Therefore, it will be very unusual for a neuropsychological phenotype to be present in all affected individuals, and some phenotypes will not be present in the majority but will be detectable only as the central tendency of the group. It is unlikely that there will be a neuropsychological profile that is diagnostic of a genetic syndrome at the individual level.

Ascertainment Bias

In trying to arrive at the core set of neuropsychological symptoms that are specific and primary in a genetic disorder, one must avoid ascertainment bias. Individuals referred for clinical services are more likely to have additional, unrelated diagnoses (Berkson 1946), which only add to our confusion in trying to sort out core symptoms. Prospective studies of infants with sex chromosome anomalies were initiated to avoid just this problem, and the phenotype results from such prospective samples did differ considerably from those reported for clinically ascertained cases (Robinson et al. 1979). In studies of fra(X) females, an affected male is usually the proband who has come to clinical attention. His male and female relatives who also have the mutation would provide a less biased sample, although it would not be as unbiased as a sample identified through population screening. Thus far, no fra(X) sample has been identified through screening of the general population, although screening has been done in special populations (e.g., retarded autistics).

Issues Specific to Fra(X)

Two aspects of this syndrome create special problems for research on the neuropsychological phenotype—the late decline in IQ in males and the extreme variation in penetrance in females. The former problem is a potential confound in studies with a wide age range of fra(X) males. If the biologic changes responsible for this decline also affect the pattern of abilities, then group data across a broad age range will be misleading not only about the levels of IQ at different ages but also about developmental changes in the patterns of abilities at different ages. The frequency and variability of psychiatric symptoms found in fra(X) samples (which can include attention problems, depression, tics, and autistic features) also complicate neuropsychological testing. Deciding which of these psychiatric symptoms are primary features of the syndrome is an important goal of phenotype analysis.

Similarly, the various mechanisms responsible for the extreme variation in penetrance in females may affect not only the level but also the pattern of abilities. As we will see, there are indications that the ability pattern in unaffected or nonimprinted fra(X) females has similarities to dyslexia, whereas the ability pattern observed in affected or imprinted females resembles that found in groups with nonverbal learning disabilities. Consequently, mixing imprinted and nonimprinted females in the same group could average out distinctive ability profiles actually present in each subgroup.

Review of Studies of Fra(X) Males

Cognitive Measures

Although the spectrum of involvement is quite variable, the fra(X) male generally functions within the moderately to severely retarded range of intelligence (Herbst 1980; Hagerman and Smith 1983; Chudley et al. 1983). Sutherland and Hecht (1985) reported findings from 21 studies in which the IQ for fra(X) males ranged from normal to profound retardation. Investigations of higher-functioning males have been reported, although these males have been described as having significant learning problems (Hagerman et al. 1985; Gold-fine et al. 1987). There have also been descriptions of nonpenetrant males (Froster-Iskenius et al. 1986; Sherman et al. 1984; Loesch et al. 1987). These males tend to be unaffected intellectually, although they may possess behavioral and psychological difficulties.

Many studies of IQ in fra(X) males were reviewed. Studies with sufficient sample size and details that provide meaningful information about mean IQ in fra(X) males are summarized in table 5.1.

Overall IQ

Considering the cross-sectional studies first, it can be seen that the mean IQ ranges from 22.0 to 65.0. However, the latter value came from a study that included only males with an IQ of 50 or greater and is not relevant to the question of the mean IQ in unselected fra(X) males. (Similarly, the sample of Dykens et al. (1988) was drawn from an institutional population.) Considering the remaining studies, the means cluster around two values, 34 and 50 approximately. The two studies with the higher value had a younger age range, suggesting age decline in IQ in fra(X) males, an issue discussed below. Thus, these results are quite consistent in indicating moderate to severe mental retardation in fra(X) males.

Table 5.1

IQ Results in Fragile (X) Males[a]

Cross-sectional Studies

Study	No.	Age (yr)	Controls	Measures	Full Scale IQ	Verbal IQ	Nonverbal IQ
Borghgraef et al. 1987	17	15–22	DD males matched on age & IQ	Wechsler SB	34.5	VIQ > PIQ for *both* groups	
Chudley et al. 1983	37	6–65	No	Wechsler SB	34.8	ND	ND
Dykens et al. 1987	14	7–28	No	SB KABC	50.0	Seq < Sim on KABC	
Dykens et al. 1988	12	23–62	fra(X)-neg. autistics, MRs	SB	MA = 3–2	—	—
Freund and Reiss 1989	17	3–24	No	SB	50.0	—	—
Kemper et al. 1988	20	4–12	fra(X)-neg. DD	KABC	65.0	62.0 (Seq)	71.0 (Sim)
Prouty et al. 1988	93	?	No	Mixed	33.0	—	—
Veenema et al. 1987	14	26–74	Normal relatives	WAIS	22.0 (4 at floor of test)	—	—

Studies of IQ Change with Age

Study	No.	Age (yr)	Controls	Measures	Prepuberty IQ	Postpuberty IQ
Borghgraef et al. 1988	40	2–25	fra(X)-neg. MR	Mixed	51.0	34.0
Hodapp et al. 1990	66	<20	No	SB	53.3	47.3

[a]*Abbreviations:* FSIQ, full-scale IQ; VIQ, verbal IQ; NVIQ, nonverbal IQ; SB, Stanford-Binet; PIQ, performance IQ; ND, not done; KABC, Kaufman Assessment Battery for Children; WAIS, Wechsler Adult Intelligence Scale-Revised.

Specific Cognitive Profile

There is not much evidence of significant verbal IQ-performance IQ (VIQ-PIQ) discrepancies on the Wechsler Scale. Borghgraef et al. (1988) found a significant VIQ-PIQ discrepancy in their fra(X) males, but a similar discrepancy was found in non-fra(X) mentally retarded (MR) male controls matched on

IQ and age. Moreover, Theobald et al. (1987) did not find a significant VIQ-PIQ discrepancy in a larger fra(X) male sample. Unfortunately, most of the existing studies do not provide data on VIQ-PIQ differences.

At a finer-grained level of analysis, there is some evidence for a pattern of cognitive strengths and weaknesses that is specific to fra(X) males. Kemper et al. (1988) identified a consistent pattern of performance on the Kaufman Assessment Battery for Children (K-ABC). This pattern includes (1) a simultaneous processing score greater than a sequential processing score, (2) an achievement standard score greater than a mental processing composite score, (3) a matrix analogy subtest score greater than a spatial memory subtest score, and (4) an arithmetic subtest score less than the mean achievement subtest score. In other words, the fra(X) males were more impaired in math and both verbal and nonverbal short-term memory than they were in spatial reasoning, reading, or verbal long-term memory.

Kemper's study included 40 boys between the ages of 4 and 12. All boys were cytogenetically tested for the presence of fra(X). Twenty boys demonstrated the fragile site and also demonstrated the physical features consistent with the identified physical phenotype. The comparison group of 20 boys were cytogenetically negative for fra(X). Significant differences in overall level of functioning were identified, with the fra(X) group scoring lower cognitively, although performance on the achievement subtests was consistently higher in fra(X) boys. The fra(X) group also demonstrated much more variation across subtests, with the comparison group demonstrating a relatively flat profile. Kemper et al. concluded that there is a cognitive phenotype possibly related to specific central nervous system deficits for males with the fra(X) syndrome.

Dykens et al. (1987) also examined the cognitive profiles on the K-ABC of 14 fra(X) boys. They identified significant weaknesses in sequential processing, short-term auditory memory, visual and motor skills, and arithmetic. Their results were similar to those reported by Kemper et al. (1988). These particular patterns of strength were noted to be unusual for mentally retarded individuals.

Thus, it seems that deficits in short-term memory and arithmetic tasks may be a specific feature of the neuropsychological phenotype in fra(X) males. These deficits could be explained by an underlying attentional deficit, as striking attention problems are frequently noted in the clinical description of fra(X) males. More data are needed to confirm these apparently specific deficits and to explore their neuropsychological significance.

Developmental Trajectory of IQ

Although IQ scores for mentally retarded children are reported to be relatively stable (Silverstein et al. 1982), a decline in the intellectual performance of fra(X) males has been described by many investigators (Chudley et al. 1983; Hagerman and Smith 1983; Partington 1984; Lachiewicz et al. 1987; Dykens et al. 1989; Hagerman et al. 1989; Hodapp et al. 1990; Borghgraef et al. 1987, 1988). Problems with many of these studies include cross-sectional data analysis, comparison of different IQ tests over time, and ascertainment bias. (The initial studies focused on institutionalized men, who tend to be low functioning, rather than on less selected samples of fra(X) males.)

Lachiewicz et al. (1987) were among the first investigators to describe the declining IQs of young fra(X) males. They identified significant declines in IQ scores over time for the study as a whole, although many individuals did not follow this pattern. Lachiewicz et al. did make reference to other groups of mentally retarded boys, but no direct comparisons were made.

Table 5.1 summarizes two studies relevant to this issue, only one of which (Hodapp et al. 1990) is a longitudinal study. This study includes data from three previously published studies. Borghgraef et al. (1987) compared pre- and postpubertal IQ cross-sectionally in fra(X) males and fra(X)-negative MR controls and found a significant difference only in the fra(X) males, whose postpubertal IQs were lower. Interestingly, the two mean fra(X) male IQ values found in this study are very similar to the two mean IQ values discussed above that were found in cross-sectional studies with varying age composition.

The most recent study of the IQ trajectory of cognitive development (Hodapp et al. 1990) analyzed longitudinal data from three major centers involved with the diagnosis and treatment of the fra(X) syndrome. Results supported a significant decrease in IQ over time, with the most marked declines during the early pubertal period.

Hodapp argued that the nature of IQ change is different for different causes of mental impairment. For example, Down syndrome children seem to develop at slower and slower rates over time (Kopf and McCall 1982). Dykens et al. (1989), whose data were included in the Hodapp sample, attempted to address the questions of when the IQ declines in fra(X) males, whether the IQ decline is steady or varies based on age, and what factors might be associated with irregular declines. The Dykens study concluded that the decline in IQ is not artifactual, that greater declines are observed in the higher-functioning, younger males, and that the most significant declines are found during the pubertal ages. However, the study of Hagerman et al. (1989) found significant declines well before puberty, which they attributed to a much greater requirement for abstract thinking in IQ items for school-age children compared with those for younger children. This study argues against only one etiologic factor being responsible for the overall decline in IQ over time.

In summary, fra(X) males as a group are moderately to severely retarded, may have specific impairments in short-term memory and arithmetic functioning, and exhibit a late decline in IQ unlike that observed in other retarded groups.

Speech

To help in understanding the terminology we will divide speech competence into segmental and nonsegmental (Crystal 1979). Segmental competence is the ability to produce the set of articulatory movements (e.g., positions and movements of tongue, lips, nasal cavities, teeth) that enable one to produce the sounds of one's native language. Nonsegmental competence is the ability to produce the prosodic elements (duration, tone, intonation, stress) of one's particular language which stretch over sound, word, and even phrase boundaries. These two competencies in turn are controlled by motor-perceptual plans at the level of the central nervous system, and all combine to create a proficient speaker of the language.

The literature describing the speech behaviors of the fra(X) male is fraught with problems. The research is anecdotal, descriptive, and based on small numbers (one child or one family). Children with varying degrees of impairment are described together, and we are not told whether there has been an effort to control and/or eliminate children with autistic disorder or atypical pervasive developmental disorder. In addition, such a minute number of the studies have control groups that we cannot even begin to address the central issue of specificity, namely, which speech problems are caused by the fra(X) syndrome and which are caused by retardation.

Abnormalities in speech production have been consistently found and described. Frequent findings include dysfluent, dyspraxic, poorly articulated speech (Jacobs et al. 1980; Herbst 1980) with "jocular," "litany-like phraseology" (Turner et al. 1980). Prouty et al. (1988) investigated the articulatory structures of fra(X) males and females and found that they "did not demonstrate abnormalities of dental structure nor asymmetry of the lips or face. Twelve males and one female had a high palate. Short frenulum was evident in one patient, tongue mobility appeared normal" (p. 129). It can be concluded that, if speech problems exist in the sample, these problems could not be attributed solely to anomalies of the articulatory structures. The fra(X) subjects demonstrated articulation errors in the form of substitutions and omissions. However, these types of errors would be consistent with the mental age of the subjects. Several of the fra(X) subjects manifested dysfluency and repetitive phrases, and 80% of the patients had hoarse or harsh voice quality. Thus, the fra(X) male is manifesting *delay* in articulation and *deviance* in prosody, which affect his intelligibility.

Paul et al. (1984), describing the language of three fra(X) males, said that they manifested (1) poorer performance on production than on receptive language, (2) poor intelligibility in connected speech, (3) the use of the phonologic simplification processes, (4) poor performance on repetition tasks, and (5) dysfluency.

In a thoughtful study by Newell et al. (1983), one aspect of the research was an investigation into the speech of fra(X) males. Most of the study subjects (90%) demonstrated unusual speech patterns characterized by dissolutions or disruptions in air flow, repetitions, inappropriate pauses, revisions, and interjections. In addition, errors in articulation were described as not being different from those manifested by nonretarded children during the normal development of articulation competence.

Niemi et al. (1985), describing the speech of Finnish males with fra(X), found that they exhibit perseveration, clutter, and repetition of initial syllables. In addition, their spontaneous speech is often unclear, incoherent, and wildly associative and also exhibits phonologic and morphologic errors. Speech-motor evaluation suggested that the client was clumsy motorically. The slow repetition of initial syllables, perseveration, unintelligibility, incoherence, and comprehension problems on verbal tasks led the authors to believe that the speech problems of the fra(X) male are analogous to those experienced by individuals with developmental apraxia of speech. They supported their argument by demonstrating that articulation is generally faultless when test words are uttered separately but that there are phonologic mistakes in spontaneous speech. In addition, they concluded that disturbances in speech rhythm, like cluttering and stammering, support the hypothesis of Paul et al. (1984) that the speech problems are suggestive of developmental dyspraxia.

Madison et al. (1986) researched the speech and language of fra(X) males and females. They used formal and informal measures to assess the communicative abilities of their sample. All fra(X) males in this study evidenced difficulty in timed motor speech tasks. The authors concluded, as did Niemi et al. (1985), that the long pauses, automatic phrases, perseveration, and inconsistent volume and prosody may be the result of apraxia.

In summary, the articles come to a consensus that the fra(X) male manifests speech behavior that is characterized by dysfluency, dysrhythmia, repetitions, and perseverations. Without control groups we do not know whether these problems are different from problems experienced by other retarded males of similar level. We also are left wondering what exactly is meant by "jocular" or "litany-like" and what is the difference between repetition and perseveration. In addition, we are left asking if all fra(X) males exhibit these behaviors and, if not, what separates the dysfluent from the fluent males. Some of these results are very important, such as the conclusion that the speech problems of the fra(X) male are suggestive of developmental apraxia of speech, but before we can take this suggestion seriously we must see more carefully designed studies with control groups.

In a descriptive article by Hanson et al. (1986), the speech of mildly impaired fra(X) males was described as "cluttered." *Cluttering* was defined as a disability of language formation that is characterized by an increased rate of speech and an erratic rhythm. The article is well conceived for what it does, which is describe speech problems in high-functioning fra(X) males. The authors can be commended for separating higher-functioning from lower-functioning fra(X) males, thereby not confounding results with males of many different levels of functioning. However, control groups should be included in studies so we can determine whether the anomaly described can be attributed to fra(X) or is somehow related to retardation. What percentage of the high-functioning non-fra(X) males present with this same behavior? If they do present with this behavior, do the fra(X) children utter significantly more cluttered speech? Is the speech more dysfluent or dysrhythmic?

In direct disagreement with the above stance that there is something different about the speech and language of fra(X) males are two articles, one by Howard-Peebles et al. (1979) and one by Dykens et al. (1988). Howard-Peebles et al. described a generalized language disability with articulation errors similar to those of patients with nonspecific delay of development. "Thus misarticulations for the present study could be the result of delayed development and does not demonstrate a distinctive pattern" (p. 219). Dykens et al. (1988), studying an institutionalized population with severe and profound retardation, found no distinctive specific profile of speech patterns among fra(X) males, autistic males, and males with cultural/familial retardation. These articles are confusing if taken together with the ones cited above. However, the seeming contradictions can be cleared up if one realizes that (1) different aspects of speech behavior were being described (articulation versus prosody) and (2) different groups comprised of fra(X) males with very different levels of functioning were used. To avoid future contradictions in the literature, we must ask for better control of definitions and methods.

Language

Language mastery can be divided into a combination of several competencies. The superordinate level consists of receptive and expressive competence. Receptive competence is the ability to receive and understand the speech/language signal and act upon the command or request in a way that suggests understanding. Expressive competence (including speech competence) is the ability to produce meaningful, intelligible sentences that say what the speaker means to say. Subordinate to both receptive and expressive skill are (1) syntactic competence, which is the ability to put words together to form questions, statements, negations, phrases, clauses, and sentences; (2) semantic competence, which is the knowledge of word meanings (e.g., that the word *girl* entails the features of female, two eyes, two legs, the ability to walk, etc.) and world knowledge (e.g., the knowledge that mountains do not fly or that trees do not talk); and (3) pragmatic competence, which is the knowledge of how to listen, how to carry on a conversation, how to initiate conversations, how and when to ask questions, how and when to answer questions, and how to maintain eye contact so that the person with whom you are talking knows that you are listening and understanding.

The deviant language behaviors that have been noted most frequently in the fra(X) male are perseveration, tangential conversational style, palilalia (direct self-repetition), and echolalia (repetition of others) (Wolf-Schein et al. 1987; Fryns et al. 1984; Newell et al. 1983; Renier et al. 1983; Sudhalter et al. 1990).

Using a variety of methods, Newell et al. (1983) assessed the speech and language behaviors of 21 fra(X) patients aged 17 months to 31 years. They found that the syntactic ability of the males (as measured by mean length of utterance) did not increase as IQ increased, suggesting that the verbal ability reached asymptote. The males generally produced perseveration, echolalia, and palilalia. Although this article made huge strides by employing standardized measures, no control groups were used, not even a control for autism and atypical pervasive developmental disorder, and there was a broad range of chronologic ages, intellectual levels, and interfering behaviors.

Wolf-Schein et al. (1987) compared two groups, 35 males with fra(X) and 15 males with Down syndrome (DS), in an attempt to answer the question of whether the language behaviors produced by the fra(X) male are indicative of retardation or of the fra(X) syndrome. These two groups had been matched for adaptive behavior score as measured on the Vineland Adaptive Behavior Scale and were rated on 16 speech and language behaviors using a measure developed by the researchers. The fra(X) males were found to be significantly more likely to talk to themselves and produce stereotyped vocalizations (e.g., "ga, ga, ga"), jargon, dysrhythmia, perseveration, echolalia, conditioned statements (i.e., stereotypic statements like "Good morning") and inappropriate/tangential remarks than were the DS males and were significantly less likely to use referential gestures and facial/head signals than were males with DS.

Madison et al. (1986), describing the conversational speech of fra(X) males, said that it contained inappropriate responses based on related or associated thoughts, perseveration on earlier topics, disinhibited responses, rambling, and frequent use of automatic phrases.

Borghgraef et al. (1987) matched 23 fra(X) and 17 non-fra(X) males. Each fra(X) boy's speech and language development was described as being delayed. Within the preschool age group, no major differences were observed between the two groups. In the 7–11 age group, significant differences were noted between the two groups (although no statistics were offered to substantiate claims). The older fra(X) males' speech and language was characterized by rapid speech rhythm, verbal unstructuredness, speech impulsiveness, and perseverative speech. The authors provided numbers, but it is not always clear to what the numbers refer. In addition, 39% of the fra(X) males were also given the behavioral diagnosis of autistic disorder. Thus, one wonders whether the language deviance described is a result of fra(X), retardation, and/or autistic disorder. The authors did state that "echolalia was not found to be of diagnostic relevance. In contrast perseverative speech was 2.5 times more frequent in the preschool fra(X) boys and was not related to their intellectual level." This contrast in the prevalence of a particular deviant language behavior as produced in fra(X) versus the language deviance produced in autistic disorder was also seen in the study of Sudhalter et al. (1990).

Sudhalter et al. (1990) compared the emergence of deviant perseverative language in 12 fra(X) males, 12 non-fra(X) autistic males, and 9 DS males. The fra(X) males had a diagnosis of mental retardation; none had a diagnosis of autism or pervasive developmental disorder. In addition, these groups had been chosen to have ages that were not significantly different and were matched on the communication, daily living, and socialization subscales of the Vineland Adaptive Behavior Scales. There was one significant finding within the subscales; as would be expected, the males with autism had significantly lower scores than had the males with either fra(X) or DS on the socialization subscale of the Vineland Scale. The particular language sample was derived from two conversations, one between the male and his parent/caretaker and one with someone whom he did not know. Each subject's language sample was then separated into three mutually exclusive pragmatic categories of direct response (answers to questions), initiation (self-initiated productions), and topic maintenance (productions that added information to a topic) for each of the two conversations. A percentage of *deviant* repetitive language was then derived for each of the categories for each conversation, resulting in six scores. The only pragmatic category on which group differences were found was topic maintenance, and these deviations were present in conversations with both parent/caretaker and an unfamiliar adult. In maintaining a topic, fra(X) males produced significantly more deviant repetitive language than did the males with DS and significantly less deviant language than did the males with autistic disorder. This suggests that fra(X) males do produce a pattern of deviant language that is distinct both from their peers with DS and from peers with autism not associated with fra(X) syndrome. The language deviance produced by the fra(X) males was perseveration, and the language deviance produced by the males with autism was echolalia, similar to the results of Borghgraef et al. (1987).

A number of articles state that the language of the fra(X) male is commensurate with his intellectual level. These articles are measuring other aspects of the fra(X) male's language ability besides pragmatics. For example, Fryns et al. (1984) stated that the delay in speech and verbal ability does not differ significantly from that observed in the mentally retarded population in general. Madison et al. (1986) stated additionally that the language skills of the affected males generally were commensurate with their cognitive skills. They thought that the deviance in both speech and language manifested by the fra(X) male is primarily caused by a generalized inability to coordinate the muscles necessary for speech and language production. Paul et al. (1987) assessed the speech and language of severely/profoundly retarded fra(X) males, autistic males, and males with cultural/familial retardation and found little difference among these groups. As an explanation for these apparently discrepant findings, Sudhalter (1991) showed how the syntactic ability of the fra(X) male would not be described as deviant, whereas his pragmatic and conversational skills would be regarded as deviant.

In summary, it can be concluded that the fra(X) male seems to present with delays in syntax, which would be expected inasmuch as the vast majority of these males present with mental retardation. However, we also can conclude that the male presents with language deviance in that he perseverates on words, phrases, and topic above and beyond what would be expected from his mental age. More research is needed to identify the underlying cognitive or linguistic cause of this deviant pragmatic language in fra(X) males and to compare their pragmatic errors with those found in other clinical groups. For instance, to what extent is the language of fra(X) males similar to schizophrenic or thought-disordered language?

Summary of the Neuropsychology of Fra(X) Males

Existing studies support the conclusions that adult fra(X) males are on average moderately to severely retarded and that there is some preliminary evidence for specificity of their neuropsychological phenotype, with regard to both domains of function and other DD groups. Specifically, in the cognitive area, there is preliminary evidence for specific deficits in attention, verbal short-term memory, and arithmetic. There also clearly seems to be a late decline in IQ that is unlike that observed in other retarded groups, but the mechanisms responsible for this decline are unclear. Because of strengths in language and long-term memory, fra(X) males can appear less retarded during the preschool years than other retarded groups.

In terms of speech and language, it seems that fra(X) males may have a developmental delay in speech praxis and specific deviance in pragmatic and conversational skills beyond what would be expected on the basis of level of retardation. In contrast, other language processing, such as syntax, seems to be at an expected level for the level of retardation. Fra(X) males do not seem to have a traditionally defined developmental dysphasia in which the main impairment is in the phonologic and syntactic domains. Their language deficit is somewhat reminiscent of the semantic-pragmatic syndrome without autism described by Rapin and Allen (1983), although children with this syndrome are more fluent than are most fra(X) males. In this syndrome, there are deficits in the social and meaning levels of language but not in phonology or syntax.

Overall, the profile of deficits and relative strengths in fra(X) males is suggestive of underlying problems in executive functions and/or social cognition, but these domains of neuropsychological function have not been specifically tested in fra(X) males. It is unlikely that there is a specific deficit in phonologic processing and reading or long-term memory in fra(X) males. In fact, reading and spelling may be significant strengths in this population based on achievement data from the K-ABC. There is also little evidence for a specific deficit in spatial reasoning.

In terms of methodologic issues, existing studies have begun to address the issues of specificity and wide age range, but the issues of discriminant validity, primacy, consistency, and ascertainment bias have generally not been addressed. The cognitive studies of fra(X) males have nearly all relied exclusively on IQ measures, and so many domains of neuropsychological function either have not been studied or have been studied with measures that are factorially complex, so the significance of patterns of strengths and weaknesses is not clear. For instance, fra(X) males seem to be impaired on number and word list memory tasks, but such tasks are vulnerable to problems with attention, verbal short-term memory, and anxiety. Nearly all of the research is descriptive rather than hypothesis driven, and there is little in the way of testable models that attempt to account for all of the speech, language, and cognitive data.

Review of Studies of Fra(X) Females

Cognitive Studies

Conflicting findings concerning psychological functioning of fra(X) females have been reported. Fra(X) females demonstrate significant variability in many features that seem to be more stable in men. The range of cognitive involvement is quite variable. Sherman et al. (1985) reported that up to one-third of fra(X) females function in the borderline or mentally retarded ranges. Loesch and Hay (1988) suggested that up to 85% of heterozygotes demonstrated some type of cognitive impairment. On the other hand, Brainard et al. (1991) described a significant difference in the overall level of functioning in fra(X)-positive versus fra(X)-negative women. They described fra(X)-negative women as being generally cognitively unimpaired. Thus, the lack of differentiation between positive and negative carrier females in many studies may have a significant influence on their results. Prouty et al. (1988) also identified a significant difference in the general level of functioning between positive and negative fra(X) women.

Many factors complicate the interpretation of the results of cognitive studies of fra(X) females. Researchers have not examined test results with reference to fragility levels, and many have not examined patterns of performance with reference to positive or negative status. The fact that most studies have not differentiated adults from children could be significant in that the inheritance pattern of fra(X) could have increasing involvement in subsequent generations (Sherman et al. 1985; Laird 1987). Many of the studies of fra(X) females have also drawn conclusions from very small samples. Issues of discriminant validity and specificity have rarely been addressed. As was true in studies of fra(X) males, most studies have used only IQ measures and have not had appropriate control groups.

The majority of research with fra(X) females has concentrated on cognitive profiles, correlations of IQ and fragility level, and prevalence of learning disabilities. Studies are fairly preliminary but are becoming more sophisticated in the attempt to identify or rule out a specific cognitive phenotype. Preliminary data do suggest that the fra(X) gene may affect physical, cognitive, and emotional development even in the normal IQ female. Some researchers have also speculated that there may be not a specific cognitive phenotype, but instead a more dispersed effect of the gene on neuropsychological domains.

Many studies of IQ functioning in fra(X) females were reviewed. Of these, eight had sufficient sample sizes and detail about measures and methods to permit a summary. These eight studies are presented in table 5.2. Results on fra(X)-negative carriers are presented separately from results of samples that mainly or exclusively consist of fra(X)-positive females. The results across studies are surprisingly consistent and warrant several conclusions.

Overall IQ

At the level of overall IQ, fra(X)-negative obligate carriers seem to be unaffected because their mean IQ in three separate studies is consistently above the population mean ($\bar{x} = 102.3–106.0$) and not different from controls in the Wolff et al. (1988) study. Similarly, there was a normal mean full scale IQ (FSIQ) in the fra(X)-negative females in the family study reported by Veenema et al. (1987). These results argue against a negative ascertainment bias in the selection of these fra(X) families, at least for IQ; if such a bias were operating, we would expect lower mean IQs in these fra(X)-negative carriers. Fra(X) families who come to clinic because of an affected male do not seem to be a biased sample with respect to IQ. (Obviously, the male probands could still be a biased sample.)

In contrast to obligate carriers, fra(X)-positive females have mean IQs that consistently fall in the low average range ($\bar{x} = 81.0–87.9$). (The sole exception is the very low mean reported by Prouty et al. [1988]; however, the women who received IQ testing were only a subset of their total sample. The study was

Table 5.2

IQ Results in Fragile (X) Females[a]

Study	N	Age (yr)	Controls	Measures	FSIQ	VIQ	NVIQ
Fra(X)-negative carriers							
Brainard et al. 1991	38	adults	No	WAIS-R	106.0	106.0	107.5
Prouty et al. 1988	10	adults	No	WAIS-R	102.3	103.6	100.8
Wolff et al. 1988	9	adults	Relatives of DS males	WAIS-R	105.2	104.2	106.1
Fra(X)-positive carriers							
Brainard et al. 1991	21	adults	No	WAIS-R	85.6	84.9	87.6
Chudley et al. 1983	32[b]	10–88		Mixed	87.9	ND	ND
Freund and Reiss 1989	11	6–20	No	SB(1988)	84.0	VIQ = PIQ	
Cronister et al. 1991	43	daughters		Mixed	81.0	ND	ND
Loesch and Hay 1988	80–81	41.3 (11.0)		PPVT, Block Design	—	82.9	62.3
	19–20	11.0 (4.0)		same	—	83.6	69.5
Prouty et al. 1988	33	?	No	Mixed, mostly SB(1972)	54.5	ND	ND
Veenema et al. 1987	11	adults	Normal relatives	WAIS-R	86.8	VIQ = PIQ	

[a]*Abbreviations:* FSIQ, full-scale IQ; VIQ, verbal IQ; NVIQ, nonverbal IQ; ND, not done; SB, Stanford-Binet; PIQ, performance IQ; PPVT, Peabody Picture Vocabulary Test; WAIS-R, Wechsler Adult Intelligence Scale-Revised.
[b]included a few fra(X)-negative females.

based on clinical data, and one suspects that more severely affected women were more likely to receive IQ testing.) There is approximately a 20-point IQ difference between fra(X)-negative obligate carriers and fra(X)-positive females, indicating a large effect on IQ of what may turn out to be imprinting.

Specific Cognitive Profile

The data on Wechsler verbal versus performance IQ differences are much better than those available for fra(X) males, and the results are uniformly negative for both fra(X)-positive females and fra(X)-negative female carriers.

There is no evidence for a specific cognitive phenotype at the level of VIQ-PIQ differences.

At the level of specific IQ subtests, however, there is some evidence for specificity. Several investigators found particular problems on several Wechsler subtests, mainly in fra(X)-positive females. These subtests include block design, arithmetic, and digit span.

Miezejeski et al. (1986) reported Wechsler intelligence test results of seven fra(X) females, including children and adults. Unlike studies with larger samples, Miezejeski et al. (1986) described significantly lower performance than verbal IQs. They also found significantly lower scores on particular subtests of the Wechsler Scales, including arithmetic, digit span, block design, and object assembly. A lower score on the arithmetic subtest of the Wide Range Achievement Test was also noted. On the basis of these findings, Miezejeski concluded that fra(X) females demonstrate dyscalculia and a visual spatial deficit.

Kemper et al. (1986) explored Wechsler profiles of 22 fra(X) females, children and adults, with varying levels of fragility. A control group of 20 learning-disabled females was included to evaluate their subtest patterns. The fra(X) group demonstrated weaknesses on the arithmetic, digit span, and block design subtests that were not seen in the comparison groups. The full scale IQ of the fra(X) subjects was in the average range. Kemper et al. (1986) identified a correlation between percentage of fragility and both verbal and full scale IQ.

Loesch et al. (1987) examined physical characteristics, reproductive history, and cognitive profiles of 113 fra(X) females. There was considerable variability in percentage of fragility, and results were not examined with reference to these different levels, which is an interpretative problem. Eighty-five percent of a selected subsample had an IQ of <85 assessed by the Peabody Picture Vocabulary Test (PPVT) and one nonverbal subtest (block design) of a standardized IQ test. Most importantly, in adults the mean IQ score on the PPVT (82.9) was similar to that for full scale IQ in other studies of fra(X)-positive females, whereas the mean IQ score for block design was about 20 points lower (62.3). A similar discrepancy was found in fra(X) female children. It was concluded from this study that fra(X) females have more well-developed verbal than nonverbal abilities. Although this conclusion is too broad, given the lack of VIQ-PIQ differences, this study certainly supports the finding of a deficit on the block design subtest. Deficient performance on this subtest could be due to executive function rather than to visuospatial problems.

Brainard et al. (1991) studied the cognitive performance of 74 adult heterozygous females (38 of whom were negative carriers). All women completed the Wechsler Adult Intelligence Scale-Revised (WAIS-R), and full scale IQ was normally distributed. For the group as a whole, significant subtest weaknesses were found in arithmetic, block design, and digit span and significant subtest strengths were found on vocabulary, comprehension, and digit symbol. The group of fra(X)-positive women had a subtest pattern that was significantly different from that of the fra(X)-negative women. In the latter group, the pattern of subtest strengths and weaknesses was similar to that of the group as a whole, except for the lack of a significant weakness on arithmetic. In the fra(X)-positive group, the only significant weakness was on arithmetic, and the only significant strength was on digit symbol. When results were analyzed individually, however, no consistent patterns emerged. The group findings were supportive of the previously discussed studies in indicating weaknesses in arithmetic, digit span, and block design.

Grigsby et al. (1987) studied a subset of 20 of the fra(X)-positive women later studied by Brainard et al. (1991) for signs of Gerstmann syndrome. One control group consisted of fra(X)-negative relatives of the experimental group; the other consisted of a mixed group of head-injured and learning-disabled females. The fra(X)-positive group did significantly worse than both control groups on measures of spatial dyscalculia, dysgraphia, finger agnosia, right-left disorientation (the four symptoms of Gerstmann syndrome), and constructional dyspraxia but not on measures of visual agnosia or ideomotor apraxia or on a screening test for aphasic symptoms. They likewise did worse on the three Wechsler subtests found to be deficient in other studies—digit span, arithmetic, and block design. However, less than half of the fra(X)-positive sample had all of the signs of full Gerstmann syndrome, which does not support the consistency of this putative phenotype at the individual level. Moreover, the range of discriminant measures was limited, and all seem to have been subject to floor effects. Finally and most importantly, both control groups had considerably higher full scale IQs than had the fra(X) females (between 10 and 19 points higher), so we do not know if the Gerstmann deficits found in the fra(X)-positive group are an effect of lower overall neuropsychological functioning or a specific effect of fra(X).

Wolff et al. (1988) assessed cognitive, linguistic, and memory functions of 15 adult heterozygous women of normal intelligence. The control group consisted of 13 mothers and 1 sister of Down syndrome males. Wolff et al. (1988) examined both groups with Wechsler intelligence tests, academic achievement tests, neuropsychological measures of receptive and expressive language, short-term auditory memory tasks, and short-term visual memory tasks. Fra(X) heterozygotes all had average or above average intelligence, and there were no significant group differences in measured intelligence on verbal, performance, or full scale IQ. Likewise, no consistent subtest patterns in either the fra(X) group or the control group were observed. However, Wolff et al. (1988) did find deficits in the fra(X) group on language and short-term memory for verbal material. The short-term memory results are consistent with previous results indicating poor performance on another measure of verbal short-term memory (digit span). The heterozygotes did relatively poorly on the arithmetic subtests, although the control group demonstrated this deficit as well. Wolff et al. concluded that the relatively low scores on the standardized tests of arithmetic may not be specific to nonretarded heterozygotes, as postulated by Miezejeski et al. (1986), Chudley et al. (1987), and Kemper et al. (1986). Wolff et al. (1988) argued that their findings support the argument that fra(X) female carriers demonstrate some functional deficits similar to those displayed by dyslexics.

Because the findings of Wolff et al. (1988) are discrepant from those of other studies of fra(X) females, it is important to point out that their sample consisted almost entirely of fra(X)-negative carriers. There may be a qualitative difference between the phenotypes of fra(X)-positive and fra(X)-negative carrier females.

Freund and Reiss (1989) described the performance of nine fra(X) females on the Stanford-Binet 4th Edition. Their subject group was intellectually normal, with a mean IQ of 95. They discussed a particular pattern of performance suggestive of strengths in inductive reasoning and semantic memory function. They postulated that the females compensated for short-term memory weaknesses to some degree with their stronger verbal processing skills. Particular weaknesses were identified in short-term memory, quantitative skills, and visual motor tasks, similar to those identified in studies using the Wechsler Scale.

In summary, the mean full scale IQ for fra(X)-positive females falls in the low average range, about 20 IQ points below the mean full scale IQ for fra(X)-negative carrier females, whose overall IQ seems to be unaffected by fra(X). Neither group of fra(X) females demonstrates significant VIQ-PIQ discrepancies. In terms of individual Wechsler subtests, several studies of fra(X)-positive females have found specific weaknesses on arithmetic, digit span, and block design subscales, suggesting that there may be a specific neuropsychological phenotype in this fra(X) female group. Unfortunately there are no data on the three Wechsler factor scores, which provide a level of analysis intermediate between VIQ-PIQ differences and subtest profiles and which have proved informative in other syndromes, such as dyslexia and Turner syndrome. There are fewer studies of fra(X)-negative carriers, and the only consistent specific weakness that has been found is in verbal short-term memory, which was evident on different measures to both Wolff et al. (1988) and Brainard et al. (1991). Wolff et al. (1988) also reported other results suggesting that fra(X)-negative carriers have developmental dyslexia, which is different from the phenotype in fra(X)-positive samples.

Speech and Language

We were able to find only one study in this area, that of Madison et al. (1986). The speech articulation of the five affected women was clear and intelligible. No oral or speech apraxia was noted in the women, but they did have hypernasal voices and were 1 SD lower on timed polysyllabic repetition tasks. The pitch, loudness, rate, and fluency (with the exception of frequent revisions) of the women were within average limits.

In terms of language, the three lower-functioning women were said not to always be appropriate in speech content and all five women were said to use conditionalized phrases. Although Madison et al. used standardized measures, they did not include control groups so it cannot be determined if the subject sample is manifesting behavior that is consistent with or different from developmental level.

Clearly, more research is needed on speech and language functions in fra(X) females, especially research on pragmatic functions to determine if they exhibit a milder form of the pragmatic deficits found in fra(X) males.

Implications for Research

Based on what is currently known about the neuropsychological phenotype in fra(X), we think that it is most similar to previously described learning disorders—autistic spectrum disorder (ASD) and nonverbal learning disorder (or right hemisphere learning disability). Before discussing these analogies, it is necessary to clarify the relation between etiologic and phenotypic diagnoses. It is already known that the fra(X) mutation is one cause of autism, and it has been speculated that it is one cause of nonverbal learning disorder. Etiologic heterogeneity is established for autism and is likely in nonverbal learning disorder, as it is for most complex behavioral disorders. Despite etiologic heterogeneity, the neuropsychological phenotype may not be heterogeneous in these two learning disorders, so that the relation between etiologic and neuropsychological subtypes is not necessarily one to one. Obviously, research on the neuropsychological phenotype in etiologically homogeneous groups like fra(X) male and females will lead to greater precision in defining syndromal constructs like ASD and nonverbal learning disorders. As we said earlier, there is a dialectic relation between phenotype definition and existing neuropsychological constructs.

In ASD, there seems to be a primary deficit in one or more aspects of basic social cognition, including imitation, emotion perception, and intersubjectivity—or theory of other minds (Rogers and Pennington 1991). This primary deficit leads to secondary deficits in symbolic play and language, especially the pragmatic aspects of language. Mental retardation and abnormalities of attention and arousal regulation are correlated symptoms. An alternative account of ASD (Dawson and Leary 1989) holds that the attention/arousal regulation deficits are primary and that the social cognitive deficits are secondary. Regardless of which theory is correct, the important point here is that the symptom complex of ASD provides a possible analogy for the neuropsychological phenotype of fra(X), especially for fra(X) males.

However, it is important to point out the ways in which the ASD analogy does not fit. First of all, it is probably a better analogy for the phenotype in fra(X) males than in fra(X) females, in whom the rate of diagnosable autism is low. Moreover, there are indications that autism in diagnosable fra(X) males may be somewhat different than typical autism, in that gaze avoidance is more prominent in fra(X) while other markers of social relatedness are less impaired. Moreover, fra(X) females seem to be impaired on spatial constructional tasks but have preserved skills in verbal comprehension, whereas autistic samples exhibit an opposite profile. These opposite cognitive profiles are another weakness of the analogy, at least for the neuropsychological phenotype of fra(X) females.

The second possible analogy is nonverbal learning disorder, on which there is much less research than on autism. Nonverbal learning disorder is a better analogy for fra(X)-positive females than it is for fra(X) males. Nonverbal learning disorder is much rarer than a learning disability like dyslexia and has a crudely estimated prevalence of 0.1–0.05%. The symptom complex subsumed under this label is less clearly defined, as is the relation among symptoms, but it includes at a minimum depressed performance IQ, poor math and handwriting (but preserved reading), and poor visuomotor skills. All of these are similar to the pattern found in fra(X) females (and to a certain extent, fra(X) males), with the very important exception of depressed performance IQ, which is not found in fra(X) females.

Early researchers (e.g., Kinsbourne and Warrington 1963; Geschwind 1974) labeled this learning disorder *developmental Gerstmann syndrome* because of the similarity to acquired Gerstmann syndrome, in which the four defining symptoms are dyscalculia, dysgraphia, right-left disorientation, and finger dysgnosia. Acquired Gerstmann syndrome is associated with lesions to the parietal cortex in the left hemisphere. The validity of acquired Gerstmann syndrome, however, has been questioned by research that failed to show a stronger association among these four symptoms than between these symptoms and other left parietal signs (Benton 1977), and so the concept of Gerstmann syndrome may not be that useful.

Later researchers (Strang and Rourke 1983; Tranel et al. 1987; Weintraub and Mesulam 1983) preferred the term *right hemisphere learning disability* because the lateralizing data that have been collected on such patients are consistent with a right rather than a left hemisphere locus of dysfunction.

The cognitive results from these three studies are very similar. Performance IQ was depressed relative to verbal IQ; nonverbal memory was depressed relative to verbal memory; performance on visuoconstructive tasks was depressed relative to performance on auditory-linguistic tasks; and motor and tactile perceptual performance was worse on the left side of the body than on the right. The subjects in all three studies also had problems with math and handwriting but not reading.

The socioemotional results from these three studies are also similar. In the study of Weintraub and Mesulam (1983), problems with shyness, depression, and social isolation were reported by a substantial majority of these adult subjects. The majority of these patients also had deficits in eye contact, gestures, and prosody. In the study of Tranel et al. (1987), all of the patients reported significant problems with shyness, depression, and social isolation, and only 2 of 11 were normal on measures of eye contact, gestures, and prosody, with no 1 subject being normal in all three areas. The subjects in these two studies were predominantly adults, and one wonders if similar social deficits would be found in children with the same nonverbal learning disorder (LD). The studies by Rourke and colleagues help to answer this question. Strang and Rourke (1983) compared maternal report of psychopathology on the Personality Inventory for Children (PIC) for different LD groups, including a nonverbal LD group. This group was significantly elevated on the PIC psychosis scale and generally elevated on the other scales that load on an internalizing factor—depression, withdrawal, anxiety, and poor social skills. Qualitatively, the children in this group had tangential speech and problems with the understanding and use of gestures and other pragmatic cues. The social symptoms seen in nonverbal learning disorder are similar to those found in both fra(X) males and females (Crowe and Hay 1990; Hagerman and Sobesky 1989).

These two potential analogies of ASD and nonverbal LD make it clear that future neuropsychological studies of fra(X) should systematically test for deficits in social cognition as well as for right hemisphere cognitive deficits. These two analogies make some overlapping predictions (e.g., deficits in social cognition), but they also make some competing ones because spatial reasoning is preserved in ASD but impaired in right hemisphere LD. Another consideration in using these analogies is that either ASD or right hemisphere LD may include executive function deficits, which have not been systematically studied in either of these developmental learning disorders or in fra(X). An executive function hypothesis might provide a better comprehensive explanation of the strengths and weaknesses in fra(X) groups because (unlike the right hemisphere hypothesis) it does not predict depressed performance IQs and because it provides a better explanation for the attention deficits and perseverative behaviors that are prominent symptoms in fra(X) males. We are currently conducting research to test these competing neuropsychological hypotheses, and preliminary studies have demonstrated significant frontal lobe deficits in affected fra(X) females compared with control subjects (Mazzocco et al. 1990).

Before concluding, it is important to comment on other genetic syndromes whose phenotypes can be used to compare and contrast with fra(X). Among retardation syndromes, fra(X) researchers have begun to use Down syndrome and retarded autistic comparison populations. The neuropsychology of both of these groups is currently better understood than that of fra(X) males. The neuropsychological characteristics of DS may be attributable to a cholinergic defect that affects language and memory systems but that leaves spatial reasoning and social cognition relatively spared. In autism, there are no specific deficits in the phonologic or syntactic levels of language, but there are severe deficits in social cognition that impair the communicative use of language. Executive function deficits also seem likely in autism. Spatial reasoning, in contrast, is often a splinter skill in autism. A third, rarer MR syndrome, Williams syndrome, has begun to be defined neuropsychologically (Bellugi et al. 1990) and provides some interesting contrasts to fra(X), DS, and autism. Briefly, children with Williams syndrome have remarkably preserved phonologic and syntactic language, high social drive, and apparently preserved social cognition but markedly impaired spatial reasoning skills. At the semantic level their language is not tangential, perseverative, or otherwise pragmatically disordered, as is the language of both fra(X) males and autistics. By systematically studying all four of these different types of MR, we could gain a much clearer understanding of developmental associations and dissociations among neuropsychological systems and a better understanding of the neuropsychology of fra(X).

Among non-MR genetic syndromes, the most obvious comparisons are with X chromosome anomalies. None of these provide a clear fit to the emerging phenotype in fra(X)-positive females. Males with a 47,XXY karyotype have a developmental dysphasia characterized by depressed verbal IQs, phonologic and syntactic problems, and dyslexia. Females with a 47,XXX karyotype have similar language problems but more widespread cognitive problems as well. Finally, 45,X females (Turner syndrome) have depressed performance IQs, other visuospatial deficits, problems in math and attention, and some diffuse neuropsychological problems, but relatively preserved reading and language skills. Although they may have subtle problems in social cognition, these are not as prominent at a clinical level as those observed in fra(X) males or females. A clearer understanding of which X chromosome loci are most important in producing the neuropsychological phenotypes in these X chromosome anomalies would be useful in furthering our understanding of their relation to fra(X). For instance, does the fra(X) locus play any role in these disorders?

To summarize, future research on the neuropsychological phenotype in fra(X) should be guided by hypotheses to test a wider domain of neuropsychological functions and to make better use of the comparison groups provided by other MR and DD syndromes. Simultaneous studies of several syndromes will be much more powerful than piecemeal studies of each syndrome in isolation.

Acknowledgments

This work was supported by National Institute of Mental Health (NIMH) Grant MH 45916, by NIMH Research Scientist Development Award Grant 00419, by NIMH Project Grant 38820, by March of Dimes Grant 12-135, and by a grant from the Orton Dyslexia Society, all awarded to Bruce F. Pennington. Vicki Sudhalter's work was supported by NIMH Grant 38201 and by the New York State Office of Mental Retardation and Developmental Disabilities.

References

Bellugi, U., A. Bihrle, D. Traurer, T. Jernigan, and S. Doharty. 1990. Neuropsychological, neurological, and neuroanatomical profile of Williams syndrome children. *Am. J. Med. Genet.* In press.

Benton, A. L. 1977. Reflections on the Gerstmann syndrome. *Brain Lang.* 4:45–62.

Berkson, J. 1946. Limitations of the application of fourfold table analysis to hospital data. *Biometrics* 2:47–51.

Borghgraef, M., J. P. Fryns, A. Dielkens, K. Pyck, and H. Van den Berghe. 1987. Fragile (X) syndrome: A study of the psychological profile in 23 prepubertal patients. *Clin. Genet.* 32:179–186.

Borghgraef, M., J. P. Fryns, K. Dyck, and H. Van den Berghe. 1988. Fragile X syndrome: A study of the psychological profile of 40 pre and postpubertal patients. Presented to the 8th World Congress of the International Association for the Scientific Study of Mental Deficiency, Dublin.

Brainard, S. S., R. A. Schreiner, and R. J. Hagerman. 1991. Cognitive profiles of the adult carrier fra(X) female. *Am. J. Med. Genet.* 38:505–508.

Chudley, A. E., J. Knoll, J. W. Gerrard, L. Shepel, E. McGahey, and J. Anderson. 1983. Fragile (X) X-linked mental retardation. I: Relationship between age and intelligence and the frequency of expression of fragile (X) (q28). *Am. J. Med. Genet.* 14:699–712.

Chudley, A. E., R. de von Flindt, and R. J. Hagerman. 1987. Cognitive variability in the fragile X syndrome. *Am. J. Med. Genet.* 28(1):13–15.

Cohen, H. 1962. Psychological test findings in adolescents having ovarian dysgenesis. *Psychol. Med.* 24:249–256.

Cronister, A., R. Schreiner, M. Wittenberger, K. Amiri, K. Harris, and R. J. Hagerman. 1991. The heterozygous fragile X female: Historical, physical, cognitive and cytogenetic features. *Am. J. Med. Genet.* 38:269–274.

Crowe, S., and D. Hay. 1990. Neuropsychological dimensions of the fragile X syndrome: Support for a non-dominant hemisphere dysfunction hypothesis. *Neuropsychologia* 28:9–16.

Crystal, D. 1979. Prosodic development. In P. Fletcher and M. Garman (eds), *Language acquisition: Studies in first language development.* Cambridge: Cambridge University Press, pp. 33–48.

Dawson, G., and A. Lewy. 1989. Arousal, attention, and the socioemotional impairments of individuals with autism. In G. Dawson (ed.), *Autism*. New York: Guilford Press.

Dykens, E. M., R. M. Hodapp, and J. F. Leckman. 1987. Strengths and weaknesses in the intellectual functioning of males with fragile X syndrome. *Am. J. Med. Genet.* 28(1):13–15.

Dykens, E. M., J. F. Leckman, R. Paul, and M. Watson. 1988. Cognitive, behavioral, and adaptive functioning in fragile X and non-fragile X retarded men. *J. Autism Dev. Disord.* 18(1):41–52.

Dykens, E. M., R. Hodapp, S. Ort, B. Finucane, L. Shapiro, and J. Leckman. 1989. The trajectory of cognitive development in males with fragile X syndrome. *J. Am. Acad. Child Adolesc. Psychiatry* 28:422–426.

Freund, L., and A. L. Reiss. 1989. Cognitive profile comparisons of fragile X males and females. Presented at the Fourth International Workshop on Fragile X Syndrome and X-linked Mental Retardation, New York, July 4–7.

Froster-Iskenius, U., B. C. McGillivray, F. J. Dill, J. G. Hall, and D. S. Herbst. 1986. Normal male carriers in the fragile (X) form of X-linked mental retardation (Martin-Bell syndrome). *Am. J. Med. Genet.* 23(1–2): 619–631.

Fryns, J. P., J. Jacobs, A. Kleczkowska, and H. Van den Berghe. 1984. The psychological profile of the fragile X syndrome. *Clin. Genet.* 25(2):131–134.

Geschwind, N. 1974. The anatomical basis of hemispheric differentiation. In S. J. Dimond and J. G. Beaumont (eds.), *Hemispheric function in the human brain*. New York: Halsted Press.

Goldfine, P. E., P. M. McPherson, V. A. Hardesty, G. A. Heath, L. J. Beauregard, and A. A. Baker. 1987. Fragile-X chromosome associated with primary learning disability. *J. Am. Acad. Child Adolesc. Psychiatry* 26:589–592.

Grigsby, J., M. B. Kemper, and R. J. Hagerman. 1987. Developmental Gerstmann syndrome without aphasia in fragile X syndrome. *Neuropsychologia* 25(6):881–891.

Hagerman, R. J., and A. C. M. Smith. 1983. The heterozygous female. In R. J. Hagerman and P. M. McBogg (eds.), *The fragile X syndrome: Diagnosis, biochemistry and intervention*. Dillon, Colo.: Spectra Publishing, pp. 83–94.

Hagerman, R. J., and W. E. Sobesky. 1989. Psychopathology in fragile X syndrome. *Am. J. Orthopsychiatry* 59(1):142–152.

Hagerman, R. J., M. Kemper, and M. Hudson. 1985. Learning disabilities and attentional problems in boys with the fragile X syndrome. *Am. J. Dis. Child.* 139(7):674–678.

Hagerman, R. J., R. A. Schreiner, M. B. Kemper, M. D. Wittenberger, B. Zahn, K. Habicht. 1989. Longitudinal IQ changes in fragile X males. *Am. J. Med. Genet.* 33:513–518.

Hanson, D. M., A. W. Jackson III, and R. J. Hagerman. 1986. Speech disturbances (cluttering) in mildly impaired males with the Martin-Bell/fragile X syndrome. *Am. J. Med. Genet.* 7:471–489.

Herbst, D. S. 1980. Nonspecific X-linked mental retardation: I. A review with information from 24 families. *Am. J. Med. Genet.* 7:443–460.

Hodapp, R. M., E. M. Dykens, R. J. Hagerman, R. A. Schreiner, A. M. Lachiewicz, and J. F. Leckman. 1990. Developmental implications of changing trajectories of IQ in males with fragile X syndrome. *J. Am. Acad. Child Adolesc. Psychiatry* 29:214–219.

Howard-Peebles, P. N., G. R. Stoddard, and M. G. Mims. 1979. Familial X-linked mental retardation, verbal disability, and marker X chromosomes. *Am. J. Hum. Genet.* 31:214–222.

Jacobs, P. A., T. W. Glover, M. Mayer, P. Fox, J. W. Gerrard, H. G. Dunn, and D. S. Herbst. 1980. X-linked mental retardation: A study of seven families. *Am. J. Med. Genet.* 7:471–489.

Kemper, M. B., R. J. Hagerman, R. S. Ahmad, and R. Mariner. 1986. Cognitive profiles and the spectrum of clinical manifestations in heterozygous fragile (X) females. *Am. J. Med. Genet.* 23(1–2):139–156.

Kemper, M. B., R. J. Hagerman, and D. Altshul-Stark. 1988. Cognitive profiles of boys with the fragile X syndrome. *Am. J. Med. Genet.* 30(1–2):191–200.

Kinsbourne, M., and E. K. Warrington. 1963. A study of finger agnosia. *Brain* 85:57–66.

Kopf, C. R., and R. McCall. 1982. Predicting later mental performance for normal, at risk, and handicapped infants. In P. Baltes and O. Brim (eds.), *Lifespan development and behavior*. New York: Academic Press, pp. 33–61.

Lachiewicz, A. M., C. M. Guillion, G. A. Spiridigliozzi, and A. S. Aylsworth. 1987. Declining IQs of young males with the fragile X syndrome. *Am. J. Ment. Retard.* 92(3):272–278.

Laird, C. D. 1987. Proposed mechanism of inheritance and expression of the human fragile X syndrome of mental retardation. *Genetics* 117:587–599.

Loesch, D. Z., and D. A. Hay. 1988. Clinical features and reproductive patterns in fragile X female heterozygotes. *J. Med. Genet.* 25(6):407–414.

Loesch, D. Z., D. A. Hay, G. R. Sutherland, J. Halliday, C. Judge, and G. C. Webb. 1987. Phenotypic variation in male-transmitted fragile X: Genetic inferences. *Am. J. Med. Genet.* 27(2):401–417.

Madison, L. S., C. George, and J. B. Moeschler. 1986. Cognitive functioning in the fragile-X syndrome: A study of intellectual, memory and communication skills. *J. Ment. Defic. Res.* 30(pt 2):129–148.

McGlone, J. 1985. Can special deficits in Turner's syndrome be explained by focal CNS dysfunction or atypical speech lateralization? *J. Clin. Exp. Neuropsychol.* 7:375–394.

Mazzocco, M. M. M., B. F. Pennington, A. E. Cronister, and R. J. Hagerman. 1990. The neurocognitive phenotype of women with fragile X. Presented at the American Society of Medical Genetics, Cincinnati, Ohio, October.

Miezejeski, C. M., E. C. Jenkins, A. L. Hill, K. Wisniewski, J. H. French, and W. T. Brown. 1986. A profile of cognitive deficit in females from fragile X families. *Neuropsychologia* 24(3):405–409.

Money, J. 1973. Turner's syndrome and parietal lobe functions. *Cortex* 9:385–393.

Newell, K., B. Sanborn, and R. J. Hagerman. 1983. Speech and language dysfunction in the fragile X syndrome. In R. J. Hagerman and P. M. McBogg (eds.), *The fragile X syndrome: Diagnosis, biochemistry, and intervention*. Dillon, Colo.: Spectra Publishing, pp. 175–200.

Niemi, J., E. Vilkman, and U. Ikonen. 1985. Fragile X speech in Finnish: Phonological observations. In J. Niemi and P. Koiveselka-Sallinene (eds.), *Neurolinguistic papers: Proceedings of the 2nd Finnish Conference of Neurolinguistics.*

Partington, M. W. 1984. The fragile X syndrome: Preliminary data on growth and development in males. *Am. J. Med. Genet.* 17:175–194.

Paul, R. E., D. Cohen, R. Greg, M. Watson, and S. Herman. 1984. Fragile X syndrome: Its relation to speech and language disorders. *J. Speech Hear. Disord.* 49:328–332.

Paul, R. E., E. Dykens, J. F. Leckman, M. Watson, W. R. Breg, and D. J. Cohen. 1987. A comparison of language characteristics of mentally retarded adults with fragile X syndrome and those with nonspecific mental retardation and autism. *J. Autism Dev. Disord.* 17:457–468.

Pennington, B. F. 1991. *Diagnosing: A neuropsychological framework.* New York: Guilford Press.

Pennington, B. F., and S. D. Smith. 1988. Genetic influences on learning disabilities: An update. *J. Consult. Clin. Psychol.* 36:817–823.

Pennington, B. F., R. K. Heaton, P. Karzmark, M. G. Pendleton, R. Lehman, and D. W. Shucard. 1985. The neuropsychological phenotype in Turner syndrome. *Cortex* 21:391–404.

Prouty, L. A., R. C. Rogers, R. E. Stevenson, J. H. Dean, K. K. Palmer, R. J. Simensen, G. N. Coston, and C. E. Schwartz. 1988. Fragile X syndrome: Growth, development, and intellectual function. *Am. J. Med. Genet.* 30(1–2):123–142.

Rapin, I., and D. A. Allen. 1983. Developmental language disorders: Nosologic considerations. In U. Kirk (ed.), *Neuropsychology of language, reading and spelling.* New York: Academic Press.

Renier, W. O., D. F. C. Smeets, J. M. J. C. Scheres, T. W. J. Hustinx, C. F. C. Hulsman, C. P. M. O. Ophey, A. J. A. M. Bomers, and F. J. M. Gabreels. 1983. The Martin-Bell syndrome: A psychological logopaedic and cytogenetic study of two affected brothers. *J. Ment. Defic. Res.* 27:51–59.

Robinson, A., H. A. Lubs, and D. Bergson. 1979. *Sex chromosomes aneuploidy: Prospective studies on children.* New York: Alan R. Liss.

Rogers, S., and B. F. Pennington. 1991. A theoretical approach to the deficits in infantile autism. *Dev. Psychopath.* In press.

Shaffer, J. W. 1962. A specific cognitive deficit observed in gonadal aplasis (Turner's syndrome). *J. Clin. Psychol.* 18:403–406.

Sherman, S. L., N. E. Morton, P. A. Jacob, and G. Turner. 1984. The marker (X) syndrome: A cytogenetic and genetic analysis. *Ann. Hum. Genet.* 48:21–37.

Sherman, S. L., P. A. Jacobs, N. E. Morton, U. Froster-Iskenius, P. N. Howard-Peebles, K. B. Nielsen, M. W. Partington, G. R. Sutherland, G. Turner, and M. Watson. 1985. Further segregation analysis of the fragile X syndrome with special reference to transmitting males. *Hum. Genet.* 69:289–299.

Silverstein, A. B., G. Legutki, S. L. Friedman, and D. L. Takayama. 1982. Performance of Down syndrome individuals on the Stanford-Binet Intelligence Scale. *Am. J. Ment. Defic.* 86:548–551.

Strang, J. D., and B. P. Rourke. 1983. Arithmetic disability subtypes: The neuropsychological significance of specific arithmetic impairment in childhood. In B. P.

Rourke (ed.), *Neuropsychology of learning disabilities: Essentials of subtype analysis*. New York: Guilford Press.

Sudhalter, V., I. L. Cohen, W. P. Silverman, and E. G. Wolf-Schein. 1990. Conversational analyses of males with fragile X, Down syndrome and autism: A comparison of the emergence of deviant language. *Am. J. Ment. Retard.* 94:431–441.

Sudhalter, V., H. S. Scarborough, and I. C. Cohen. 1991. Syntactic delay and pragmatic deviance in the language of fragile X males. *Am. J. Med. Genet.* 38:493–497.

Sutherland, G. R., and F. Hecht. 1985. *Fragile sites on human chromosomes*. New York: Oxford University Press.

Theobald, T. M., D. A. Hay, and C. Judge. 1987. Individual variation and specific cognitive deficits in the fra(X) syndrome. *Am. J. Med. Genet.* 28(1):1–11.

Tranel, D., L. E. Hall, S. Olson, and N. N. Tranel. 1987. Evidence for a right-hemisphere developmental learning disability. *Dev. Neuropsychol.* 3:113–127.

Turner, G., A. Daniel, and M. Frost. 1980. X-linked mental retardation, macroorchidism and the Xq27 fragile site. *J. Pediatr.* 96:837–841.

Veenema, H., T. Veenema, and J. P. Geraedts. 1987. The fragile X syndrome in a large family: II. Psychological investigations. *J. Med. Genet.* 24(1):32–38.

Waber, D. P. 1979. Neuropsychological aspects of Turner syndrome. *Dev. Med. Child Neurol.* 21:58–70.

Weintraub, S., and M. Mesulam. 1983. Developmental learning disabilities of the right hemisphere. *Arch. Neurol.* 40:436–468.

Wolff, P. H., J. Gardner, J. Lappen, J. Paccia, and D. Meryash. 1988. Variable expression of the fragile X syndrome in heterozygous females of normal intelligence. *Am. J. Med. Genet.* 30(1–2):213–225.

Wolf-Schein, E. G., V. Sudhalter, I. L. Cohen, G. S. Fisch, D. Hanson, A. G. Pfadt, R. Hagerman, E. Jenkins, and W. T. Brown. 1987. Speech-language and the fragile X syndrome: Initial findings. *ASHA* 29(7):35–38.

CHAPTER 6

Other Disorders with X-Linked
Mental Retardation:
A Review of Thirty-three Syndromes

J. Fernando Arena, M.D., Ph.D.,
and Herbert A. Lubs, M.D.

In 1938, Penrose suggested that the higher frequency of mental retardation in males compared to females was due to social factors rather than X-linked genes. In the early 1940s, however, families with mental retardation and an X-linked pattern of inheritance were reported by Martin and Bell (1943) and Allan et al. (1944). No specific clinical findings within these families were reported in either paper. The few other publications before 1970, including the report by Renpenning et al. (1962), were generally referenced under the term "nonspecific X-linked mental retardation." In the late 1960s and early 1970s, Lehrke (1974) also promulgated the idea of the significance of X-linked genes in mental retardation. This concept was later reviewed and confirmed by Morton et al. (1977), Herbst and Miller (1980), and others who suggested that a total of 17 to 19 specific disorders accounted for this sex difference.

Progress in understanding X-linked mental retardation (XLMR) was delayed, not only by the apparent nonspecific clinical features and the absence of laboratory diagnoses for these entities but also because the X-linked inheritance was obscured by the frequent occurrence of mildly affected females in many families. The report by Lubs in 1969 of the marker X chromosome (now known as the fragile X) in a family with mental retardation in four males provided a laboratory basis for the diagnosis of one important type of XLMR. Giraud et al. (1976) and Harvey et al. (1977) reported additional cases, and Sutherland (1977) demonstrated the requirements for low folate and low thymidine in culture media for consistent detection of the fra(X) and indicated that the condition had a high incidence. These reports allowed the subsequent separation of XLMR families into several groups based on a combination of labora-

202

tory and clinical findings. The pace of reports of additional XLMR syndromes also accelerated significantly after 1969.

Most studies have shown that only 30–40% of unselected families with "nonspecific" X-linked mental retardation have the fra(X). Of the 345 X-linked disorders listed in the McKusick catalogue, *Mendelian Inheritance in Man,* approximately 80 involve mental retardation in at least some affected family members or as a variable manifestation. The majority of these disorders have a clear clinical picture, have a known metabolic basis, or have been localized to a specific chromosome band. Although several of the better-known disorders, such as the Coffin-Lowry syndrome, are included in this review because they were originally found in the "nonspecific" XLMR category, the general basis for inclusion is that the disorders are still emerging from this category (i.e., their clinical manifestations are still being defined and there is no diagnostic laboratory test). Linkage studies will play a critical role in syndrome delineation in many of these disorders.

The present review excludes the fra(X) syndrome, because the clinical features are well described elsewhere and addresses 33 other syndromes: in 11, two or more cases have been reported, but in 22 syndromes only a single family has been reported. About half (Neri et al. 1991) have tentative gene localizations. In addition, other families that have no obvious clinical problem except mental retardation have been reported (Neri et al. 1991). In still others, the findings vary widely and no "syndrome" has yet emerged. These families will not be discussed except in reference to the gene localization studies.

Unfortunately, no contemporary study is available in which all cases of XLMR in a region or country have been adequately studied, so it is difficult to estimate the proportion of the XLMR families with each of these disorders or those that are truly nonspecific. Even if current population data were available, it is likely that cases, particularly in males, would only have been identified as X-linked in large families and that many cases would remain undetected. A battery of direct DNA tests is needed before a definitive answer to these questions can be obtained. The frequency of female carriers with either minor clinical manifestations or impaired intelligence also remains to be investigated in most instances.

The Present Compilation of Syndromes and Database

Description of the Database and Terminology

Literature reports of these various syndromes were acquired through standard literature searches and stored in a computer system especially designed to

Table 6.1

Facial and Other Clinical Features of 33 X-linked Mental Retardation Syndromes

BD or OMIM Number[a]	Syndrome	Distinctive Features	Other Features
Coarse facies (4)			
2640	Coarse facies & normal stature (Clark and Baraitser [1987])	Normal stature Hypotelorism Broad nose & coarse facies Large testes	Large head (males) & square forehead
2840	Coarse facies & short stature (Atkin et al. [1985])	Short stature Hypertelorism Broad nose and coarse facies Large testes (? familial)	Large, square forehead; may have large head (? familial) & ears
2826 312870 **	Coarse facies and overgrowth (Simpson et al. [1975]; Golabi et al. [1984]; Behmel et al. [1984, 1988])	Striking coarse facies Macrostomia Pre- + postnatal growth Coccygeal skin tags Midline notching lower lip	Submucous cleft Bone anomalies Cystic kidney Hepatosplenomegaly Early death in some
0190 303600 **	Coarse facies Muscle weakness Progressive skeletal & growth abnormalities (Coffin and Lowry; Hunter et al. [1982]; Partington et al. [1988a])	Downslanting palpebral fissures Mild hypertelorism Prominent brow Broad nose	Thick, soft skin Large hands with tapering fingers
Distinct facies (18)			
——	Distinctive facies Short stature Small head (2–20 %ile) Brachydactyly (Carpenter et al. [1988])	Moderate MR Expressive language delay Broadening of distal phalanges	Bushy eyebrows Depressed nasal bridge & widening tip of nose Widely spaced teeth
——	Distinctive facies	Small head	Bitemporal narrowing

(continued)

204

Table 6.1 (*Continued*)

BD or OMIM Number[a]	Syndrome	Distinctive Features	Other Features
	Short stature Obesity Gynecomastia Hypogonadism (Vasquez et al. [1979])	Structural abnor- malities of hands Skeletal defects	Almond-shaped pal- pebral fissures
3147 309490	Facial dysmorphia Short stature Obesity Hypogonadism (Chudley et al. [1988])	Moderate to severe MR Mild obesity—infancy onset Distinct facial features Short neck	Bitemporal narrowing Almond-shaped pal- pebral fissures Flat nasal bridge Inverted V-shaped up- per lip Short upper lip
3250 **	Xq duplication Short stature Somatomedin C deficiency (Thode et al. [1988])	Growth deficiency Short stature (<3%ile) Delayed bone age Peculiar face	Small palpebral fissure Bilateral ptosis Tented upper lip Full lower lip Down-turned corners of the mouth
2340 308830	Keratosis follicularis Dwarfism Cerebral atrophy (Cantú et al. [1974])	Delayed somatic growth Microcephaly Seizures	Absence of hair and eyelashes Micrognatia Delayed dentition
2272 301900	Dwarfism Epilepsy Endocrine disorders (Börjeson et al. [1962])	Short stature (<3%ile) Narrow palpebral fissures Large ears, hypo- gonadism Seizures	Obesity and swelling of subcutaneous face Hypometabolism Short, upturned nose
2480 309590 **	Growth, hearing, & genital defects (Juberg and Marsidi [1980])	Small stature & de- layed bone age Mild–severe deafness Small scrotum & penis Cryptorchidism	Severe mental retar- dation Small palpebral fis- sures Flat nasal bridge Poor survival

(*continued*)

Table 6.1 (*Continued*)

BD or OMIM Number[a]	Syndrome	Distinctive Features	Other Features
——	Distinctive facies Microcephaly Postnatal growth retardation Skeletal dysplasia (Miles and Carpenter [1991])	Severe MR Long palms & hands Hyperextensible joints Syndactyly Proximately placed thumbs Thoracic scoliosis Hallux valgus	Facial asymmetry Midface hypoplasia Exotropia Obtuse mandibular angle High, narrow palate Distal muscle wasting
0754 305450 **	FG syndrome (Opitz et al. [1982])	Hypotonia Slow motor development Short stature Abnormal skull/relative macrocephaly High, prominent forehead Frontal cowlick Micrognathia	Hypertelorism/telecanthus Abnormal (mostly antimongoloid) palpebral slant Long philtrum High, arched palate Abnormal dermatoglyphics Striking personality
2830 312840 **	Choreoathetosis (Schimke et al. [1984])	Choreoathetosis in first year; often constant; later spasticity, ophthalmoplegia & deafness Postnatal growth retardation & microcephaly	Normal appearance at birth; later sunken eyes & pinched lower nose
3199	Craniofacial anomalies & postnatal growth deficiency (Golabi-Ito-Hall) (Golabi et al. [1984])	Postnatal growth deficiency Microcephaly Narrow, triangular face Anteverted ears	Epicanthal folds ASD Brittle, dry hair

(*continued*)

Table 6.1 *(Continued)*

BD or OMIM Number[a]	Syndrome	Distinctive Features	Other Features
		Upslanted palpebral fissures Laterally displaced inner canthi	
2921 309520 **	Marfanoid habitus (Lujan et al. [1984])	Tall (>90%ile), thin Connective tissue abnormalities with pectus & long, thin hands; long, narrow face with thin, high nasal bridge, small chin Large testes (≥90%ile)	Agenesis corpus callosum in some
2904 309620	Skeletal dysplasia & abducens palsy (Christian et al. [1977])	Ridging of metopic suture Fused & hemivertebrae Scoliosis & sacral hypoplasia Short midphalanges Abducens palsy	Antimongoloid slant & epicanthic folds Broad nasal bridge
3248 309610	Subcortical atrophy Facial dysmorphia Clinodactyly (Prieto et al. [1987])	Ear malformations High nasal bridge Patella luxation Febrile convulsion Abnormalities of fundus of eye	Abnormal teeth Skin dimple of back Limb malformation
3200	Craniofacial abnormalities Microcephaly & clubfoot (Holmes and Gang [1984])	Peculiar facies (coarse) Large anterior fontanel Clubfoot deformity Early death	Epicanthic folds Flat nasal bridge Anteverted nostrils Abnormal teeth Hypotonia

(continued)

207

Table 6.1 *(Continued)*

BD or OMIM Number[a]	Syndrome	Distinctive Features	Other Features
——	Distinctive facies Early hypotonia (Pettigrew et al. [1991])	Severe MR Spasticity, contractures & seizures	Long narrow face with coarse features
3252 309480	MR, seizures Psoriasis (Tranebjaerg I) (Tranebjaerg et al. [1988])	Normal growth Ataxic gait	Apparent hypertelorism Large ears Macrostomia Long philtrum
2845 309580 **	Microcephaly Short stature Unusual facial appearance (Smith-Fineman-Myers) (Smith et al. [1980])	Micrognathia Narrow face Patulous lower lip	Minor foot deformities Hyperreflexia Seizures
Normal facies (11)			
2920 309500 **	Small head Short stature Small testes (Renpenning syndrome)	Head, stature, testes in 2–25%ile	All features are highly variable & may fall in normal range in some family members
—— 309470	Microcephaly Short stature Small testes Spastic diplegia (4/5) (Sutherland et al. [1988])	Lean body build Brachycephaly Unusual appearance (3/5) Moderate retardation	Prominent ears Limited joint extension
—— **	Dyspraxia Psychosis Clubfoot (Tranebjaerg II)	Macroorchidism	Seizures
2479	MR & seizures	Probably X-linked	

(continued)

Table 6.1 *(Continued)*

BD or OMIM Number[a]	Syndrome	Distinctive Features	Other Features
121250	(Juberg and Hellman [1971])	dominant inheritance; expression limited to females Seizures with onset at 6–18 mo Half also retarded	
2841 31151	Basal ganglia disorder (Laxova et al. [1985])	Persistent frontal lobe reflexes, cogwheel rigidity, abnormal gait, & parkinsonian tremor Frontal bossing & large head	Strabismus Seizures
3253 314580	Muscle atrophy Congenital contractures Oculomotor apraxia (Wieacker-Wolff) (Wieacker et al. [1985])	Weakness of upper and lower limbs Distal muscle atrophy Dyspraxia of the eye, face and tongue muscles Swallowing difficulties	Overlap of toes Manifestations apparently more restricted to nervous system
3247 309560	Spastic paraplegia Palmoplantar hyperkeratosis (Fitzsimmons et al. [1983])	Pes cavus deformity Abnormal gait	Peculiar face (may be familial)
3251 309510	MR Dystonic spasms of hands Dysarthria (Partington et al. [1988b])	Normal growth	No special facial features
2291 303350	Clasped thumb (Gareis and Mason	Bilateral absence of extensor pollicis	Usually normal appearance; may

(continued)

Table 6.1 (*Continued*)

BD or OMIM Number[a]	Syndrome	Distinctive Features	Other Features
**	[1984])	brevis tendons with thumb flexion deformity	have growth retardation, lordosis & microcephaly
——— 309640	Normal facies (?) Dysarthria Spastic quadriparesis Muscle wasting (mild) Clubfoot (equinovarus) (Davis et al. [1981])	Spastic gait Pseudobulbar signs Ankle clonus & active deep tendon reflex	Characteristic body habitus & posture Scoliosis
3249 30960	Limber neck (Allan-Herndon-Dudley) (Allan et al. [1944])	Severe MR Hypotonia Joint contractures Delayed, clumsy walking Awkward, wide-based gait	Hyporeflexia Marked speech defect No special facial features described

[a]*Abbreviations:* BD, *Birth Defects Encyclopedia* (Buyse [1990]).
**Two or more families reported.

function as a databank on XLMR syndromes. This has been reported in detail (Arena and Lubs 1991). This information is summarized in table 6.1 and constitutes much of the raw material of the present review. Where only one or two families have been reported, the literature presented is complete. In the few instances in which many families have been reported, the original reports and only the more useful later summary reports were included. Those syndromes that include two or more reported families in the literature are indicated by an asterisk and are discussed in more detail in the next section. The brief descriptions in table 6.1 refer to the descriptive numbers in the *Birth Defects Encyclopedia* and McKusick's *Mendelian Inheritance in Man* and include a summary of the most distinctive and other important features. Since most syndromes have not yet evolved a characteristic name, we give a brief description of the several most significant features and the first author of the original or most representative paper. In a few cases, such as the Simpson-Golabi-Behmel or

Coffin-Lowry syndrome, several authors' names that have come to be closely associated with the syndrome have been used in the tables and text.

Comments on Classification

The syndrome reported by Juberg and Hellman (1971) with seizures and mental retardation in affected females is classified as autosomal dominant in the McKusick catalogue, but the pattern of inheritance may be equally well explained by an X-linked gene with manifestations only in females. It is, therefore, tentatively included in the present list of XLMR disorders.

Very likely, certain of the apparently similar XLMR disorders will be delineated as entities by combined clinical, linkage, and localization studies and others will prove to be overlapping descriptions of a syndrome described under several names by different authors. For example, the syndromes described by Atkin et al. (1985) and by Clark and Baraitser (1987) are listed as separate entities, although the facial features are quite similar. The distinguishing features are the presence of hypertelorism and short stature in the Atkin family compared to possible hypotelorism (as shown by the original illustrations) and normal stature in the Clark-Baraitser family. These and other pairs of syndromes with many similarities are summarized in table 6.2.

Differential Diagnosis of XLMR Syndromes

Since certain clinical features, such as coarse facies, short stature, and small or large testes, occurred in a number of syndromes, a series of flow diagrams was developed within the Macintosh II system. These are illustrated in figures 6.2 to 6.9 and were designed both to highlight common features in various syndromes and to provide an organized approach to the diagnosis of families that may be ascertained with a diagnosis that is not initially clear.

In table 6.1, for example, we grouped disorders according to three classes of facial appearance: coarse facies, distinct facies, or normal facies. Using these data, we developed a flow chart showing syndromes with coarse facies (fig. 6.1). In addition to these four syndromes with an overall appearance of coarse facies, however, several other syndromes have specific coarse features. For example, FG syndrome and families reported by Thode et al. (1988), Smith et al. (1980), Tranebjaerg et al. (1988), and Holmes and Gang (1984) have thick lower lips but do not have other features of coarse facies. Distinct facies were noted in 18 syndromes and, in more than one-half of the cases (11 of 18), short stature was also present (fig. 6.2). Normal facies were noted in 11 syndromes (fig. 6.3). The large number of syndromes with only neuromuscular findings and normal facies is of interest. These 11 syndromes are probably due to

Table 6.2

Three Pairs of Syndromes with Similarities

BD or OMIM Number[a]	Syndrome	Distinctive Features	Other Features
2920 309500	Small head Short stature Small testes (Renpenning et al. [1962])	Head, stature, testes in 2–25%ile	All features are highly variable & may fall in normal range in some family members
309470	Microcephaly Short stature Small testes Spastic diplegia (4/5) (Sutherland et al. [1988])	Lean body build Brachycephaly Unusual appearance (3/5) Moderate retardation	Prominent ears Limited joint extension
2840	Coarse facies & short stature (Atkin et al. [1985])	Short stature Hypertelorism Broad nose and coarse facies Large testes (? familial)	Large, square forehead; may have large head (? familial) & ears
2640	Coarse facies & normal stature (Clark and Baraitser [1987])	Normal stature Hypotelorism Broad nose & coarse facies Large testes	Large head (males) & square forehead
3147 309490	Facial dysmorphia Short stature Obesity Hypogonadism (Chudley et al. [1988])	Moderate to severe mental retardation Mild obesity—infancy onset Distinct facial features Short neck	Bitemporal narrowing Almond-shaped palpebral fissures Flat nasal bridge Inverted V-shaped upper lip Short upper lip
——	Distinctive facies Short stature Obesity Gynecomastia Hypogonadism (Vasquez et al. [1979])	Mental retardation & developmental delay Small head Structural abnormality of hands Skeletal defects	Bitemporal narrowing Almond-shaped palpebral fissures

[a]*Abbreviations:* BD, *Birth Defects Encyclopedia* (Buyse [1990]).

212

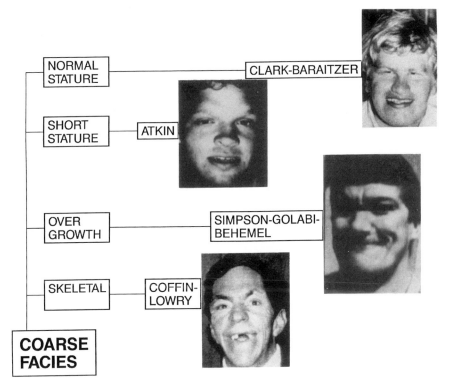

Figure 6.1 Syndromes with coarse facies. Note the hypotelorism in Clark-Baraitser syndrome and the hypertelorism in Atkin-Flaitz syndrome. Ears are large in only these two syndromes.

specific single gene mutations. Others remain candidates for small duplications or deletions.

Flow diagrams based on other frequently observed abnormalities, such as large testes and short stature, are shown in figures 6.4 through 6.6. Large testes have been reported in XLMR syndromes other than fra(X) (fig. 6.4). Extreme enlargement (over 60 ml) is less common in these syndromes than in fra(X) families. The upper limit of normal testicular size is still not adequately documented by age, race, or measurement technique; therefore, the definition of syndromes with only slight testicular enlargement remains difficult. There is, for example, significant variation in size in both affected and normal family members in the Atkin syndrome (i.e., both normals and affecteds have testes larger and smaller than 30 ml). This casts some doubt on the inclusion of this syndrome in this category.

Eight syndromes include both small testes and short stature (fig. 6.5) and

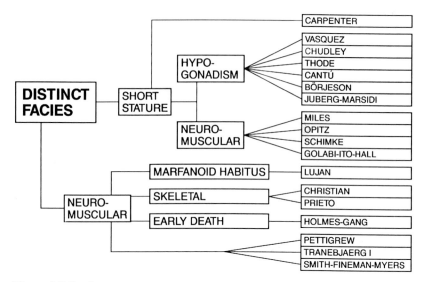

Figure 6.2 Syndromes with distinct facies (Other features are described in table 6.1)

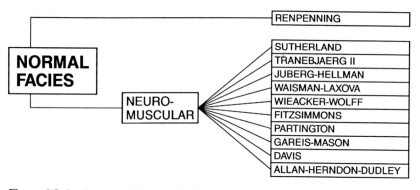

Figure 6.3 Syndromes with normal facies (Other features are described in table 6.1)

warrant specific comments. In addition, the families reported by Sutherland et al. (1988) and by Thode et al. (1988) have similar localizations (Xq13-21). The similarities between Renpenning syndrome and the family reported by Sutherland et al. (1988) are noted in table 6.2. No localization data are available for the remaining syndromes. The possibility that genes affecting both stature and testicular development might be present in this region deserves investigation. Decreased somatomedin was reported in one family by Thode et al (1988), but the gene for somatomedin has been localized to 12q22-q24.1 and the relationship of somatomedin to the syndrome is not clear. Short stature was present in a

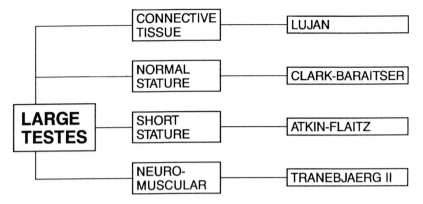

Figure 6.4 Syndromes with large testes

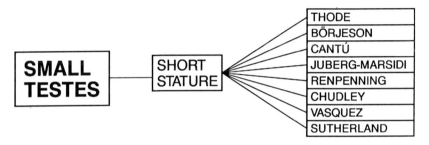

Figure 6.5 Syndromes with small testes

total of 14 syndromes (fig. 6.6). Twelve of 14 syndromes with short stature also had distinct facies, and 6 of 12 with distinct facies and short stature also had hypogonadism.

Twenty-four of the 33 syndromes had neurologic manifestations. These are shown in figure 6.7. Significant neuromuscular findings occur in 5 of 14 syndromes with short stature. Only a few reports include brain imaging studies. The neuromuscular abnormalities vary widely in their level of description; these should be better and more precisely documented in future studies, and the involvement of a neurologist is desirable.

Many other combinations of these differential diagnosis charts have been developed for syndromes with common features. These charts may also be useful in planning additional genetic studies. For example, the four syndromes shown in figure 6.8 all have short stature, neuromuscular involvement, hypogonadism, and a different but distinct facies. The syndrome reported by Thode et al. (1988) was due to a small duplication that mimicked X-linked recessive

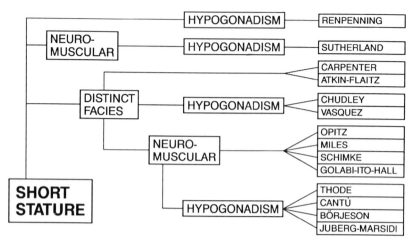

Figure 6.6 Syndromes with short stature

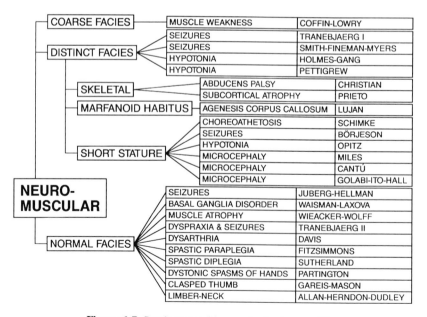

Figure 6.7 Syndromes with neurologic abnormalities

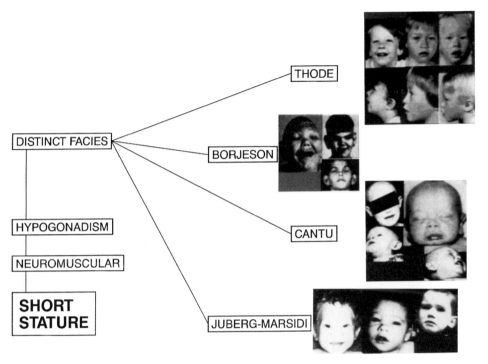

Figure 6.8 Syndromes with short stature, neuromuscular abnormalities, hypogonadism, and a distinct facies. Small palpebral fissures; a short, usually upturned nose; and a full lower lip occur in all. Large ears were also present, except in Thode syndrome.

inheritance; therefore, high resolution chromosome studies in families with similar features should be carried out. Ultimately, DNA studies should also be carried out in these syndromes to rule out duplications and possible deletions as gene localization studies progress.

In present practice, most families with XLMR who do not have the fra(X) remain without a specific diagnosis. As a result, specific prenatal counseling and diagnosis are generally not available to these families.

Comments on Specific Syndromes in Which Two or More Cases Have Been Reported

General Comments

Synthesis of data from reports that are disparate in time, quality, and ethnic origin is difficult. In some cases, the clinical features are clearly defined and adequately summarized in table 6.1. In others, the definition of the syndrome or, indeed, the validity of lumping family reports into a syndrome is in doubt and considerable additional study is required.

In a few cases, the history of the syndromes has included several redefinitions of names; comments are included to help clarify these otherwise confusing descriptions. The statement that linkage studies will be extremely useful in resolving these questions is applicable in all cases. These studies, however, may not resolve all problems until the gene is precisely characterized and a direct test is available because small families may provide incomplete linkage information. Better clinical reports, including both adequate photographs and measurements, as well as editorial requirements for reporting both positive and negative results for pertinent features of each family member, will be of equal importance in the further delineation of these syndromes.

Specific Syndromes

Simpson-Golabi-Behmel (SGB) Syndrome

The seven initial or follow-up reports (Simpson et al. 1975; Behmel et al. 1984; Golabi and Rosen 1984; Opitz 1984; Neri et al. 1988; Behmel et al. 1988; Opitz et al. 1988a) illustrate most of the problems listed above. This syndrome in the past was also referred to as Golabi-Rosen syndrome. The consistent and common feature in these families is pre- and postnatal overgrowth as manifested by large size, coarse features, broad hands, and early death in about one-half of reported cases. Intelligence, however, varies widely and was either normal or borderline in the majority of cases. In one family (Opitz 1984), however, the intellectual impairment was severe. Other distinctive features, such as midline notching of the lower lip, were only irregularly present. The genetics are of particular interest in that some presumed female heterozygotes had decreased intelligence, and the syndrome was described as an incompletely recessive X-linked disorder. In addition to the relatively distinctive or common features shown in table 6.1, a great variety of other abnormalities were reported, including hypertelorism; cleft uvula and cleft lip; a high, arched palate; branchial arch anomalies including preauricular tags; helacine fistulas; deep voice; enlarged tongue; large maxilla and jaw; short, broad neck; vertebral segmentation defects such as posterior fusion of C-2 and C-3; scoliosis; pectus excavatum; partial atrioventricular block; intestinal malrotation; Meckel diverticulum; extra nipples; postaxial hexadactyly; tibial clinodactyly of the second toe; hypoplasia or absence of nails; sudden infant death; seizures; deafness; and possible cortical blindness. Metabolic abnormalities have not been found. In isolated cases, Beckwith-Wiedemann and Soto syndromes must be included in the differential diagnosis.

Coffin-Lowry Syndrome

This disorder is perhaps the best-characterized syndrome reviewed here. The main features are shown in table 6.1, and a typical appearance is given in figure 6.2. The characteristic fat, tapering fingers; happy temperament; down-slanting eyes; and coarse facies make the syndrome relatively easy to diagnose correctly.

The genetics are of particular interest in that there is a high proportion of manifesting heterozygotes and that the mode of inheritance might best be characterized as X-linked dominant with incomplete penetrance. The recent report by Partington et al. (1988a) provided the first evidence of localization to Xp22.2–Xp22.1 with DXS43. The lod score was 2.71 with theta equal to 0.00. Hanauer et al. (1988) also reported linkage studies to DXS43 and S41 with a lod score of 3.4. Thus, the localization has been confirmed in a second family by an independent group of investigators. Cloning and sequencing of the gene, however, remain to be carried out before definitive diagnosis and a full understanding of the disorder can be accomplished.

No biochemical abnormality has been found, and the mechanism by which the high frequency of manifesting heterozygotes occurs also remains to be investigated. Intellectual deterioration does not occur. Recent references include those of Hunter et al. (1982) and Hanauer et al. (1988).

Thode Syndrome

Thode et al. (1988) reported an important new syndrome with duplication of Xq13.1–Xq21.1 in three affected males: each had a characteristic and similar facial appearance, including small palpebral fissures, bilateral epicanthic folds, ptosis, tented upper lip, and down-turned corners of the mouth (fig. 6.8). Based on this report, it was possible to predict the presence of the duplication in another family with a similar appearance [see addendum to report by Thode et al. (1988) by Leonard (1987) and to find previous reports, such as those by Vejerslev et al. (1985), with similar clinical findings and similar duplications]. The molecular biology of this disorder is of great significance because the duplication, which has been well documented in biochemical and molecular terms using phosphoglycerate kinase (PGK) and a complementary DNA probe localized to this region, mimics X-linked inheritance. In carrier females the abnormal X was late replicating and their phenotype was normal. The significance of the low somatomedin C levels found in each of the three patients reported by Thode et al. (1988) is unclear, particularly because somatomedin C has been localized to 12q22–24.1. In these families the duplication behaves like an X-linked recessive trait.

Juberg-Marsidi Syndrome

The families reported by Juberg and Marsidi (1980) and by Mattei et al. (1983) present a uniform picture of clinical findings. These are outlined in table 6.1. The absence of subsequent reports, in view of an apparently clearly defined syndrome, is puzzling.

FG Syndrome

Opitz et al. (1988b) provided a review of the genetic and clinical findings in this complex syndrome. Roughly 46 patients have been reported. It also was described as an incompletely recessive X-linked syndrome with variable expressivity. The appearance is characterized by a high, prominent forehead; a frontal cowlick; hypertelorism; antimongoloid slant; long filtrum; and micrognathia. Severe manifestations involved the anus (60%), other gastrointestinal defects (33%), hypospadias (25%), and cleft palate (6%). Central nervous system manifestations included hypotonia, seizures, and agenesis of the corpus callosum in about one-quarter of the patients. The behavioral phenotype was summarized by Opitz et al. (1988b) as follows: "FG syndrome boys tend to be busy and willful lads with much mischievousness, impulsiveness and great affability, who were very demanding of attention, occasionally aggressive, excessively hyperactive, impatient, gregarious, and competitive." At least three manifesting heterozygotes have been described. No positive linkage studies have yet been reported.

Schimke Syndrome

The report by Schimke et al. (1984) included three boys in one family and an isolated case. In addition to choreoathetosis, manifestations included microcephaly and a poor course with death by a relatively early age in two of four cases (at 4 years and 14 years). Central nervous system manifestations were severe and included external ophthalmoplegia and deafness.

Marfanoid Habitus

Two families with X-linked mental retardation and the marfanoid habitus are known. The first was reported by Lujan et al. (1984) and the second (four males in two families) by Fryns and Buttiens (1987). In both reports, the syndrome included a long, narrow facies together with a marfanoid habitus; long, slender fingers; and pectus excavatum. Testicular size was borderline or large in the family reported by Lujan but was normal and very small in the report by Fryns and Buttiens. IQ ranged from 49 to 65. Hyperactivity was noted in four of eight patients.

Smith-Fineman-Myers Syndrome

The two reports in the literature of this syndrome included two affected brothers (Smith et al. 1980) and a third unrelated male (Stephenson and Johnson 1985). Features not listed in table 6.1 include small size for gestational age, lightly pigmented skin with freckles, chest deformity, prominent maxilla, prominent upper central incisors, flat philtral pillars, decreased nasolabial folds, decreased frontonasal angle, hyperopia, dolichocephaly, and hypotonia.

Renpenning Syndrome

Nine members of the family reported by Renpenning et al. in 1962 with nonspecific XLMR were restudied by Fox et al. in 1980. This family proved not to have the fra(X) chromosome but did show a moderately consistent pattern of findings, including low mean measurements (usually less than 20%) for height, weight, head circumference, and testicular volume. This combination of findings is used in this paper to define Renpenning syndrome. Several other families that may have Renpenning syndrome have been reported but were not reported with this definition in mind and, hence, had insufficient clinical detail to allow a retrospective diagnosis. One family is known to our program (J. E. Lujan and H. Lubs, Clinical Variation in Renpenning Syndrome, personal communication), and two of the families reported by Archidiacono et al. (1987) also seem to have Renpenning syndrome. It is, therefore, very likely a common syndrome. Sutherland et al. (1988) reported a family with these and other findings, with possible localization to Xq13–21.1, which may represent a family with Renpenning syndrome, but the presence of additional clinical abnormalities precludes a firm decision. Linkage studies in families classified as having Renpenning syndrome will resolve the issue. (Most of the reports in the older literature referring to Renpenning syndrome used this term only in the sense of nonspecific mental retardation and are not classifiable by the present definition.)

Tranebjaerg II Syndrome

In the Fourth Conference on Fragile X and XLMR, Tranebjaerg (1991) reported a second syndrome with X-linked mental retardation in two families. As shown in table 6.1, manifestations included dyspraxia, psychosis, clubfoot, macroorchidism, and seizures.

Clasped Thumb Syndrome (Gareis-Mason Syndrome)

Two Mexican-American and two Anglo-American families with 41 affected males have been reported (Bianchine and Lewis 1974; Gareis and Mason 1984). Thumb contractures were present in all 13 reported individuals; these were symmetric and included a hyperplastic thenar eminence. Mild short stature, lordosis or kyphosis, and pes planus were less frequently present. There was lower extremity spasticity in 5 and a shuffling gait in 2. Microcephaly was present in 4 of 13. Intelligence ranged from severely delayed to normal.

Recent Gene Localizations

Few linkage studies were reported until 1988. In the series of papers reported at the Third Conference on Fragile X and XLMR in 1988, only one study reported a lod score greater than 3 (the usual acceptance for a significant linkage), but a number of suggestive linkages were reported. These and more recent tentative localizations are summarized in table 6.3. There may be clustering of these loci in the mid-short arm and Xc-Xq2 regions, but minimal data and lack of precise localization of the probes preclude any firm decisions. Samanns et al. (1988), however, provided a combined maximal lod score of 4.37 with no recombi-

Table 6.3

Current Gene Localization Data for XLMR Syndromes

Band Localization	Probe/ Technique	Lod Score/ Recombination Fraction	Reference
Xpter –Xp21	DXS41	2.11 ($\theta = 0$)	Partington et al. (1988b)
Xp22.3–Xp22.2	DXS85	2.62 ($\theta = 0.06$)	Arveiler et al. (1988)/(Proops et al. 1983)[a]
Xp22.2–Xp22.1	DXS43	2.71 ($\theta = 0.00$)	*Partington et al. (1988a)/ (Procopis and Turner 1972)[a]
Xp22.2–Xp22.1	DXS41, DXS43	3.41(multipoint)	*Hanauer et al. (1988)
Xp21.1–Xq21.3	DXS159	4.37 ($\theta = 0$)[b]	Samanns et al. (1988)
Xp11.3–Xq21.1	DXS14	2.12 ($\theta = 0$)	Suthers et al. (1988)/(Turner et al. 1971)[a]
Xp11.3–Xp21.1		1.15 ($\theta = 0$)	Prieto et al. (1987)
Xp11 –Xq22	DXS162/[c]	1.63 ($\theta = 0$)	Carpenter et al. (1988)
Xq12 –Xq13	DXS159	2.53 ($\theta = 0$)	Arveiler et al. (1988)
Xq13.1–Xq21.1	Cytogenetic	—	Thode et al. (1988)
Xq13 –Xq21.1	DXYS1	2.10 ($\theta = 0.01$)	Sutherland et al. (1988)
Xq13 –Xq21	DXYS1	3.22 ($\theta = 0$)	Wieacker et al. (1987)
Xq21.31	DXYS1	2.78 ($\theta = 0$)	Miles and Carpenter (1991)
Xq26.3–Xq27.1	F9	1.63 ($\theta = 0.09$)	Glass et al. (1988)
Xq27 –Xqter	DXS52	3.27 ($\theta = 0$)	Dlouhy et al. (1987)

*Coffin-Lowry syndrome.
[a]Previous clinical reports
[b]Compiled lod score with families reported by Arveiler et al. (1988) and Suthers et al. (1988).
[c]And DXSY1/DXS101.

nants with DXS159 (Xp21.1-Xq21.3). This included the data reported by Arveiler et al. (1988) and Suthers et al. (1988). It is, therefore, possible that a gene leading to one form of nonspecific XLMR is in this region. Nearly all of these studies were carried out on a single large family, and these suggestive lod scores (roughly equal to 2) were generally obtained by restudying large families that had been known to investigators either in Europe or Australia/New Zealand as a result of long-term programs in XLMR. The Coffin-Lowry localization (Partington et al. 1988a), in contrast, was confirmed by a second report (Hanauer et al. 1988). Many more families must be available for study in genetics centers throughout the world. Collaborative efforts among these centers and the several programs carrying on linkage studies in these disorders are critical to further progress.

References

Allan, W., C. N. Herndon, and F. C. Dudley. 1944. Some examples of the inheritance of mental deficiency: Apparently sex-linked idiocy and microcephaly. *Am. J. Ment. Defic.* 48:325–334.

Archidiacono, N., M. Rocchi, A. Rinaldi, and G. Filippi. 1987. X-linked mental retardation. II. Renpenning syndrome and other types (report of 14 families). *J. Genet. Hum.* 35:381–398. (Note: only 2 of these families appear to have Renpenning syndrome.)

Arena, J. F., and H. A. Lubs. 1991. Computerized approach to X-linked mental retardation syndromes. *Am. J. Med. Genet.* 38:190–199.

Arveiler, B., Y. Alembik, A. Hanauer, P. Jacobs, L. Tranebjaerg, M. Mikkelsen, H. Puissant, L. Larget Piet, and J. L. Mandel. 1988. Linkage analysis suggests at least two loci for X-linked non-specific mental retardation. *Am. J. Med. Genet.* 30:473–483.

Atkin, J. F., K. Flaitz, S. Patil, and W. Smith. 1985. A new X-linked mental retardation syndrome. *Am. J. Med. Genet.* 21:697–705.

Behmel, A., E. Plochl, and W. Rosenkranz. 1984. A new X-linked dysplasia gigantism syndrome: Identical with the Simpson dysplasia syndrome? *Hum. Genet.* 67:409–413.

―――. 1988. A new X-linked dysplasia gigantism syndrome: Follow up in the first family and report on a second Austrian family. *Am. J. Med. Genet.* 30:275–285.

Bianchine, J. W., and R. G. Lewis. 1974. The MASA syndrome: A new heritable mental retardation syndrome. *Clin. Genet.* 5:298–306.

Börjeson, M., H. Forssman, and O. Lehmann. 1962. An X-linked, recessively inherited syndrome characterized by grave mental deficiency, epilepsy, and endocrine disorder. *Acta Med. Scand.* 171:13–21.

Buyse, M. L. (ed.). 1990. *Birth Defects Encyclopedia.* Cambridge, Mass.: Blackwell Scientific Publications.

Cantú, J. M., A. Hernandez, J. Larracilla, A. Trejo, and E. Macotela-Ruiz. 1974. A new X-linked recessive disorder with dwarfism, cerebral atrophy, and generalized keratosis follicularis. *J. Pediatr.* 84:564–567.

Carpenter, N. J., M. Waziri, J. Liston, and S. R. Patil. 1988. Studies on X-linked mental retardation: Evidence for a gene in the region Xq11-q22. *Am. J. Med. Genet. (Suppl.)* 43:A139.

Christian, J. C., W. DeMyer, E. A. Franken, J. S. Huff, S. Khairi, and T. Reed. 1977. X-linked skeletal dysplasia with mental retardation. *Clin. Genet.* 11:128–136.

Chudley, A. E., R. B. Lowry, and D. I. Hoar. 1988. Mental retardation, distinct facial changes, short stature, obesity, and hypogonadism: A new X-linked mental retardation syndrome. *Am. J. Med. Genet.* 31:741–751.

Clark, R. D., and M. Baraitser. 1987. Letter to the editor: A new X-linked mental retardation syndrome. *Am. J. Med. Genet.* 26:13–15.

Davis, J. G., G. Silverberg, M. K. Williams, A. Spiro, and L. R. Shapiro. 1981. A new X-linked recessive mental retardation syndrome with progressive spastic quadriparesis. *Am. J. Hum. Genet.* 33:75A.

Dlouhy, S. R., J. C. Christian, J. L. Haines, P. M. Conneally, and M. E. Hodes. 1987. Localization of the gene for a syndrome of X-linked skeletal dysplasia and mental retardation to Xq27-qter. *Hum. Genet.* 75:136–139.

Dunn, H. G., H. Renpenning, J. W. Gerrard, J. R. Miller, T. Tabata, and S. Federoff. 1963. Mental retardation as a sex-linked defect. *Am. J. Ment. Defic.* 67:827–848.

Fitzsimmons, J. S., E. M. Fitzsimmons, J. I. McLachlan, and G. B. Gilbert. 1983. Four brothers with mental retardation, spastic paraplegia and palmoplantar hyperkeratosis. A new syndrome? *Clin. Genet.* 23:329–335.

Fox, P., D. Fox, and J. W. Gerrard. 1980. X-linked mental retardation: Renpenning revisited. *Am. J. Med. Genet.* 7:491–495.

Fryns, J. P., and M. Buttiens. 1987. X-linked mental retardation with marfanoid habitus. *Am. J. Med. Genet.* 28:267–274.

Gareis, F. J., and J. D. Mason. 1984. X-linked mental retardation associated with bilateral clasp thumb anomaly. *Am. J. Med. Genet.* 17:333–338.

Giraud, F., S. Ayme, J. F. Mattei, and M. G. Mattei. 1976. Constitutional chromosome breakage. *Hum. Genet.* 34:125–136.

Glass, I. A., L. A. Pirrit, F. Cockburn, and J. M. Connor. 1988. Linkage analysis in a large family with non-specific X-linked mental retardation. *Clin. Genet.* 34:397.

Golabi, M., and L. Rosen. 1984. A new X-linked mental retardation-overgrowth syndrome. *Am. J. Med. Genet.* 17:345–358.

Golabi M., M. Ito, and B. D. Hall. 1984. A new X-linked multiple congenital anomalies/mental retardation syndrome. *Am. J. Med. Genet.* 17:367–374.

Hanauer, A., Y. Alembik, S. Gilgenkrantz, P. Mujica, A. Nivelon Chevallier, M. E. Pembrey, I. D. Young, and J. L. Mandel. 1988. Probable localisation of the Coffin-Lowry locus in Xp22.2-p.22.1 by multipoint linkage analysis. *Am. J. Med. Genet.* 30:523–530.

Harvey, J., C. Judge, and S. Wiener. 1977. Familial X-linked mental retardation with an X chromosome abnormality. *J. Med. Genet.* 14:46–50.

Herbst, D. S., and J. R. Miller. 1980. Nonspecific X-linked mental retardation. II. The frequency in British Columbia. *Am. J. Med. Genet.* 7:461–469.

Holmes, L. B., and D. L. Gang. 1984. Brief clinical report: An X-linked mental retardation syndrome with craniofacial abnormalities, microcephaly and club foot. *Am. J. Med. Genet.* 17:375–382.

Hunter, A. G. W., M. W. Partington, and J. A. Evans. 1982. The Coffin-Lowry syndrome: Experience from four centres. *Clin. Genet.* 21:321–335.

Juberg, R. C., and C. D. Hellman. 1971. A new familial form of convulsive disorder and mental retardation limited to females. *J. Pediatr.* 79:726–732.

Juberg, R. C., and I. Marsidi. 1980. A new form of X-linked mental retardation with growth retardation, deafness and microgenitalism. *Am. J. Hum. Genet.* 32:714–722.

Laxova, R., E. E. S. Brown, K. Hogan, K. Hecox, and J. M. Opitz. 1985. An X-linked recessive basal ganglia disorder with mental retardation. *Am. J. Med. Genet.* 21:681–689.

Lehrke, R. G. 1974. X-linked mental retardation and verbal disability. *Birth Defects* 10:1–100.

Leonard, C. 1987. Unknown cases. Presented at the 6th Annual David Smith Workshop on Malformations and Morphogenesis, Greenville, South Carolina, August 15–19.

Lubs, H. A. 1969. A marker-X chromosome. *Am. J. Hum. Genet.* 21:231–244.

Lujan, J. E., M. E. Carlin, and H. A. Lubs. 1984. A form of X-linked mental retardation with marfanoid habitus. *Am. J. Med. Genet.* 17:311–322.

Martin, J. P., and J. Bell. 1943. A pedigree of mental defect showing sex-linkage. *J. Neurol. Psychiatry* 6:154–157.

Mattei, J. F., P. Collignon, S. Ayme, and F. Giraud. 1983. X-linked mental retardation, growth retardation, deafness and microgenitalism. A second familial report. *Clin. Genet.* 23:70–74.

McKusick, V. A. 1988. *Mendelian inheritance in man.* Baltimore: Johns Hopkins University Press.

Miles, J. H., and N. J. Carpenter. 1991. Unique X-linked mental retardation syndrome with fingertip arches and contractures mapped to Xq21.31. *Am. J. Med. Genet.* 38:215–223.

Morton, N., D. Rao, H. Lang-Brown, C. Maclean, R. Bart, and R. Lew. 1977. Colchester revisited: A genetic study of mental defect. *J. Med. Genet.* 14:1–9.

Neri, G., R. Marini, M. Cappa, P. Borrelli, and J. M. Opitz. 1988. Simpson-Golabi-Behmel syndrome: An X-linked encephalo-trophoschisis syndrome. *Am. J. Med. Genet.* 30:287–299.

Neri, G., F. Gurrieri, A. Gal, and H. A. Lubs. 1991. XLMR Genes: Update 1990. *Am. J. Med. Genet.* 38:186–189.

Opitz, J. M. 1984. The Golabi-Rosen syndrome—report of a second family. *Am. J. Med. Genet.* 17:359–366.

Opitz, J. M., K. G. Kaveggia, W. N. Adkins, Jr., E. F. Gilbert, C. Viseskul, J. C. Pettersen, and B. Blumberg. 1982. Studies of malformation syndromes of humans: XXXIIIC. The FG syndrome—further studies on three affected individuals from the FG family. *Am. J. Med. Genet.* 12:147–154.

Opitz, J. M., J. Herrmann, E. F. Gilbert, and R. Matalon. 1988a. Simpson-Golabi-Behmel syndrome. *Am. J. Med. Genet.* 30:301–308.

Opitz, J. M., A. Richieri-da Costa, J. M. Aase, and P. J. Benke. 1988b. FG syndrome update 1988: Note of 5 new patients and bibliography. *Am. J. Med. Genet.* 30:309–328.

Partington, M. W., J. C. Mulley, G. R. Sutherland, A. Thode, and G. Turner. 1988a. A family with the Coffin-Lowry syndrome revisited: Localization of *CLS* to Xp21-pter. *Am. J. Med. Genet.* 30:509–521.

Partington, M. W., J. C. Mulley, G. R. Sutherland, A. Hockey, A. Thode, and G. Turner. 1988b. X-linked mental retardation with dystonic movements of the hands. *Am. J. Med. Genet.* 30:251–262.

Penrose, L. S. 1938. A clinical and genetic study of 1,280 cases of mental defect. *Ment. Res. Council Spec. Rep. Ser.* 229.

Pettigrew, A. L., L. G. Jackson, and D. H. Ledbetter. 1991. New X-linked mental retardation disorder with Dandy Walker malformation, basal ganglia disease & seizure. *Am. J. Med. Genet.* 38:200–207.

Prieto, F., L. Badia, F. Mulas, A. Monfort, and F. Mora. 1987. X-linked dysmorphic syndrome with mental retardation. *Clin. Genet.* 32:326–334.

Procopis, P. G., and B. Turner. 1972. Mental retardation, abnormal fingers and skeletal anomalies: Coffin's syndrome. *Am. J. Dis. Child.* 124:258–261.

Proops, R., M. Mayer, and P. A. Jacobs. 1983. A study of mental retardation in children in the island of Hawaii. *Clin. Genet.* 23:81–96.

Renpenning, H., J. W. Gerrard, W. A. Zaleski, and T. Tabata. 1962. Familial sex-linked mental retardation. *Can. Med. Assoc. J.* 87:954–956.

Richards, B. W., P. E. Sylvester, and C. Brooker. 1981. Fragile X-linked mental retardation: The Martin-Bell syndrome. *J. Ment. Defic. Res.* 25:253–256.

Samanns, C., R. Albrecht, M. Neugebauer, N. Fraser, I. Craig, and A. Gal. 1988. Gene of X-linked non-specific mental retardation is closely linked to DXS159. *Am. J. Hum. Genet. (Suppl.)* 43:A157.

Schimke, R. N., A. H. Williams, D. L. Collins, and L. Therou. 1984. A new X-linked syndrome comprising progressive basal ganglion dysfunction, mental and growth retardation, external ophthalmoplegia, postnatal microcephaly and deafness. *Am. J. Med. Genet.* 17:323–332.

Simpson, J. L., S. Landey, M. New, and J. German. 1975. A previously unrecognized X-linked syndrome of dysmorphia. *Birth Defects* 11:18–24.

Smith, R. D., R. M. Fineman, and G. G. Myers. 1980. Short stature, psychomotor retardation, and unusual facial appearance in two brothers. *Am. J. Med. Genet.* 7:5–9.

Stephenson, L. D., and J. P. Johnson. 1985. Smith-Fineman-Myers syndrome: Report of a third case. *Am. J. Med. Genet.* 22:301–304.

Stevenson, R. E., H. O. Goodman, C. E. Schwartz, R. J. Simensen, W. T. McLean, Jr., and C. N. Herndon. 1990. Allan-Herndon syndrome. I. Clinical studies. *Am. J. Hum. Genet.* 47:446–453.

Sutherland, G. R. 1977. Fragile sites on human chromosomes: Demonstration of their dependence on the type of tissue culture medium. *Science* 197:265–266.

Sutherland, G. R., A. K. Gedeon, E. A. Haan, P. Woodroffe, and J. C. Mulley. 1988. Linkage studies with the gene for an X-linked syndrome of mental retardation, microcephaly and spastic diplegia (*MRX2*). *Am. J. Med. Genet.* 30:493–508.

Suthers, G. K., G. Turner, and J. C. Mulley. 1988. A non-syndromal form of X-linked mental retardation (XLMR) is linked to *DXS14*. *Am. J. Med. Genet.* 30:485–491.

Thode, A., M. W. Partington, M. Y. Yip, C. Chapman, V. F. Richardson, and G.

Turner. 1988. A new syndrome with mental retardation, short stature and an Xq duplication. *Am. J. Med. Genet.* 30:239–250.

Tranebjaerg, L., and P. Kurc. 1991. Prevalence of fra(X) and other specific diagnoses in autistic individuals in a Danish county. *Am. J. Med. Genet.* 38:212–214.

Tranebjaerg, L. A., A. Svegjaard, and G. Lykkesfeldt. 1988. X-linked mental retardation associated with psoriasis: A new syndrome? *Am. J. Med. Genet.* 30:263–273.

Turner, G., B. Turner, and E. Collins. 1971. X-linked mental retardation without physical abnormality: Renpenning's syndrome. *Dev. Med. Child Neurol.* 13:71–78.

Turner, G., J. M. Opitz, W. T. Brown, K. E. Davies, P. A. Jacobs, E. C. Jenkins, M. Mikkelsen, M. W. Partington, and G. R. Sutherland. 1986. Conference report: Second International Workshop on the Fragile X and on X-linked Mental Retardation. *Am. J. Med. Genet.* 23:11–67.

Vasquez, S. B., D. L. Hurst, and J. F. Sotos. 1979. X-linked hypogonadism, gynecomastia, mental retardation, short stature, and obesity: A new syndrome. *J. Pediatr.* 94:56–60.

Vejerslev, L. O., M. Rix, and B. Jespersen. 1985. Inherited tandem duplication dup(X)(q131-q212) in a male proband. *Clin. Genet.* 27:276–281.

Wieacker, P., G. Wolff, T. F. Wienker, and M. Sauer. 1985. A new X-linked syndrome with muscle atrophy, congenital contractures, and oculomotor apraxia. *Am. J. Med. Genet.* 20:597–606.

Wieacker, P., G. Wolff, and T. F. Wienker. 1987. Close linkage of the Wieacker-Wolff syndrome to the DNA segment DXYS1 in proximal Xq. *Am. J. Med. Genet.* 28:245–253.

CHAPTER 7

Modeling the Inheritance and Expression of Fragile X Syndrome, with Emphasis on the X-Inactivation Imprinting Model

Charles D. Laird, Ph.D., Mary M. Lamb, Ph.D.,
John Sved, Ph.D., and Jeffrey Thorne, Ph.C.

The fragile X syndrome has very complex patterns of inheritance and expression. These patterns are so unusual that the syndrome and its underlying mutation have been characterized as an "enigma" (Sutherland 1985) and as "unique" (Nussbaum and Ledbetter 1986). The purpose of this chapter is to summarize genetic peculiarities associated with the fra(X) syndrome, to provide a brief guide to the different models that have been offered to explain the fra(X) syndrome, and to describe recent progress in developing and testing the model proposed by Laird (1987).

Peculiarities of Inheritance and Expression

Extensive analysis of pedigree data (Sherman et al. 1985) has uncovered a remarkable number of peculiarities in the inheritance and expression of the fra(X) syndrome. These are summarized in the following questions.

Why Is the Fragile Site at Xq27.3 Correlated with a Major Human Disorder?

The locus for the fra(X) syndrome maps at or near Xq27.3, as determined most precisely by analysis of DNA polymorphisms relative to known genetic loci in this band (Brown et al. 1989). In fra(X) families, the phenotype of mental retardation in males almost always cosegregates with the cytogenetic marker, the fragile site at Xq27.3, as was originally proposed by Lubs (1969). It therefore seems that the same mutation that leads to this fragile site also leads to a major syndrome that includes mental retardation. Why is this fragile site correlated with a major syndrome while other fragile sites seem not to be (Sutherland and Hecht 1985)?

Why Are There Nonpenetrant Males Who Are Carriers of the Fra(X) Mutation (fig. 7.1, Individual I-2)?

Nonpenetrant, or asymptomatic, carrier males (also called transmitting males) frequently transmit the fra(X) mutation to their progeny. In contrast, affected fra(X) carrier males seldom reproduce. (We use the term carrier to refer to any male or female who is hemizygous, heterozygous, or homozygous for the fra(X) mutation, regardless of whether the individual is classified as affected or normal.) Estimates of the fraction of carrier males who are nonpenetrant range from 0.2 (Sherman et al. 1985) to about 0.5 (Sved and Laird 1990), with the latter being a prediction from population genetic calculations, to be discussed below.

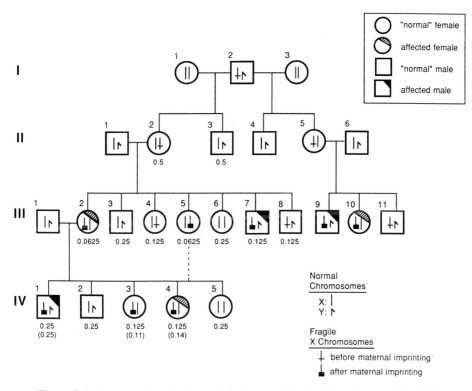

Figure 7.1 A proposed mechanism of inheritance of the fra(X) syndrome. [Reprinted with permission from Laird (1987), copyright Genetics Society of America]

Why should there be *any* carrier males who are nonpenetrant? This is, after all, an X-linked mutation that shows virtually complete penetrance in males of some families, namely those in which the mother is affected. Other X-linked diseases are not reported to have such a large class of nonpenetrant males.

Why Are Carrier Daughters of Nonpenetrant Males Classified as Mentally Normal, Whereas Carrier Granddaughters of Such Males Frequently Are Classified as Mentally Retarded?

The observation that daughters of nonpenetrant males are classified as mentally normal led to suggestions that the fra(X) mutation must first be passed through a female before its effects are manifested (Sherman et al. 1985; Pembrey et al. 1985). The various models account for this important finding in different ways.

What Accounts for the Peculiarities Termed *Clustering* (Sherman et al. 1985) and the *Sherman Paradox* (Opitz 1986) That Have Been Uncovered in Segregation Analysis?

The former term refers to the observation that there are clusters of nonpenetrant carrier males in some families; the latter term refers to markedly different penetrances of mental retardation among carrier brothers of transmitting males (penetrance = 0.18) compared with carrier brothers of affected grandsons of transmitting males (penetrance = 0.74; fig. 7.2). With standard genetic models, there is no basis for markedly different penetrances in these different pedigree situations.

Why Are Only One-Half of Carrier Daughters of Affected Females Classified as Mentally Affected?

In contrast to the observed 50% penetrance of mental retardation in carrier daughters of affected females, virtually all carrier sons of affected females are classified as mentally retarded.

Why Does the Expression of the Syndrome Vary between Affected Individuals?

There is considerable variability in the spectrum of abnormal physical phenotypes of individuals classified as mentally affected (Loehr et al. 1986). Could there be a novel source of phenotypic variation in the fra(X) syndrome?

Why Has It Been so Difficult to Identify Individuals Who Represent New Mutations?

New mutations should be plentiful at equilibrium. They should balance the loss of mutant alleles from affected males, who usually do not reproduce. Most models predict that about a third of fra(X) carriers should represent new muta-

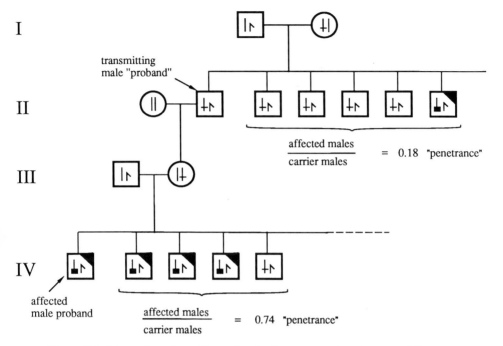

Figure 7.2 Schematic pedigree illustrating the Sherman paradox. Apparent differences in the penetrance of the fra(X) syndrome among carrier brothers of a transmitting male, compared with the penetrance among carrier brothers of an affected grandson of a transmitting male, are illustrated (see fig. 7.1 for definitions of symbols). These apparent differences in penetrance are interpreted here as reflecting differences in the average frequency of imprinting among mothers who have at least one transmitting (nonimprinted) son, compared with mothers who have at least one affected (imprinted) son. This schematic pedigree summarizes data from Sherman et al. (1985), based on many smaller families; noncarrier sibs and carrier sisters of carrier males are not represented here.

tions, following Haldane's result (Haldane 1935; Sherman et al. 1985; Winter 1987; Sved and Laird 1990). Individuals representing new mutations are not, however, readily identified (Sherman et al. 1985).

Why Does the Cytogenetic Manifestation of the Fra(X) Syndrome Essentially Disappear in Daughters of Affected Males?

Laird (1991) identified, from the fra(X) literature, seven daughters of affected fra(X) males. In all of these daughters, the high level of cytogenetic expression associated with the deleterious form of the mutation has disappeared. This change in the level of cytogenetic expression is almost never observed when the fra(X) chromosome is transmitted through affected females.

An Overview of Different Models of the Fra(X) Syndrome

Many different models have been proposed to explain some or all of the genetic peculiarities summarized above. We divide models explaining the fra(X) syndrome into those that do and those that do not involve a second genetic change.

Models That Involve a Second Genetic Change

The important unifying feature of this class of models is that a second genetic event in females is postulated to change further the DNA sequence at or near the fra(X) site. Within the context of these models, the fra(X) mutation is sometimes called a *premutation* (Sherman et al. 1985; Pembrey et al. 1985). In a female carrying such a putative premutation, a second genetic change leads to a *full mutation* at the fra(X) site. The models in this class differ in the details of this postulated second change. For example, some authors propose that a genetic crossing-over event is necessary to convert the initial benign mutation into a deleterious one (Pembrey et al. 1985; Siniscalco 1986; Ledbetter et al. 1986). Warren (1988) proposed that breakage of the fra(X) chromosome occurs in somatic cells, leading to mosaic nullisomy for genes distal to the fra(X) site. Other models in this class involve transposable elements that genetically modify the fra(X) mutation (Friedman and Howard-Peebles 1986; Hoegerman and Rary 1986).

Models That Do Not Require a Second Genetic Change

Models in this class accommodate peculiarities of fra(X) inheritance and expression by the postulated occurrence of a conditional event that is necessary for the mutation to have deleterious effects. One proposed conditional event is the co-occurrence, with the fra(X) mutation, of a particular genotype at an autosomal locus that modifies the expression of the fra(X) mutation (Steinbach 1986; Israel 1987). Another proposal is that the fra(X) mutation has a strong maternal-effect component (Van Dyke and Weiss 1986). In this case, the conditional event would be oogenesis.

The X-inactivation imprinting model (Laird 1987), which is the primary subject of this chapter, may also be included in this category of models that do not require a second genetic change. The conditional event that occurs in females and is necessary for the deleterious effects of the fra(X) mutation to be expressed is inactivation of the mutant X chromosome. The mutation then exerts its effect by blocking reactivation of this mutant X chromosome before female meiosis.

Some of the models described above were discussed and evaluated by Nussbaum and Ledbetter (1986) and by Brown (1989, 1990). In this chapter, we consider in detail the X-inactivation imprinting model of Laird (1987). To our knowledge this is the only model that has been developed comprehensively to consider the cytogenetic, developmental, and population genetic implications of the fra(X) syndrome. This model successfully accommodates the peculiarities of inheritance and expression described above, and makes novel molecular and genetic predictions.

The X-Inactivation Imprinting Model

Background

As a possible solution to these genetic and cytogenetic peculiarities, Laird (1987) proposed that the fra(X) syndrome results from abnormal chromosome imprinting. The term *chromosome imprinting* refers to a stable, nongenetic alteration to a chromosome that affects a chromosome's function at some future developmental stage or generation. The term was introduced by Crouse (1960) to describe unusual chromosome behavior in the dipteran *Sciara* and was extended to mammalian chromosomes by Chandra and Brown (1975). Examples of normal chromosome imprinting in the mouse were described by McGrath and Solter (1984) and Cattanach and Kirk (1985); experiments with transgenic mice also identified chromosome regions that may be subject to chromosome or gene imprinting (Sapienza et al. 1987; Reik et al. 1987; Swain et al. 1987).

For the fra(X) syndrome, Laird proposed that the imprint was established by failure of a fra(X) chromosome to be reactivated completely, before meiosis in females, after it had been inactivated for dosage compensation. The fra(X) mutation causes the block to reactivation (fig. 7.3). According to this model, the gene or genes that fall within the putative domain of imprinting are functionally inactivated; their inactivity is the cause of the phenotypic manifestations of the fra(X) syndrome. The mutant fra(X) allele can thus exist in two states, nonimprinted and imprinted.

What kind of mutation would block reactivation of an inactive X chromosome? Laird et al. (1987) proposed that a fragile site represents a *cis*-acting mutation that delays replication of DNA at that site. (*Cis*-acting refers to a mutation that acts only on the homolog with the mutant allele and not on the homolog with the normal allele.) There are many possible mutational—and epimutational—mechanisms that could lead to delayed DNA replication. This proposal is independent of the X-inactivation imprinting model (i.e., the acceptance or rejection of each model is independent of the acceptance or rejection of the other). If both models are correct, however, together they lead to the prediction that the mechanism of X-chromosome reactivation is tightly coupled to the timing of DNA replication (fig. 5 of Laird et al. 1987).

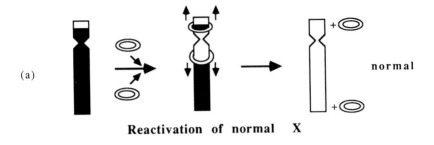

(a)

Reactivation of normal X

normal

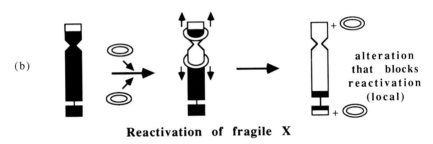

(b)

alteration
that blocks
reactivation
(local)

Reactivation of fragile X

Figure 7.3 The reactivation of an inactivated normal X chromosome (*a*) and an inactivated fra(X) chromosome (*b*) before oogenesis: proposed local block to reactivation of the fra(X). [After Laird (1987), modified to show that the distal tip of the short arm of the X chromosome escapes inactivation]

If more than one gene is functionally inactivated by the failure to reactivate completely an inactive fra(X) chromosome, then the fra(X) syndrome can be viewed as a contiguous gene syndrome of considerable novelty. Unlike other described contiguous gene syndromes (Schmickel 1986), genes affected in the fra(X) syndrome are postulated to be functionally inactivated rather than deleted or in extra copies. In addition, the boundary between the region of persistent inactivation and the region of normal activity on the fra(X) chromosome is expected to be variable. Such variability is seen in "position-effect variegation" in *Drosophila* (Spofford 1976) and in the mouse (Cattanach and Perez 1970). A central feature of this variability is that it leads to mosaicism within an individual for cells that express and cells that do not express the gene or genes subject to the inactivation. Differences in the extent of chromosomal inactivation within and between individuals could account for a wide variation in expression of the phenotypes that characterize the syndrome. Thus, the variability in phenotypes associated with the fra(X) syndrome (Loehr et al. 1986) may have an additional basis that is not predicted from previously described contiguous gene syndromes.

Another source of phenotypic variability among females with an imprinted fra(X) chromosome is expected to be the somatic component of X chromosome inactivation, or lyonization (Lyon 1961). A female who inherited an imprinted fra(X) chromosome was assumed to be at risk for mental retardation if the fra(X) chromosome was inactivated in less than one-half of her somatic cells (Laird 1987). Although initial reports of X-inactivation patterns provided contradictory evidence for this assumption, a recent analysis using glucose 6-phosphate dehydrogenase (G6PD) polymorphisms to assess active X chromosomes showed a "significant inverse correlation between the IQ level (as measured by the Wechsler-Bellevue test) and the percentage of fibroblast cells with an FRA-X active chromosome" (Rocchi et al. 1990). IQ scores in the normal range for the population under study were reported for individuals in whom the fra(X) chromosome was inactivated in about 50% of fibroblasts. Thus, these data for fibroblasts support the initial assumptions concerning the effects of somatic X chromosome inactivation on clinical classification of imprinted fra(X) females. Rocchi et al. (1990) suggested that, in contrast to fibroblasts, precursors of red blood cells exhibit selection against cells with an active fra(X) chromosome.

In the X-inactivation imprinting model, two classes of fra(X) carriers are predicted, imprinted and nonimprinted. With respect to carrier females, imprinted and nonimprinted mothers are expected to have different distributions of imprinted and nonimprinted carrier progeny: the carrier progeny of imprinted females are almost always imprinted (fig. 7.1). For carrier mothers who were classified as mentally normal and included in the analysis of Sherman et al. (1985), it was estimated that about one-half had the imprinted and one-half had the nonimprinted fra(X) chromosome. This estimate provided a good fit between expected and observed frequencies of the various classes of carrier progeny (table 1 of Laird 1987).

Another aspect of the distinction between imprinted and nonimprinted carrier females not classified as mentally retarded was examined by Reiss et al. (1989). These authors concluded that fra(X)-positive carrier females have more frequent psychological disabilities than do fra(X)-negative carrier females. As described in the following section, we expect that an even stronger correlation between clinical symptoms and fra(X) expression would be found if a distinction were made between individuals exhibiting high cytogenetic expression (greater than 9% usually reflects an imprinted state) and those exhibiting low or zero cytogenetic expression (less than 7% usually reflects a nonimprinted state). Among females who cytogenetically express the fragile site at high frequencies, no correlation is expected between the degree of impairment and the percentage of cytogenetic expression. As a first-order approximation, the imprinting event is expected to be an all-or-none phenomenon.

A key prediction of the X-inactivation imprinting model is that females who inherit a nonimprinted but mutant fra(X) chromosome will imprint the mutant chromosome in only one-half of their primary oocytes, namely the half that descended from oogonial cells in which it was the fra(X) chromosome that was inactivated. The other half of their primary oocytes descended from oogonial cells in which it was the normal X chromosome that was inactivated; in these lineages, the fra(X) mutation has no effect because the event that the mutation blocks has not occurred. (In this model the mutation is a *cis*-acting block; i.e., it affects reactivation of its own chromosome but not that of the normal homolog.) Thus, the frequency of imprinting in females who inherit a nonimprinted fra(X) should average 0.5. But what should be the variability in this imprinting frequency among individual females? The model makes no prediction about the extent of this variability. If the variability is large, however, the model could explain the clustering of nonpenetrant (nonimprinted) males in some sibships (Sherman et al. 1985). If the X-inactivation imprinting model is correct, however, clustering of nonimprinted carrier individuals would have to be balanced by a comparable amount of clustering of imprinted carrier progeny in other sibships (Laird 1987). As described below, the pedigree data are consistent with this latter prediction. An important analytical tool was required for this analysis, to which we now turn.

Assigning States of Imprinted or Nonimprinted to the Mutant Fra(X) Allele

According to the X-inactivation imprinting model, the imprinted state of the mutant fra(X) allele leads to mental retardation in almost all males and about one-half of the females who carry this allelic state. The nonimprinted state is thought to have few if any phenotypic correlates, although further work on this topic is necessary. The imprinted state was predicted to be correlated with high cytogenetic expression in lymphocytes of the fragile site at Xq27; the nonimprinted state was correlated with low or zero expression of the fra(X) site (Laird 1987). We have quantified this correlation and found that it holds for a large set of data representing pedigrees from nine publications (Laird et al. 1990). For this data set, most fra(X) carriers could be classified as having the imprinted or nonimprinted state of the mutant allele solely on the basis of cytogenetics: individuals with an imprinted fra(X) chromosome usually expressed the fra(X) site in more than 9% of their lymphocytes; individuals with a nonimprinted fra(X) usually expressed the fra(X) site in less than 7% of their lymphocytes. (A few imprinted and nonimprinted individuals expressed the fra(X) site at percentages between 6% and 10%.) This correlation was established for individuals for whom DNA polymorphism [restriction fragment length polymorphism (RFLP)], cytogenetic, and clinical data were available, and it was used to assess the frequency with which individual females, all of whom were interpreted as having inherited a nonimprinted fra(X), have imprinted the fra(X) in their primary oocytes.

Why is it useful to use the level of cytogenetic expression to assess the state of the mutant fra(X) allele? Because fra(X) carrier females who are classified as mentally normal may have either the imprinted or the nonimprinted state of the mutant allele (Laird 1987), criteria other than mental function must be used to assign the state of their mutant allele. As mentioned above, the level of cytogenetic expression is usually sufficient for this assignment (Laird et al. 1990). Thus, female as well as male carrier progeny of mothers who are potentially able to imprint a fra(X) allele were used to assess the apparent frequency of imprinting in individual women. This method provided a more complete analysis than if the mental status of carrier males had been the sole criterion for imprinting. We emphasize that this approach is useful for research purposes but that further data collection and analysis may be necessary before applying the cytogenetic approach to clinical situations (Shapiro et al. 1988). It will be important to quantify data from prenatal cytogenetic analysis, coupled with RFLP and postnatal clinical evaluation, to learn whether there is a useful demarcation between percentages of cytogenetic expression for fetuses with imprinted and with nonimprinted fra(X) chromosomes.

A potential alternative to the cytogenetic assessment of the state of the mutant allele would depend on finding a molecular signature of the imprinted state. The predicted abnormal pattern of DNA methylation (Laird 1987), for example, would probably provide a more reliable assessment of the deleterious state of the mutant allele than does cytogenetic analysis. Progress toward this goal will be described in the final sector.

Proposed Solution to Clustering and the Sherman Paradox

The above-described data set (Laird et al. 1990) includes 39 mothers who were interpreted as having inherited a nonimprinted fra(X) and who had two or more fra(X) carrier progeny. Twenty-five of these mothers had only imprinted carrier progeny; 5 mothers had only nonimprinted carrier progeny; 9 mothers had both imprinted and nonimprinted carrier progeny. Our interpretation is that this last class of mothers represents the predicted class of females who imprinted at intermediate frequencies of 0.5 and that the first two classes represent clusters of nonimprinted carriers in some families and imprinted carriers in other families. From these data, we conclude that imprinting frequencies in primary oocytes of individual females who inherited a nonimprinted fra(X) range from 0.0 to 1.0 (fig 7.4). This very large range of apparent imprinting frequencies indicated to us that another biological variable must be considered.

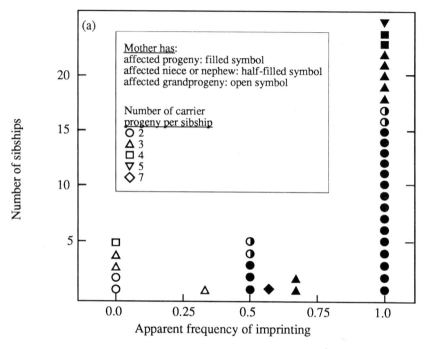

Figure 7.4 Apparent frequencies of imprinting in women who inherited a nonimprinted fra(X) chromosome. [Reprinted with permission from Laird et al. (1990), copyright American Society of Human Genetics]

If imprinting depends on a cycle of X-chromosome inactivation and attempted reactivation, then variations in imprinting frequencies can be viewed as a consequence of oogonial mosaicism (Laird 1987); this would represent a special case of mosaicism in mammals caused by X-inactivation (Lyon 1961). The extent of variation in mosaicism among individuals and among tissues of an individual can be used to estimate the number of embryoblasts present at the time of X chromosome inactivation and the number of progenitor cells for various organs and tissues (Gandini et al. 1968; Nesbitt 1971). For humans, Fialkow (1973) has estimated that there are 15–20 embryoblasts at the time of X-inactivation and that, after many subsequent divisions of these embryoblasts, 50–100 progenitor cells are set aside for each of the individual somatic lineages. No estimate was available for the number of progenitor cells for the human germ line, although there are reasons to expect this number to be much smaller than the number estimated for somatic lineages. One reason is that even after some differentiation there are only a small number of germ-line precursor cells in the human (about 10) (Van Wagenen and Simpson 1965). In

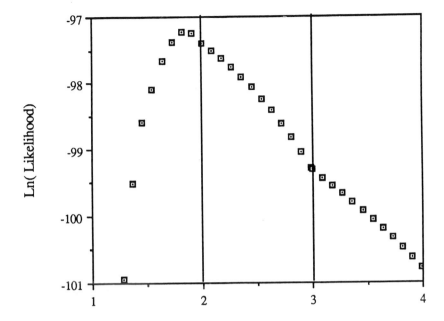

Estimate of Oogonial Progenitor Cell Number

Figure 7.5 The probability of the pedigree data, given models of 1–4 progenitor cells. [Reprinted with permission from Laird et al. (1990), copyright American Society of Human Genetics]

addition, analysis in the mouse has led to estimates of 3 to 8 progenitors for the germ line (Russell 1964; Mintz 1974; Searle 1978; Soriano and Jaenisch 1986). If there is a small number of oogonial progenitors after the time of X-inactivation in human embryos, then a large variation in imprinting frequencies in individual women would be expected.

We used our data set, interpreted within the context of the X-inactivation imprinting model, to estimate the number of oogonial progenitor cells in humans. The best integer estimate is two progenitor cells (Laird et al. 1990). One progenitor cell for oogonia in all females can be excluded by the data; three or more progenitor cells are unlikely (fig. 7.5).

With only two progenitor cells after the time of X-inactivation, one would expect three classes of females who imprint at frequencies of 0.0, 0.5, and 1.0, corresponding to those whose oogonia were derived from zero, one, or two progenitor cells that had the mutant fra(X) as the inactivated X chromosome (fig. 7.6). This estimate explains the broad distribution of apparent imprinting frequencies in figure 7.4. With complete ascertainment and with families of

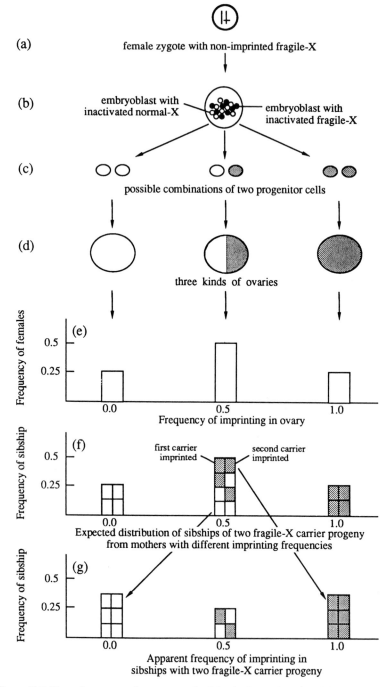

Figure 7.6 From the zygote of a woman who inherited a nonimprinted fra(X) chromosome to her progeny. [Reprinted with permission from Laird et al. (1990), copyright American Society of Human Genetics]

four progeny that include two carrier progeny, a 3:2:3 distribution would be observed for females who imprint with apparent frequencies of 0.0, 0.5, and 1.0. The marked excess of females who imprint at an apparent frequency of 1.0 is attributed to ascertainment biases. Mothers who imprint at frequencies of 0.0 and 0.5 are less readily ascertained than are mothers who imprint at a frequency of 1.0. Mothers in imprinting classes of 0.0 and 0.5 have, on average, fewer affected progeny than do mothers in the 1.0 imprinting class.

The conclusion that there are mothers whose imprinting frequencies vary widely about a mean of 0.5 leads to a proposed explanation for the Sherman paradox. Mothers who give birth to nonpenetrant carrier males must have imprinting frequencies of 0.0 or 0.5; mothers who give birth to affected males must have imprinting frequencies of 0.5 or 1.0 (fig. 7.6). Thus, the potential mosaicism of the oogonial population leads to an unusual form of ascertainment bias that results from variations in imprinting frequencies in individual mothers.

We also used the data that led to the Sherman paradox—penetrances of 0.18 and 0.74 for carrier males in different pedigree situations (fig. 7.2)—to provide an estimate of the number of oogonial progenitor cells after the time of the initial event that leads to chromosome imprinting. Our best estimate is two, in agreement with our other estimates (Laird et al. 1990). In addition to providing a possible resolution to the Sherman paradox, this analysis may provide the most accurate available estimate of the number of oogonial progenitor cells in humans at the development stage marked by X chromosome inactivation.

Evaluation of Ascertainment in the Fra(X) Syndrome

Sved and Laird (1988) estimated the relative ascertainment frequencies in the data set that Sherman et al. (1985) used as the basis of their analysis. If the X-inactivation imprinting model and the inference that there are two progenitor cells for human oogonia after the imprinting event are correct, the data are consistent with an ascertainment frequency of 0.18 for carrier females who have no primary oocytes with imprinted fra(X) chromosomes (imprinting frequency of 0.0) relative to females who have imprinted the fra(X) in all of their oocytes (imprinting frequency of 1.0). This analysis by Sved and Laird (1988) is consistent with an intermediate frequency of ascertainment (0.6) for females who imprinted with frequencies of 0.5.

The relative ascertainment frequency for nonpenetrant males was estimated to be about 0.2, according to population genetic calculations discussed below. Thus, there is close correspondence between the estimates of 0.18 and the 0.2 for the relative ascertainment frequencies of female and male fra(X) carriers who do not have affected children.

Population Genetic Predictions

Sved and Laird (1990) modeled the population genetics of the fra(X) syndrome on the X-inactivation imprinting model. They concluded that at equilibrium there should be about twice as many nonimprinted carrier females as there are imprinted carrier females. Using the above-described estimates of ascertainment frequencies and the cytogenetic criterion for imprinting (Laird et al. 1990), Sved and Laird (1990) concluded that the data of Sherman et al. (1984, 1985) are consistent with the fra(X) syndrome being at or near equilibrium. The approach to equilibrium would be rapid, however. Frequencies indistinguishable from equilibrium would be attained within 5 to 10 generations after the establishment of the predicted high rate of mutation (see below) (fig. 7.7).

At equilibrium, the frequencies of imprinted and nonimprinted carrier males are predicted to be approximately equal (Sved and Laird 1990). As mentioned above, the current estimate of 20% of carrier males being nonpenetrant (Sherman et al. 1985) is probably low because of ascertainment bias. Thus, Sved and Laird (1990) expect that there are more than twice as many nonpenetrant males in the human population as has been estimated by others.

In accord with others who modeled the genetics of the fra(X) syndrome (Sherman et al. 1985; Vogel 1984; Winter 1987), Sved and Laird (1990) predicted that a very high mutation rate is needed to balance the loss of mutations due to low reproductive success of affected (imprinted) males. Assuming a prevalence of affected males of 10^{-3} (Brown et al. 1989), equal mutation rates in males and females, and a 20% reduction in fertility of affected females (Sherman et al. 1985), a mutation rate of 4×10^{-4} would be required to maintain equilibrium. This would be an extraordinarily high mutation rate—the highest rate yet estimated for a human mutation (Vogel and Motulsky 1986). If this estimate is correct, it suggests that the fra(X) mutation, as well as the proposed imprinting event, is very unusual.

Possible Erasure of the Imprint When Transmitted through Males

If the fra(X) syndrome is a disorder of chromosome imprinting, then the question of stability of the imprint when transmitted through males becomes of considerable interest. Normal chromosome imprints are erased when the chromosome is transmitted by the parental gender opposite the one that established the imprint (Cattanach and Kirk 1985). This erasure avoids permanent inactivation of a chromosome or chromosome site that has been inactivated in one gender. Several examples of imprinting have been observed for *trans*-genes in which the imprint on the gene is erased when transmitted through parents of the gender opposite that of the imprinting parent (Sapienza et al. 1987; Swain et al. 1987; Reik et al. 1987). From data on some of these *trans*-genes, it seems

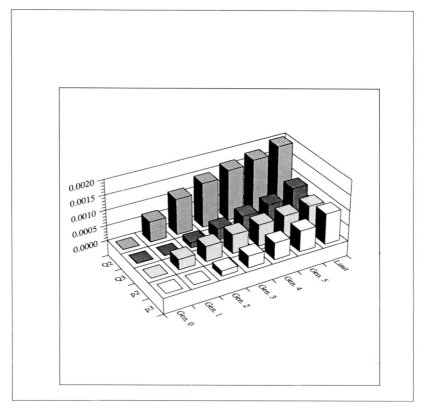

Figure 7.7 Predicted frequencies of fra(X) genotypes at various generations in a population starting without mutations. *Q2* and *Q3* represent the frequencies of nonimprinted and imprinted females, respectively; *p2* and *p3* represent the frequencies of nonimprinted and imprinted males, respectively. [Reprinted with permission from Sved and Laird (1990), copyright American Society of Human Genetics]

that the erasure is either initiated or completed in the germ line rather than in somatic cells of the parental gender that erases the imprint.

Although most imprinted fra(X) males do not reproduce, Laird (1991) concluded that four such males with daughters have been reported (Moric-Petrovic and Laca 1983; Voelckel et al. 1989; Loesch et al. 1987; Yu et al. 1990). From cytogenetic data, Laird concluded that the imprint is erased in all seven daughters of these imprinted males. For one of these seven daughters, probable paternity is established by blood group markers; for another three of the daughters, probable paternity is established by the daughters' having affected sons diagnosed as fra(X). The occurrence of these affected sons (grandsons of the affected males) also establishes that the change in the fra(X) allele that is here called erasure was not due to a permanent alteration to the fra(X) mutation: it was capable of being reimprinted.

The possible erasure of the fra(X) imprint is useful in evaluating different models of the fra(X) syndrome. As is described elsewhere, the X-inactivation imprinting model is compatible with erasure in males and with occasional erasure in females; most other models are not readily compatible with these results (Follette and Laird 1991).

Summary of Proposed Answers to the Peculiarities of Fra(X) Inheritance and Expression

Based on the X-inactivation imprinting model and our subsequent analysis, we propose the following answers to the questions raised by the peculiarities of inheritance and expression of the fra(X) syndrome.

The Fra(X) Mutation, Like Other Fragile Site Mutations, Results in Unusually Late DNA Replication at the Mutant Site

This late replication interferes with condensation of DNA, which leads to the appearance of a fragile site. Unlike other fragile sites, the fragile site mutation at Xq27.3 also interferes with one aspect of the process of dosage compensation in females. The reactivation of an inactivated fra(X) chromosome is blocked locally, before female meiosis. After attempted reactivation, the mutant fra(X) allele is termed *imprinted*. The imprinted state is the cause of the fra(X) phenotypes; genes in the imprinted region are functionally inactivated. A high frequency of cytogenetic expression of the fra(X) site Xq27.3 is indicative of the imprinted state of the mutant allele; low or zero cytogenetic expression is indicative of the nonimprinted state. Thus, individuals with high cytogenetic expression of the fra(X) site are at risk for mental retardation. Individuals who have low or zero expression of the fra(X) site usually are not at risk for fra(X) mental retardation; subsequent imprinting of the mutant fra(X) allele can occur in females, however, putting at risk the carrier descendants of a nonimprinted carrier.

Nonpenetrant Carrier Males Are Classified as Normal because They Have Inherited the Mutant Fra(X) Allele in its Nonimprinted State

The nonimprinted state does not lead to readily detected phenotypes because genes at or near the fra(X) site can be appropriately expressed. For some nonpenetrant males, their nonimprinted allele arose as a new mutation. For other nonpenetrant males, the nonimprinted fra(X) allele was inherited from a mother who, by chance, did not imprint the mutant fra(X) allele in the oogonial lineage that led to such a male.

Daughters of Nonpenetrant Carrier Males Are Classified as Normal because They always Inherit the Nonimprinted State of the Mutant Allele

Males do not inactivate an X chromosome for dosage compensation; hence, nonpenetrant carrier males cannot imprint the mutant fra(X) allele.

The Sherman Paradox Quantifies a Peculiar Clustering of Affected Individuals in Some Families and of Unaffected Carriers in Other Families

This clustering is caused by extreme variation in imprinting frequencies in different females. The extreme variation is a consequence of there being only two progenitor cells for human oogonia after the imprinting event in female embryos. Sibships ascertained by an affected (imprinted) grandprogeny of a nonpenetrant male will have mothers who imprinted with frequencies of 0.5 or 1.0. Sibships ascertained by a nonpenetrant (nonimprinted) male will have mothers who imprinted at frequencies of 0.0 or 0.5. These different ascertainment criteria will lead to marked ascertainment biases. The clustering of nonpenetrant carrier males in some families (Sherman et al. 1985) is a reflection of the latter ascertainment bias.

Virtually All Carrier Progeny of Imprinted Females Have the Imprinted State of the Fra(X) Mutation because the Imprinted State Is Not Readily Erased when It Is further Passed through a Female

Because the penetrance of the syndrome is estimated to be 1.0 among sons of affected females (Sherman et al. 1985), the imprint must be very stable when transmitted by imprinted females (Laird 1987). Therefore, most carrier daughters of imprinted mothers must have the imprinted state. Only about one-half of imprinted females are classified as affected, however, because of "lyonization" of the imprinted fra(X) chromosome (Lyon 1961). Imprinted females who have by chance inactivated the fra(X) chromosome in more than one-half of their somatic cells are likely to be classified as normal; imprinted females who have by chance inactivated the fra(X) chromosome in less than one-half of their somatic cells are likely to be classified as mentally affected.

The Imprinted State of the Fra(X) Mutation Leads to Especially Marked Phenotypes, in Addition to the Cytogenetic Phenotype, because the Region of Inactivation May Be Mosaic

The X-inactivation imprinting model thus predicts an unusual source of phenotypic variation: the boundaries between functionally active and functionally inactive genes at the fra(X) site may vary from cell to cell and from individual to individual. This phenotypic variation will be in addition to the variation in females due to somatic X chromosome inactivation and, for both males and females, due to genetic background effects.

New Mutations Are Difficult to Identify because They Are Not Detectable until After Imprinting Has Occurred

New mutations that arise in males and new mutations that arise during meiosis in females are not expected to be detected in them or in their progeny. Once imprinting occurs in females, however, all carrier progeny are at risk; therefore, there should be no sporadic fra(X) cases other than those accounted for by random segregation and by small family size. This aspect of the X-inactivation imprinting model would explain the reported paucity of sporadic fra(X) cases (Sherman et al. 1985) that would have provided evidence for new mutations. Detection of new mutations that first appear in males is also difficult because there will be a delay of at least one generation in the expression of a mutant phenotype in a family (i.e., the mutant phenotype could first occur in grandprogeny rather than progeny of males who inherited or produced a new mutation).

Erasure of the Imprint Is Proposed to Occur When the Imprinted Fra(X) Mutation Is Passed through Affected Males to Their Daughters; Reimprinting Can Occur in Oogonia of These Daughters

Erasure is consistent with an imprinting model but is inconsistent with most models in which a second genetic change is necessary before the deleterious effects of the fra(X) mutation are expressed.

The X-inactivation imprinting model, extended to consider the question of oogonial progenitor cells, thus accounts for the available pedigree and cytogenetic information, including the special peculiarities of the fra(X) syndrome. We now turn to experimental approaches that provide more direct tests of this model.

Proposed Direct Tests of the X-Inactivation Imprinting Model

The above arguments are consistent with the conclusion that the fra(X) syndrome is a disorder of abnormal chromosome imprinting and that the imprinting event occurs in females with an average frequency of about 0.5. This imprinted state is generally stable when transmitted through females but is erased when transmitted through males. The last point provides support for an epigenetic rather than genetic change that leads to the deleterious state of the fra(X) mutation. A direct test of this central feature of the X-inactivation imprinting model requires searching for an epigenetic change to DNA at the fra(X) site in the imprinted allele. Such an epigenetic change for the fra(X) site was predicted to be abnormal methylation of DNA that precludes transcriptional activity of genes (Laird 1987; Laird et al. 1987). This suggestion has been tested in several laboratories using DNA restriction endonucleases that are sensitive to methylation. Data consistent with the predicted methylation change have been reported by Vincent et al. (1991); Heitz et al. (1991); and Bell et al. (1991).

Even if an epigenetic change at the fra(X) site can be identified in affected individuals, one must test directly the second component of the X-inactivation imprinting model. Does a cycle of inactivation and attempted reactivation of the mutant fra(X) chromosome in a female establish the imprint? Molecular evidence is consistent with this component of the model: the altered methylation that is observed in DNA of affected males compared with DNA of normal males appears to be at the same CpG island that is methylated in females as a consequence of X-chromosome inactivation (Oberlé et al., 1991).

The molecular basis of the fragile-X mutation has recently been proposed to be an insertion or expansion of a few hundred base pairs of DNA (Oberlé et al., 1991; Yu et al., 1991). The site of insertion or expansion is the same CpG island whose methylation persists abnormally in affected males. A remarkable instability of the mutation has been observed, in that there appears to be an increase in the size of DNA restriction fragments that span the site of mutation (Oberlé et al., 1991; Yu et al., 1991); this instability, for which the molecular basis is unknown, appears to occur primarily after the mutant fra(X) allele is passed through a female. Within the context of the X-inactivation imprinting model, we suggest that this instability is a consequence of the imprinted state of the mutant allele. How can a mutation lead to a fragile site and to the putative chromosome imprinting?

Our proposal that the mutation leads to late replication of DNA at the fra(X) site and that this late replication is further accentuated by imprinting (Laird et al. 1987) was tested cytogenetically by Yu et al. (1990). Preliminary data in support of this proposal were presented by these authors for the imprinted fra(X) allele. Studies at the molecular level on the timing of DNA replication at the fra(X) site are necessary to test this proposal in more detail.

It will be of interest to apply the apparently novel principles learned from the fra(X) syndrome to other genetic mutations, including those of humans. These principles may appear unusual only because of the particular mechanism of chromosome imprinting in the fra(X) syndrome. The underlying genetic and epigenetic phenomena may well be general ones (Holliday 1987).

Acknowledgments

Research support for the analyses we summarized in this chapter was provided by grants from the National Institutes of Health (General Medical Sciences), the National Science Foundation (Eukaryotic Genetics), and the Joseph P. Kennedy, Jr., Foundation.

248 / *Diagnosis and Research*

References

Bell, M. V., M. C. Hirst, Y. Nakahori, R. N. MacKinnon, A. Roche, T. J. Flint, P. A. Jacobs, N. Tommerup, L. Tranebjaerg, U. Froster-Iskenius, B. Kerr, G. Turner, R. H. Lindenbaum, R. Winter, M. Pembrey, S. Thibodeau, and K. E. Davies. 1991. Physical mapping across the fragile X: Hypermethylation and clinical expression of the fragile X syndrome. *Cell* 64:861–866.

Brown, W. T. 1989. The fragile X mutation. *Nucleus* 32:102–109.

———. 1990. Invited editorial: The fragile X: Progress toward solving the puzzle. *Am. J. Hum. Genet.* 47:175–180.

Brown, W. T., E. C. Jenkins, M. S. Krawczun, K. Wisniewski, R. Rudelli, I. L. Cohen, G. Fisch, E. Wolf-Schein, C. Miezejeski, and C. S. Dobkin. 1989. The fragile-X syndrome. *Ann. N.Y. Acad. Sci.* 477:129–150.

Cattanach, B. M., and M. Kirk. 1985. Differential activity of maternally and paternally derived chromosome regions in mice. *Nature* 315:496–498.

Cattanach, B. M., and J. N. Perez. 1970. Parental influence on X-autosome translocation-induced variegation in the mouse. *Genet. Res.* 15:43–53.

Chandra, H., and S. Brown. 1975. Chromosome imprinting and the mammalian X chromosome. *Nature* 253:165–168.

Crouse, H. V. 1960. The controlling element in sex chromosome behavior in *Sciara*. *Genetics* 45:1429–1443.

Fialkow, P. J. 1973. Primordial cell pool size and lineage relationships of five human cell types. *Ann. Hum. Genet.* 37:39–48.

Follette, P. J., and C. D. Laird. 1991. Estimating the stability of the proposed imprinted state of the fragile-X mutation when transmitted by females. Submitted for publication.

Friedman, J. M., and P. N. Howard-Peebles. 1986. Inheritance of fragile-X syndrome: An hypothesis. *Am. J. Med. Genet.* 23:701–713.

Gandini, E., S. M. Gartler, G. Angioni, N. Argiolas, and G. Dell'Acqua. 1968. Developmental implications of multiple tissue studies in glucose-6-phosphate dehydrogenase-deficient heterozygotes. *Proc. Natl. Acad. Sci. U.S.A.* 61:945–948.

Haldane, J. B. S. 1935. The rate of spontaneous mutation of a human gene. *J. Genet.* 31:317–326.

Hoegerman, S. F., and J. M. Rary. 1986. Speculation on the role of transposable elements in human genetic disease with particular attention to achondroplasia and the fragile-X syndrome. *Am. J. Med. Genet.* 23:685–699.

Holliday, R. 1987. The inheritance of epigenetic defects. *Science* 238:163–170.

Israel, M. 1987. Autosomal suppressor gene for fragile-X: An hypothesis. *Am. J. Med. Genet.* 26:19–31.

Laird, C. D. 1987. Proposed mechanism of inheritance and expression of the human fragile-X syndrome of mental retardation. *Genetics* 117:587–599.

———. 1991. Possible erasure of the imprint on a fragile-X chromosome when transmitted through a male. *Am. J. Med. Genet.* 38:391–95.

Laird, C. D., E. Jaffe, G. Karpen, M. Lamb, and R. Nelson. 1987. Fragile sites in human chromosomes as regions of late-replicating DNA. *Trends Genet.* 3:274–281.

Laird, C. D., M. M. Lamb, and J. L. Thorne. 1990. Two progenitor cells for human oogonia inferred from the pattern of chromosome imprinting in the fragile-X syndrome. *Am. J. Hum. Genet.* 46:696–719.

Ledbetter, D. H., S. A. Ledbetter, and R. L. Nussbaum. 1986. Implications of fragile X expression in normal males for the nature of the mutation. *Nature* 324:161–163.

Loehr, J. P., D. P. Synhorst, R. R. Wolfe, and R. J. Hagerman. 1986. Aortic root dilation and mitral valve prolapse in the fragile-X syndrome. *Am. J. Med. Genet.* 23:189–194.

Loesch, D. Z., D. A. Hay, G. R. Sutherland, J. Halliday, C. Judge, and G. C. Webb. 1987. Phenotypic variation in male-transmitted fragile X: Genetic inferences. *Am. J. Med. Genet.* 27:401–417.

Lubs, H. A. 1969. A marker-X chromosome. *Am. J. Hum. Genet.* 21:231–244.

Lyon, M. 1961. Gene action in the X chromosome of the mouse (*Mus musculus* L.). *Nature* 190:372–373.

McGrath, J., and D. Solter. 1984. Completion of mouse embryogenesis requires both the maternal and paternal genomes. *Cell* 37:179–183.

Mintz, B. 1974. Gene control of mammalian differentiation. *Annu. Rev. Genet.* 8:411–470.

Moric-Petrovic, S., and Z. Laca. 1983. A father and daughter with fragile-X chromosome. *J. Med. Genet.* 20:476–478.

Nesbitt, M. N. 1971. X chromosome inactivation mosaicism in the mouse. *Dev. Biol.* 26:252–263.

Nussbaum, R. L., and D. H. Ledbetter. 1986. Fragile-X syndrome: A unique mutation in man. *Annu. Rev. Genet.* 20:109–145.

Opitz, J. 1986. On the gates of hell and a most unusual gene. Editorial comment. *Am. J. Med. Genet.* 23:1–10.

Pembrey, M. E., R. Winter, and K. Davies. 1985. A premutation that generates a defect at crossing over explains the inheritance of fragile-X mental retardation. *Am. J. Med. Genet.* 21:709–717.

Reik, W., A. Collick, M. L. Norris, S. C. Barton, and M. A. Surani. 1987. Genomic imprinting determines methylation of parental alleles in transgenic mice. *Nature* 328:248–251.

Reiss, A. L., L. Freund, S. Vinogradov, R. Hagerman, and A. Cronister. 1989. Parental inheritance and psychological disability in fragile X females. *Am. J. Hum. Genet.* 45:697–705.

Rocchi, M., N. Archidiacono, A. Rinaldi, G. Filippi, G. Bartolucci, G. S. Fancello, and M. Siniscalco. 1990. Mental retardation in heterozygotes for the fragile-X mutation: Evidence in favor of an X inactivation-dependent effect. *Am. J. Hum. Genet.* 46:738–743.

Russell, L. B. 1964. Genetic and functional mosaicism in the mouse. In M. Locke (ed.), *Role of chromosomes in development.* New York: Academic Press, pp. 153–181.

Sapienza, C., A. C. Peterson, J. Rossant, and R. Balling. 1987. Degree of methylation of transgenes is dependent on gamete of origin. *Nature* 328:251–254.

Schmickel, R. D. 1986. Contiguous gene syndromes: A component of recognizable syndromes. *J. Pediatr.* 109:231–241.

Searle, A. G. 1978. Evidence from mutable genes concerning the origin of the germline. In L. B. Russell (ed.), *Genetic mosaics and chimeras in mammals.* New York: Plenum Press, pp. 209–224.

Shapiro, L. R., P. L. Wilmot, P. D. Murphy, and W. G. Breg. 1988. Experience with multiple approaches to the prenatal diagnosis of the fragile-X syndrome: Amniotic fluid, chorionic villi, fetal blood and molecular methods. *Am. J. Med. Genet.* 30:347–354.

Sherman, S. L., N. E. Morton, P. A. Jacobs, and G. Turner. 1984. The marker (X) syndrome: A cytogenetic and genetic analysis. *Ann. Hum. Genet.* 48:21–37.

Sherman, S. L., P. Jacobs, N. E. Morton, U. Froster-Iskenius, P. N. Howard-Peebles, K. B. Nielsen, M. W. Partington, G. R. Sutherland, G. Turner, and M. Watson. 1985. Further segregation analysis of the fragile-X syndrome with special reference to transmitting males. *Hum. Genet.* 69:289–299.

Siniscalco, M. 1986. Genetic recombination and disease. *Cold Spring Harbor Symp. Quant. Biol.* 51:191–194.

Soriano, P., and R. Jaenisch. 1986. Retroviruses as probes for mammalian development: Allocation of cells to the somatic and germ-cell lineages. *Cell* 46:19–29.

Spofford, J. B. 1976. Position effect variegation in *Drosophila*. In M. Ashburner and E. Novitski (eds.), *The genetics and biology of Drosophila*. London: Academic Press, pp. 955–1018.

Steinbach, P. 1986. Mental impairment in Martin-Bell syndrome is probably determined by interaction of several genes: Simple explanation of phenotypic differences between unaffected and affected males with the same X chromosome. *Hum. Genet.* 72:248–252.

Sutherland, G. R. 1985. The enigma of the fragile-X chromosome. *Trends Genet.* 1:108–112.

Sutherland, G. R., and F. Hecht. 1983. *Fragile sites on human chromosomes*. Oxford: Oxford University Press.

Sved, J. A., and C. D. Laird. 1988. The X-inactivation imprinting model can explain the incidence of the fragile-X syndrome of mental retardation in mother-offspring pairs. *Brain Dysfunction* 1:245–254.

———. 1990. Population genetic consequences of the fragile-X syndrome based on the X-inactivation imprinting model. *Am. J. Hum. Genet.* 46:443–451.

Swain, J. L., T. A. Stewart, and P. Leder. 1987. Parental legacy determines methylation and expression of an autosomal transgene: A molecular mechanism for parental imprinting. *Cell* 50:719–727.

Van Dyke, D. L., and L. Weiss. 1986. Maternal effect on intelligence in fragile-X males and females. *Am. J. Med. Genet.* 23:723–737.

Van Wagenen, G., and M. E. Simpson. 1965. *Embryology of the ovary and testis, Homo sapiens and Macaca mulatta*. New Haven, Conn.: Yale University Press.

Vincent, A., D. Heitz, C. Petit, C. Kretz, I. Oberlé, and J. Mandel. 1991. Abnormal pattern detected in fragile X patients by pulsed field gel electrophoresis. *Nature* 349:624–626.

Voelckel, M. A., N. Philip, C. Piquet, M. C. Pellissier, I. Oberlé, F. Berg, M. G. Mattei, and J. F. Mattei. 1989. Study of a family with a fragile site of the X chromosome at Xq27–28 without mental retardation. *Hum. Genet.* 81:353–357.

Vogel, F. 1984. Mutation and selection in the marker (X) syndrome: A hypothesis. *Ann. Hum. Genet.* 48:327–332.

Vogel, F., and A. G. Motulsky. 1986. *Human genetics: Problems and approaches*, 2d ed. Berlin: Springer-Verlag.

Warren, S. T. 1988. Fragile X syndrome: A hypothesis regarding the molecular mechanism of the phenotype. *Am. J. Med. Genet.* 30:681–688.

Winter, R. M. 1987. Population genetics implications of the premutation hypothesis for the generation of the fragile-X mental retardation gene. *Hum. Genet.* 75:269–271.

Yu, W.-D., S. L. Wenger, and M. W. Steele. 1990. X chromosome imprinting in fragile X syndrome. *Hum. Genet.* 85:590–594.

Note Added in Proofs

A DNA sequence that encodes a putative candidate gene (designated FMR-1) for the fra(X) syndrome has been described by Verkerk et al. (1991). The 5′ end of this gene, which is expressed in brain tissue of normal individuals, appears to be within several hundred nucleotides of the CpG island whose hypermethylation persists in affected males. No information was presented concerning the expression of this gene in brain cells of affected individuals. The X-inactivation imprinting model predicts that a critical gene or genes at the fra(X) site is silenced by the persistent state of inactivation, presumably mediated by the hypermethlated CpG island (Laird, 1987; Laird et al., 1987). Prediction of gene silencing as a mechanism that leads to the fra(X) syndrome is in contrast to the prediction of an abnormal gene product. The X-activation model would be consistent with the inactivation of more than one gene in the fra(X) region, although the model does not require the involvement of more than one gene.

References Added in Proof

Heitz, D., R. Rousseau, D. Devys, S. Saccone, H. Abderrahim, D. LePaslier, D. Cohen, A. Vincent, D. Toniolo, G. Della Valle, S. Johnson, D. Schlessinger, I. Oberlé, and J. L. Mandel. 1991. Isolation of sequences that span the fragile X and identification of a fragile X-related CpG island. *Science* 251:1236–1239.

Oberlé, I., F. Rousseau, D. Heitz, C. Kretz, D. Devys, A. Hanauer, J. Boué, M. F. Bertheas, and J. L. Mandel. 1991. Instability of a 550-base pair DNA segment and abnormal methylation in fragile X syndrome. *Science* 252:1097–1102.

Verkerk, A. J. M. H., M. Plerettl, J. S. Sutcliffe, Y.-H. Fu, D. P. A. Kuhl, A. Pizzuti, O. Reiner, S. Richards, M. F. Victoria, F. Zhang, B. E. Eussen, G.-J. B. van Ommen, L. A. J. Blonden, G. J. Riggins, J. L. Chastain, C. B. Kunst, H. Galjaard, C. T. Caskey, D. L. Nelson, B. A. Oostra, and S. T. Warren. 1991. Identification of a gene (FMR-1) containing a CGG repeat coincident with a breakpoint cluster region exhibiting length variation in fragile X syndrome. *Cell* 65:905–914.

Yu, S., E. Kremer, M. Pritchard, M. Lynch, J. Nancarrow, E. Baker, K. Holman, J. C. Mulley, S. T. Warren, D. Schlessinger, G. R. Sutherland, and R. I. Richards. 1991. Fragile X genotype characterized by an unstable region of DNA. *Science* 252:1179–1181.

PART II
Treatment and Intervention

CHAPTER 8

Genetic Counseling

Amy Cronister Silverman, M.S.

Many families find relief in finally knowing the cause of their child's problems. At last there is a diagnosis, possible treatment, and, most important, answers. As with all inherited conditions, fragile X parents must face the difficult and emotionally charged issue that one of them may have passed this gene on to their child. Explaining the hereditary aspects of fra(X) syndrome, and helping families cope with and resolve feelings of guilt, anger, and denial are primary goals of the genetic counseling session. Additionally, available testing and family planning options are discussed and other relatives are approached.

Perhaps when the gene(s) is localized or the underlying defect is recognized, a better understanding of fra(X) inheritance will follow. In the meantime, clearly explaining nonpenetrance, variable expressivity, baffling recurrence risks, and imperfect carrier and prenatal testing remains a challenge for the genetic counselor. Helping families grasp these concepts is essential because it enables families to appreciate how the fra(X) gene is traveling through their family.

Genetic Aspects of Fra(X) Syndrome

Inheritance

The gene(s) responsible for the fra(X) phenotype is located on the long arm of the X chromosome in the region of Xq27.3. Although authors have proposed X-linked recessive (Sherman et al. 1984), X-linked dominant (Mulley and Sutherland 1987), and X-linked semidominant (Brown et al. 1987a) modes of transmission, paradoxic aspects of this condition's inheritance have left geneticists perplexed, intrigued, and unable to fit fra(X) syndrome succinctly into any previously described model.

A preponderance of males affected by fra(X) syndrome is expected because the fra(X) gene(s) is on the X chromosome. Similarly, variable expressivity among females is not uncommon in X-linked conditions. Minimal or no expression may be due to lyonization with inactivation of the fra(X) chromosome. Deletions or monosomy of the X chromosome have also led to overt expression of X-linked diseases in occasional females. With an estimated one-third of fra(X) carrier females being cognitively impaired (Turner et al. 1980; Sherman et al. 1984, 1985) and perhaps as many as half of the remaining normal IQ females having learning disabilities (Wolff et al. 1988; Kemper et al. 1986; Miezejeski et al. 1986), the penetrance of the gene in females is more often the rule rather than the exception. Additionally, Sherman et al. (1985) demonstrated that mental impairment (an IQ estimated to be <85) in a woman in some way influences penetrance of the fra(X) gene in her offspring. This has important implications for genetic counseling because a mentally impaired fra(X) woman carrying a male fetus has a 50% risk of having an affected son compared to a 38% risk for a normally functioning mother. Mental impairment, similarly, is present in 28% of daughters of mentally impaired mothers versus only 16% of daughters of normally functioning mothers (Weaver and Sherman 1987).

Another intriguing observation, repeatedly documented in the literature (Martin and Bell 1943; Jacobs et al. 1980; Brondum-Nielson et al. 1981; Fryns and Van den Berghe 1982; Camerino et al. 1983; Froster-Iskenius et al. 1986; Brown et al. 1987a), is of families in which the gene has been passed through phenotypically normal males. These transmitting or nonpenetrant males, as they are called, are not rare. At least 20% of the males who carry the fra(X) gene are normal physically and mentally (Sherman et al. 1985; Sved and Laird 1990).

Understanding the concept of nonpenetrance may be the key to understanding fra(X) inheritance. It has already been mentioned that a mentally impaired fra(X) mother has a 50% risk of having a son affected by fra(X) syndrome. In other words, the penetrance of mental impairment in carrier sons is 100%. Mentally impaired heterozygous women, therefore, are not expected to have nonpenetrant male offspring. On the other hand, limited data suggest that all mothers of nonpenetrant males are intellectually normal and so, for reasons not yet clearly understood, are the daughters of nonpenetrant men. One curious piece to the puzzle, referred to as the Sherman paradox (Opitz 1986), is the observation that the daughters of nonpenetrant men are more likely to have affected offspring than are the mothers of nonpenetrant males. The analysis of many pedigrees suggests that mothers of nonpenetrant males have approximately a 7% chance of having an affected child compared to approximately a 28% chance for daughters of nonpenetrant men (Sherman et al. 1985).

Various models of fra(X) inheritance have been presented in the literature and are discussed in chapter 7. These include a two-step mechanism where the premutated fra(X) chromosome must pass through a female before expression is possible (Pembrey et al. 1985; Sherman et al. 1985; Sutherland 1985; Laird

1987), theories that imply autosomal interaction (Friedman and Howard-Peebles 1986; Steinbach 1986; Israel 1987), theories that involve recombinational events (Pembrey et al. 1985; Nussbaum et al. 1986), and a model of X-linked dominance with incomplete penetrance (Mulley and Sutherland 1987). Laird's two-step model of imprinting (1987) is the most precise in predicting the penetrance figures and other inheritance patterns noted above.

Recurrence Risks

After identifying fra(X) syndrome in a family, some relatives seek genetic counseling because they are uncertain whether they have any risk at all. Others may arrive at the genetic counseling session with the perception that their risk is far greater than it actually is. One person might view a 10% risk as high, and another might view it as low (Pearn 1973). In any case, because of the hereditary nature of fra(X) syndrome, all at-risk relatives or concerned family members should receive genetic counseling.

A woman who carries the fra(X) gene on one of her X chromosomes (a heterozygous fra[X] female) has a 50% risk of passing the fra(X) gene to future offspring. If a man carries the fra(X) gene (either nonpenetrant or affected with the fra[X] syndrome), he will pass the fra(X) chromosome to all of his daughters (100% risk) but none of his sons (0% risk). These risks, however, may be modified given specific information regarding the sex, mental functioning, and cytogenetic or DNA linkage results of the parent, child, or fetus. Because the inheritance pattern of fra(X) syndrome is poorly understood and data are limited, recurrence risks should be provided with caution, especially when considering isolated cases.

For the empiric risks listed in tables 8.1 and 8.2, we consider only familial cases of fra(X) syndrome. It is assumed that penetrance of mental impairment in males who carry the fra(X) gene is 100% if the mother is affected, approximately 76% if the carrier mother is mentally normal, and 80% if cognitive functioning in the carrier mother is unknown. The penetrance of mental impairment in females who carry the fra(X) gene is assumed to be 55% if the carrier parent is an affected mother, approximately 32% if the carrier mother is normal, 35% if cognitive functioning in the mother is unknown, and 0 to 0.07% if the carrier parent is a transmitting man (Sherman et al. 1985). It is also assumed that mothers of affected males are obligate carriers (Sherman et al. 1984, 1985; Nussbaum et al. 1986; Laird 1987; Mulley and Sutherland 1987). Although Navajas et al. (1987) question otherwise, most authors hypothesize that mental impairment in females is expressed only if the fra(X) chromosome has been passed through the mother (Pembrey et al. 1985; Sherman et al. 1985; Sutherland 1985; Nussbaum et al. 1986; Laird 1987). Accordingly, mothers of affected females are also assumed to be obligate carriers. Negative cytogenetic

Table 8.1

Probability of Being a Fragile (X) Gene Carrier and Empical Risk
of Having Mentally Impaired (MI), Nonpenetrant (NP) Male, and Normal (NL)
Heterozygous Female Offspring[a]

| | Gene Carrier | Offspring | | | |
		MI Male	MI Female	NP Male	NL Heterozygous Female
Females					
Obligate carrier or known heterozygote[b]					
NL IQ	100	19	8	6	17
MI	100	25	14	0	11
NL functioning daughter of heterozygous fra(X) woman [fra(X) negative or untested]					
NL IQ carrier mother	40	8	3	3	7
MI carrier mother	31	6	3	2	6
Males					
Nonpenetrant	100	0	0	0	50
Unaffected son of hetero-zygote fra(X) woman					
NL IQ carrier mother	19	0	0	0	9.5
Mentally impaired carrier mother	0	0	0	0	0
Affected fra(X) male	100	0	*	0	*

Source: Data from Weaver and Sherman (1987).
[a]For this data set, IQ was crudely estimated. Mental impairment implies IQ < 85. All values are given as percentages.
[b]Heterozygosity determined by pedigree position, cytogenetics, or DNA linkage analysis.
*Too little data available. All daughters are obligate carriers.

studies were not used to modify recurrence risks because the frequency of fra(X) females who test cytogenetically positive may vary from laboratory to laboratory (Sherman et al. 1984, 1985; Navajas et al. 1987).

Females

Reurrence risks for heterozygous fra(X) females and their daughters are listed in tables 8.1 and 8.2. Daughters of nonpenetrant men are frequently counseled as normal IQ obligate carrier females (a 19% risk to have an affected male and an 8% risk to have an affected female). Sisters of affected females, assuming mothers of affected females are obligate carriers, should be given

Table 8.2

Empirical Risk That Male Fetus Will Be Mentally Impaired (M_{MI})
or Nonpenetrant (M_{NP}) and Empirical Risk that Female Fetus
Will Be Mentally Impaired (F_{MI}) or Normal Gene Carrier (F_{NL})[a]

	Risk			
	M_{MI}	M_{NP}	F_{MI}	F_{NL}
Females				
Obligate carrier or a known heterozygote[b]				
NL IQ	38	12	16	34
MI	50	0	28	22
NL-functioning daughter of heterozygous fra(X) woman [fra(X) negative or untested]				
NL IQ carrier mother	15	5	6	14
MI carrier mother	12	4	5	11
Males				
Nonpenetrant	0	0	0	100
Unaffected son of heterozygote fra(X) woman				
NL IQ carrier mother	0	0	0	19
MI carrier mother	0	0	0	0
Affected fra(X) male	0	0	*	*

Source: Data from Weaver and Sherman (1987).
[a]For this data set, IQ was crudely estimated. Mental impairment implies IQ < 85. All values are given as percentages.
[b]Heterozygosity determined by pedigree position, cytogenetics, or DNA linkage analysis.
*Too little data available. All daughters are obligate carriers.

identical risk figures as daughters of heterozygous women. If the father's side of the family tree looks suspicious, however, one should not rule out the possibility that the father is, in fact, a fra(X) gene carrier.

Bayesian analysis was used to calculate probabilities. For those readers interested in the specific bayesian calculations, an example follows.

Example: The probability of a normally functioning sister having an affected son can be calculated using the following variables:

0.5 = the probability that the sister did not inherit the fra(X) chromosome

0.5 = the probability that the sister inherited the fra(X) chromosome from her mother

$(0.5)(1-0.32)$ = the probability that she inherited the fra(X) chromosome from her mother and that she and her mother are intellectually normal

$(0.5)(1–0.55) =$ the probability that she inherited the fra(X) gene from her mother, given that her mother is mentally impaired and she is intellectually normal

$(0.5)(0.38) =$ the risk that a normally functioning, heterozygous carrier female will have a mentally impaired son.

Assuming that her mother functions normally, the bayesian equation used to calculate the sister's risk of being a gene carrier would be

$$\frac{(0.5)(1 - 0.32)}{(0.5) + (0.5)(1 - 0.32)} = 0.40 = 40\%$$

The sister's risk to have an affected son is then $(0.40)(0.5)(0.38) = 8\%$. If prenatal ultrasound shows that a woman is carrying a male fetus, the risk that the baby will be affected increases to approximately 15%. Other similar risk calculations were outlined by Weaver and Sherman (1987).

From tables 8.1 and 8.2 one can see that mental impairment in heterozygotes does influence recurrence risks. For example, a normally functioning hetero- zygous fra(X) woman has an overall risk of 27% of having a child, male or female, with fra(X) syndrome, compared to a 39% risk if she is mentally impaired. A normal sister of a fra(X) male has a 40% chance of being a carrier if her mother is normal, compared to a 31% chance if her mother is mentally impaired. On the other hand, it is highly likely that a normal son of a mentally impaired fra(X) mother does not carry the fra(X) gene. In general, recurrence risks may be further reduced by a negative cytogenetic result. Because of variability from laboratory to laboratory, these modifications are not included in tables 8.1 and 8.2.

More distant relatives, such as first and second cousins or great aunts and uncles, may contact the genetic counseling clinic to learn their specific risks. In general, the risk of having affected offspring is the probability that one parent is a carrier, that the parent passes the fra(X) chromosome to a daughter or son, and that this child is mentally impaired. In other words, the probabilities of the three independent events are multiplied together. For example, a woman who has a brother and a maternal uncle with fra(X) may be concerned about her daughter's risk of having affected children. In this case the consultand has a 40% chance of being a carrier. If, in fact, she is a carrier, her daughter's risk is also 40%. Therefore, her daughter's empiric risk of being a carrier is the probability that both she and her daughter inherited the fra(X) gene, or $0.4 \times 0.4 = 16\%$. If this daughter is pregnant and is shown by ultrasound to be carrying a male fetus, her risk of having an affected son is $(0.16)(0.5)(0.76) = 6\%$. Again, this is an empiric risk. Chromosome testing and prenatal diagnosis could increase this risk to as high as 95%.

Males

Because the vast majority of nonpenetrant males by definition are clinically normal and negative cytogenetically, pedigree position and/or deoxyribonucleic acid (DNA) linkage studies are the only reliable means of carrier detection in normal men. Probabilities and recurrence risks for at-risk men are listed in tables 8.1 and 8.2. Using bayesian analysis, normal brothers of affected siblings have approximately a 19% chance of being nonpenetrant males if the obligate carrier mother is mentally normal.

$$\frac{(0.5)(1 - 0.76)}{(0.5) + (0.5)(1 - 0.76)} = 0.19$$

As previously discussed, nonpenetrant males pass the gene to all of their daughters but none of their sons. The risk that these daughters are carriers, therefore, is 100% if their father is a known nonpenetrant male and 19% if he is a brother of an affected male. Regardless of a man's risk of being a carrier, the risk that a normal man's daughters will be mentally impaired seems to be negligible. Three cases of mental impairment have been reported among daughters of nonpenetrant males (Sherman et al. 1985). Two daughters were fra(X) positive in ≤2% of the cells counted, and the third daughter was not tested. It is unclear from these reports, therefore, whether mental impairment was due to expression of the fra(X) gene(s). One also has to question whether the fathers were truly nonpenetrant males or instead high-functioning, but nevertheless affected, fra(X) males.

In general, affected fra(X) males are not expected to reproduce (Sherman et al. 1984). Brown et al. (1987b), however, suggested that perhaps 1% will father children. Surprisingly, Laird (1991) proposes erasure of fra(X) expression when the gene is passed from an affected male to his daughter (see chapter 7). Further case studies are indicated to clarify this issue.

Isolated Cases

The inheritance risks are unclear for families of isolated fra(X) males or females (Navajas et al. 1987; Mulley and Sutherland 1987; Sherman et al. 1988a). In chapter 7, Laird et al. discusses the uncertainties regarding the de novo mutation rate and the mutation process in general. Originally, Sherman et al. (1984) reported a lack of sporadic cases and concluded that mutations occurred only in sperm. Consequently, all mothers of affected males were counseled as obligate carriers. More recent analysis (Sherman et al. 1988a) has suggested that this assumption may not be true. Our understanding of the parental origin of the de novo mutational process is still unclear. Until the mutation rate, de novo mutation process, and mode of transmission are determined, counseling isolated cases will remain problematic.

Mulley and Sutherland (1987), Navajas et al. (1987), and Sherman et al. (1988a) calculated recurrence risks for relatives of isolated cases. Navajas et al. (1987) estimate a 9% risk for mental impairment in siblings and a 5% risk in first cousins. Sherman et al. (1988a) calculated a 17% risk for siblings and a 4% risk for first cousins, whereas Mulley and Sutherland (1987) recommended 27% as the recurrence risk for siblings and 1% as an approximate risk for first cousins.

In their calculations, Mulley and Sutherland (1987) and Navajas et al. (1987) assumed that mental impairment can be present in any individual with a de novo mutation regardless of whether it occurred in the egg or sperm. Sherman et al. (1988a), on the other hand, assumed that mental impairment is present only when the de novo mutation occurs in the mother's egg. Also, Navajas et al. (1987) did not use actual mutation rates or gene frequencies in their calculations. These factors, in combination with varying penetrance figures used by each group of authors, account for the difference in recurrence risks. Because no one model has been substantiated, Sherman et al. (1988a) suggested that genetic counselors should present a range of recurrence risks. Also, because recurrence risks involving isolated cases are lower, an exhaustive effort to rule out fra(X) syndrome or cytogenetic expression in other family members is essential.

Working Up the Family

Pedigree Analysis

Once an individual in a family is diagnosed with fra(X) syndrome, the next step is the evaluation and cytogenetic assessment of other family members. If the diagnosis is confirmed in a son, the primary focus is the mother's side of the family. If a daughter is diagnosed with fra(X) syndrome, both sides of the family are scrutinized. Outlining the family history is perhaps the most efficient way to identify relatives at risk. Although a simple task in theory, gathering accurate and pertinent family information requires skill and experience.

Frequently parents are so focused on their child's specific problems that they overlook other family members who have more variable or minimal expression of the fra(X) gene. Broader, more open-ended questions can help families explore the wide spectrum of fra(X) features and behaviors. For example, specifically asking how each relative did in school, whether anyone was slow in speaking or walking, what level of education was completed, and what jobs family members hold is more useful than simply asking who in a family is mentally retarded or developmentally delayed. Similarly, one should ask an open-ended question, "How is your health?" rather than one requiring only a yes or no response "Are you healthy?"

Having asked a more general question regarding the medical history, one can then ask more specific questions related to fra(X), such as "Has anyone ever had seizures, strabismus, heart murmurs, or multiple ear infections? Has anyone had any psychologic difficulties or behavioral problems? Is anyone taking medication on a regular basis? If so, which medication and for what purpose?" Sometimes asking the same question in multiple ways is more effective. For example, to see if any relatives have any of the physical features common among fra(X) individuals, one can ask, "Does anyone resemble your son? Does anyone look unusual in any way? Does anyone have larger ears, a longer face, or loose joints? Do you have any photographs of your family?"

It is not unusual to be counseling a mentally impaired parent or relative. These clients may be confused by questions that are too general. For these counseling situations, therefore, yes/no questions and either/or questions are recommended (Raeburn 1989). In some instances, with consent of the client, it may be more appropriate to invite a normally functioning relative to the genetic counseling session. If this is not possible, other relatives can be contacted for a more complete family history. In addition to identifying other affected relatives, the pedigree can also help identify potential carriers. Fra(X) phenotypic expression in normal heterozygous females has been suggested by a number of authors (Fryns 1986; Loesch and Hay 1988; Cronister et al. 1991a). This work, although still at the investigative stage, suggests that a long face, prominent jaw, hyperextensible finger joints, double-jointed thumbs, and shyness are frequent findings in the heterozygous female (chapter 1). Similar investigation of phenotypic expression in the nonpenetrant male population is also warranted. In the meantime, subtle clinical features suggestive of fra(X) observed among normally functioning relatives should always alert the clinician. Table 8.3 lists symptoms that should be questioned when taking the family history.

Chromosome Analysis

After targeting affected individuals and potential carriers by pedigree analysis or clinical assessment, the genetic counselor should recommend chromosome analysis. Cytogenetic studies prepared using specialized culture techniques (see chapter 3) are a definitive means of diagnosing affected males (99%) and the vast majority (90%) of affected females (Sherman et al. 1984). Although cytogenetic analysis is an important screening tool among intellectually normal individuals, the testing does have limitations. Sherman et al. (1984), in their study of fra(X) pedigrees, found that 44% of all heterozygous fra(X) females were both intellectually normal and fra(X) negative, whereas 26% had normal

Table 8.3

Symptoms To Be Questioned When Taking the Family History

Long face	Heart murmur, mitral valve prolapse
Long or prominent ears	Strabismus
Hyperextensible joints	Seizures
Joint dislocation	Hyperactivity
Hypotonia	Attention deficit hyperactivity disorder
Cerebral palsy	Obsessive/compulsive behavior
Poor eye contact	Motor or vocal tics
Autism	Ovarian dysfunction
Hernias	Premature menopause
Developmental delay	Depression
Special education	Shyness
Difficulty in math	Panic attacks/anxiety
Speech/language delay	Violent outbursts
Recurrent ear infections	

IQs but were fra(X) positive. Thus, according to these data, 44 of 70, or 63% of all normally functioning heterozygous fra(X) females test negative cytogenetically. Similarly, nonpenetrant males and their daughters, who thus far have all been classified as mentally normal, frequently exhibit a lack of expression or occasionally a low level of fra(X) expression (see table 8.4). For a more detailed discussion of cytogenetic testing, refer to chapter 3.

DNA Linkage Analysis

Carrier status remains a critical issue for many phenotypically normal, fra(X)-negative relatives, especially those in their reproductive years. Questionable, nonpenetrant males may find comfort in understanding that their risk of having affected children is negligible. Others, however, may opt not to have children because the implication for grandchildren is too burdensome. Fra(X) cytogenetically negative women, especially those raised with a fra(X) brother, may postpone pregnancy hoping for the day they are definitively shown to be noncarriers. The identification and sequencing of the fra(X) gene(s) should clarify these issues with a specific DNA diagnosis. In the meantime, DNA linkage analysis is a reliable means of carrier detection in some families. Used in conjunction with clinical evaluation, cognitive assessment, and chromosome analysis, it may increase the accuracy of carrier detection to as high as 99%.

Because researchers have not identified the exact locus of the fra(X) gene(s), we must rely on DNA linkage analysis and the use of restriction fragment length polymorphisms (RFLPs), as described in chapter 4. Several criteria are essential to improving the accuracy of this testing. First, DNA linkage analysis

Table 8.4

Percentage of Known Fragile (X) Carriers
Who Are Expected to Express the Fra(X) Site
on Chromosome Analysis

	Cytogenetic Expression	
	Positive	*Negative*
Males		
Affected	99	1
Normal[a]	Occasional	>99
Females		
Affected	90	10
Normal	37	63

Source: Percentages are calculated from data collected by Sherman et al. (1984, 1985).

[a]Data regarding normal males is theoretical and based on minimal data collected to date (see Laird [1990]; Turner and Partington [1988]). All values are given as percentages.

requires multiple family member participation. Key participants are a cytogenetically fra(X)-positive affected male; his mother; and ideally the maternal grandparents. Second, RFLPs must be informative. In other words, in females the allele of a specific RFLP on one X chromosome must be distinguishable from the corresponding allele on the other X chromosome.

Recombination between chromosomes of the same pair is a naturally occurring phenomenon among the normal population. In fra(X) families, recombination frequencies between certain loci are high and vary from family to family (Davies et al. 1985; Brown et al. 1987c; Oberlé et al. 1987; Thibodeau et al. 1988). Recombination, although not always problematic, can hamper the reliability of DNA testing. If informative markers are identified on only one side of the fra(X) locus, crossovers may go undetected. Fortunately, a number of flanking markers have been isolated which not only are polymorphic and likely to be informative, but also may prove beneficial in detecting recombinational events (Oberlé et al. 1985; Hofker et al. 1987; Veenema et al. 1987; Brown et al. 1988; Thibodeau et al. 1988). If, however, recombination occurs between flanking markers closest to the fra(X) locus, results are difficult to interpret and often inconclusive.

Despite these advances, some families will be uninformative and results on certain relatives will remain inconclusive until the fra(X) gene is cloned. For best assessment of the usefulness of DNA linkage analysis for any given family, participation and cooperation by multiple family members is required and preconceptional counseling is recommended so that studies will not be rushed.

Prenatal Diagnosis

Prenatal diagnosis is available to all at-risk relatives of fra(X) families. More than 500 prenatal diagnoses have successfully been completed on pregnancies with a known or suspected family history of fra(X) syndrome. Experience with prenatal fra(X) detection has included amniocentesis, chorionic villus sampling (CVS), and percutaneous umbilical blood sampling (PUBS). Although these prenatal procedures are available throughout the country, only a handful of laboratories in the United States are proficient in the cytogenetic and DNA techniques essential for fra(X) detection.

Shapiro et al. (1982) were the first to report prospective prenatal diagnosis of an affected fetus. Significant work and collaboration since that time have led to improved quality of cell culture techniques and improved fra(X) detection. Recommendations regarding induction systems, cell culture conditions, and appropriate protocols are described in chapter 3. Despite such advances, limitations still exist. Many issues problematic for cytogenetic expression in the liveborn are further confused by the lack of understanding of fra(X) expression in fibroblasts. For this reason prenatal diagnosis should be approached with caution.

Amniocentesis

The largest experience with prenatal fra(X) detection has been with amniocentesis, a test offered to women during the second trimester (14–18 weeks). Amniocentesis carries a low procedural risk, less than 0.5% (Tabor et al. 1986), and is widely available. When used to detect fra(X) cytogenetically in a fetus it is considered 91–95% accurate (Jenkins et al. 1986; Brown et al. 1987a).

Four percent fragility confirms the fra(X) diagnosis in the male fetus (Jenkins et al. 1986; Webb et al. 1987). If the fetus is a heterozygous female, approximately one-third are expected to be affected. Work by Cronister et al. (1991b) examined mental impairment in cytogenetically positive ($\geq 2\%$) daughters of heterozygous fra(X) females. In this study 56% of these daughters had an IQ below 85, and 23% had an IQ in the mentally retarded range. Sherman et al. (1984) also found that approximately 50% of cytogenetically positive heterozygotes were mentally impaired. These reports suggest that, if a female fetus is cytogenetically positive prenatally, there is a 50–56% risk of mental impairment. Further collaborative work in this area is in progress.

Also of concern are false negatives and false positives (all below 4% fragility) which have been reported (Rocchi et al. 1985; Tommerup et al. 1986; Turner et al. 1986; Wilmot and Shapiro 1986; Jenkins et al. 1988). Low-expressing ($<2\%$) or cytogenetically negative female fetuses are more likely to function normally. However, mental impairment cannot be ruled out. Cytogenetically low-expressing male fetuses are perhaps more problematic as these prenatal results are more difficult to interpret (Moric-Petrovic and Laca 1983; Tommerup et al. 1986; Shapiro et al. 1988). In these instances a male fetus could represent a false positive; a nonpenetrant male; a higher functioning, learning-disabled fra(X) male; or a mentally retarded fra(X) male (see chapter 1). Further testing, specifically percutaneous umbilical blood sampling and DNA linkage studies (discussed below) is recommended to confirm a negative or low-expressing amniocentesis result.

Chorionic Villus Sampling (CVS)

CVS is an appealing prenatal procedure because it is offered during the first trimester of pregnancy ($9^1/_2$–12 weeks) and is considered safe. The total loss of pregnancy with CVS has been reported as low as 1.2% and seems dependent upon the experience of the center performing the procedure (reviewed by Rhoads et al. 1989). Although promising to be the method of choice in the future (Tommerup et al. 1985; Purvis-Smith et al. 1988; Evans et al. 1989; Jenkins et al. 1991; Shapiro et al. 1991), researchers are hesitant to quote reliability for CVS fra(X) detection. Again, experience using this procedure is clouded by false positives and false negatives (Tommerup et al. 1985, 1986; Purvis-Smith et al. 1988; Jenkins et al. 1991; Kennerknecht et al. 1991). As a consequence, negative or questionable results on CVS require confirmation in a second tissue (Jenkins et al. 1988; Kennerknecht et al. 1991; Shapiro et al. 1991) or confirmation by DNA probe studies.

Percutaneous Umbilical Blood Sampling

PUBS or fetal blood sampling, a prenatal procedure that specifically examines fetal lymphocytes, is the method of choice for accurate prediction of postnatal percentage of fragility. Until recently it had been considered an excellent means of confirming inconclusive CVS or amniocentesis results because no false positives or false negatives had been reported (Webb et al. 1987; McKinley et al. 1988; Butler et al. 1988). A recent paper by Webb et al. (1989) was the first report of a false negative. Although these authors suggested reasons for this error, it has raised concern about the reliability of fetal blood sampling. Other drawbacks of this testing include a greater procedural risk than that of CVS or amniocentesis (2–4%). Additionally, the procedure is not typically offered until 20 weeks of gestation. Butler et al. (1988) and Webb et al. (1987), however, have successfully completed this procedure as early as 17 weeks.

Investigators have performed PUBS, because of its accuracy, simultaneously with amniocentesis (Webb et al. 1987; Butler et al. 1988; McKinley et al. 1988). These authors think that the risk of doing both of these procedures simultaneously is less than the cumulative risk of doing each separately. Similarly, McKinley et al. (1988) performed CVS and PUBS simultaneously at 18 weeks. Although this negates the benefit of performing CVS during the first trimester, the combined approach is another means of optimizing accuracy and allowing a simultaneous analysis of DNA prenatal studies, as discussed below.

Prenatal DNA Linkage Analysis

Another important prenatal diagnostic tool is DNA linkage analysis. This testing, performed on amniocytes or chorionic villi, can increase reliability to as high as 99% (Brown et al. 1987a; Jenkins et al. 1988; Oberle et al. 1985; Shapiro et al. 1988). DNA linkage analysis is not possible from blood obtained by PUBS. The sample is too small to perform this type of analysis. PUBS performed simultaneously with amniocentesis or CVS at 18–20 weeks, on the other hand, would enable testing of lymphocytes, fibroblasts, and DNA. It cannot be overemphasized that prenatal DNA linkage analysis is possible only if family studies have been completed. If DNA testing is discussed and initiated preconceptionally, the limitations of this testing (described previously) can be explored and its usefulness for prenatal diagnosis can be determined.

Several reports (Oberle et al. 1985; Forster-Gibson et al. 1986; Brown et al. 1987a; Jenkins et al. 1988; Purvis-Smith et al. 1988; Shapiro et al. 1988; Cronister et al. 1990) have discussed the applicability of DNA techniques prenatally. Usually, prenatal DNA linkage studies confirm prenatal cytogenetic findings. Complementary DNA linkage studies can also rule out potential false positives. A male fetus with low fra(X) expression by CVS or amniocentesis, for example, could be shown not to have the fra(X) mutation on DNA. False negatives may also be ruled out as well but are somewhat more problematic. Shapiro et al. (1988) and Cronister et al. (1990), however, point out that a cytogenetically negative but DNA-positive male fetus could represent an affected fra(X) male, a high-functioning fra(X) male, or a nonpenetrant male. Families depending on DNA results, therefore, must be aware that inconclusive results or results that require interpretation are a possibility.

Preconceptional Counseling

Families contemplating future pregnancies are best counseled before conception. At this time all factors that influence reproductive decisions can be discussed. Meryash and Abuelo (1988) found that the majority of women at risk of having a fra(X) child would consider pregnancy termination. Moreover, 81% of the women studied would opt for prenatal diagnosis during future pregnancies. Perception of burden has also been shown to influence reproductive decisions (Sorenson et al. 1981; Wertz et al. 1984). Meryash (1989) examined perception of burden among women at risk of having fra(X) children. Although mothers who have a fra(X) child seem to be coping well with the fra(X) offspring, they are also more likely to consider pregnancy termination than are women without an affected child (Meryash and Abuelo 1988). This suggests that the apparent burden of having cared for and raised a fra(X) child must in some way influence a woman's willingness to risk having another. Other variables, such as education, financial considerations, personal beliefs, and perceived social consequences should not be overlooked because they may also dramatically influence reproductive decisions (Lipperman-Hand and Fraser 1979; Wertz et al. 1984).

Exploration of these issues and of other family planning options are critical in helping families make informed reproductive decisions. Once families have reached a decision to pursue a future pregnancy, preconceptional genetic counseling is recommended. At this time all prenatal procedures and available testing can be discussed. Benefits and drawbacks of the testing should be outlined to help families decide whether they are willing to accept the limitations of the existing prenatal technology.

If a couple contacts the genetic counselor when the mother is already pregnant, which is frequently the case, all options may not be available. First, gestational age should be determined accurately by prenatal ultrasound. Depending on the gestational age, fetal sexing may also be possible. If a woman is in her first trimester, CVS, amniocentesis, and PUBS may all be considered. DNA linkage analysis is usually possible as well. Even if a woman is in her second trimester, however, laboratories performing DNA linkage studies and prenatal cytogenetic analysis should be approached immediately to determine what testing is available and at which center. Regardless of gestational age and regardless of whether a couple would consider pregnancy termination, all couples should be encouraged to have prenatal genetic counseling so they more fully understand their risks and options.

Prenatal Diagnosis for Relatives with a Suspected Family History of Fra(X) Syndrome

Taking a family history has become a routine aspect of obstetric health care. Thus, clinicians may learn that their patient has a relative who is mentally retarded. On the other hand, a pregnant couple or a couple planning a future pregnancy may ask their physician whether they need to be concerned about their family history of mental retardation. Given the multitude of genetic causes for mental impairment, further genetic evaluation of a mentally impaired relative with no clear diagnosis is highly recommended. Certain circumstances, such as death of the affected relative, however, can make this impossible.

How one counsels a couple with a suspected family history of fra(X) syndrome will vary from case to case. If available relatives display any physical or cognitive features characteristic of fra(X) syndrome, they should be tested immediately. Cytogenetic testing of any normal individuals can be pursued with the understanding that a negative result does not rule out the fra(X) diagnosis. DNA linkage analysis, however, is impossible if the affected individual is unavailable. The major question, therefore, remains whether prenatal diagnosis is recommended for couples with no definitive fra(X) diagnosis. No clear answer exists and, therefore, laboratories vary in their willingness to accept such cases.

Other Prenatal Concerns

Twinning

In 1986, Fryns was the first to report an increase in twins (1 in 35 live births) among heterozygous fra(X) women. He suggested that this may be due to a disturbed hypothalamic hypophyseal ovarian axis. Cronister et al. (1991a) showed an increased rate of ovarian problems, including cysts, tumors, and premature menopause in heterozygous women compared to controls. Sherman et al. (1988b), in a study of fra(X) families in New South Wales, reported 17 twin births (both monozygotic and dizygotic) among 752 total births. This twinning rate of 1 in 44 was significantly different from that found in the general population (1 in 96). Sherman et al. (1988b), however, questioned whether superovulation is related to the fra(X) mutation or instead is due to the advanced maternal age noted in the obligate carrier females studied.

Nondisjunction

There have been at least ten reports in the literature of the concurrence of Klinefelter syndrome and the fra(X) chromosome (Wilmot et al. 1980; Froster-Iskenius et al. 1982; O'Brien et al. 1982; Filippi et al. 1983; Fryns et al. 1983; Fryns et al. 1984; Schnur et al. 1986; Filippi et al. 1988; Fryns and Van den Berghe 1988; Kupke et al. 1991). Fryns and Van den Berghe (1988) in Belgium found that 3 of 465 fra(X)-positive males also had Klinefelter syndrome (1 in 155). Importantly, several of these reports have suggested that nondisjunction was maternal in origin (Filippi et al. 1983; Fryns et al. 1984; Kupke et al. 1991). Down syndrome has also been shown to occur simultaneously with the fra(X) mutation (reviewed by Turner et al. 1986), and Watson et al. (1988) reported that 6 of 931 fra(X) children from 236 carrier females had trisomy 21. How the fra(X) mutation might interfere with chromosomal separation at meiosis is unclear. Additional data are necessary to confirm suspicions, but clinicians should be aware that heterozygous fra(X) females may have an increased risk for meiotic nondisjunctional events over and above their age-dependent risks.

Psychosocial Implications of the Fra(X) Diagnosis

Having a child with a genetic disease has many social and psychologic ramifications. The level of burden and the number of psychologic dilemmas faced are dependent upon a complex mixture of interpersonal skills, past experiences, philosophical beliefs, and perceived social consequences (Reif and Baitsch 1985). Little work has examined the psychosocial issues specific to fra(X) families. One must rely, at least for now, on information gathered from studying parents and families coping with a variety of genetic disorders.

Unquestionably, having a child with a genetic problem can have serious but often temporary effects on self-esteem. Feelings of blame, guilt, embarrassment, and stigmatization are commonly experienced (Shore 1975; Kiely et al. 1976; Falek 1984). A considerable amount has been written regarding the "stages" of the grief response noted in families who have a child born with mental retardation (Mercer 1974; Drotar et al. 1975; Kelly 1976; Emde and Brown 1978). When families are faced with the crisis of having a handicapped child, they initially experience shock, which is followed by denial. Then begins the more emotionally laden phase when feelings of grief, guilt, anger, disappointment, and low self-esteem prevail. Eventually, parents who have received information and ongoing support become focused on their child's needs and other concerns specific to the genetic diagnosis. This period of acceptance is considered the healthy outcome of parental coping and adjustment. Importantly, however, the past may never be totally forgotten. As a consequence, chronic sorrow (recalling past hardships and grief) is a common characteristic among parents coping with genetic disease (Schild and Black 1984; Wikler et al. 1981).

The psychologic ramifications discussed above are not infrequent among fra(X) parents and should be discussed during the genetic counseling session. Additional psychosocial implications, however, may be more specific to the fra(X) diagnosis. The study of parents of children with mental impairment (Drillien and Wilkenson 1964; Carr 1970; Watkins et al. 1989) showed that parents wish to be told about their child's diagnosis and prognosis as soon as possible. The grief response for the loss of a healthy child may be worsened when information is postponed (Schild 1981). Many fra(X) children appear normal at birth and are undiagnosed until aged 3 years or later. Thus, the initial grief response is delayed. On the other hand, many parents who recognized their child's disability early but were never given a diagnosis find relief in at last having an answer.

Meryash's work (1989) suggests that fra(X) mothers learn to cope and adjust to their child's special needs and, therefore, that their perception of burden eases with time. The families reported in this study had an experienced and supportive fra(X) network available to them. For families in isolated communities where the professionals are unfamiliar with the fra(X) diagnosis, issues such as appropriate medical treatment and educational intervention often remain problematic, and the perceived burden may be greater.

Financial considerations also affect the perceived burden for parents of handicapped children (Gath 1972; Nihira et al. 1980). Meryash (1989) found that, among at-risk women without fra(X) children, education level correlated with magnitude of perceived burden. Education, however, did not correlate with level of burden in mothers who had fra(X) children, suggesting that more highly educated women, once faced with an affected son or daughter, are able to readjust and adapt to the problems and challenges inherent in raising a fra(X) child. The mean number of years of education among the mothers studied was 12.7. It would be of particular interest to examine the adjustment process and perception of burden among mildly affected females who have fra(X) children to see if the psychologic effects of the fra(X) gene, including shyness, depression, or poor self-image (Hagerman and Sobesky 1989), in any way influence the coping process.

Another important counseling issue regarding mildly affected fra(X) females is patient compliance and willingness to participate in the genetic evaluation. The genetic counseling session is typically stressful for any individual. Fears about doctors, fears of being labeled, and fears of stigmatization (Watkins et al. 1989) may be exacerbated in a retarded or learning-disabled fra(X) woman who has a poor self-concept. For these women, coming to the clinic for an evaluation or even genetic counseling may be too stressful. An appreciation of the special needs of these women is critical if the genetic counselor wants to be emotionally supportive.

The same psychologic stress that affects personal feelings of self-worth can also influence interpersonal relationships. Having a child with a genetic disease may either strengthen or disrupt marital relationships and family dynamics. Although this probably depends on preexisting variables, uncertainty or confusion about the diagnosis can negatively affect interpersonal relationships. Similarly, an inherited genetic disease that can elicit feelings of blame or guilt is especially burdensome (Gath 1977; Schild 1981).

Meryash (1989) is the only author who has examined marital relationships in fra(X) couples. He found that 81% of fra(X) syndrome mothers were still married to the child's father. This enhanced marital stability compared to the general population may be a characteristic of this specific group studied; however, our experience is similar. Further studies are indicated to explore the possibility of enhanced coping strategies in fra(X) families.

As already mentioned, affected fra(X) female relatives may be less compliant. Testing and physical evaluations may be threatening to individuals who are unwilling to consider that they or their children may be at risk for this disorder. Parents may feel the need to protect their learning-disabled child from an evaluation that may be stressful to the child's self-esteem. Others, in denial, may refuse to acknowledge that their child's problems relate in any way to the fra(X) child already diagnosed in the family.

When family members are resistant to coming in for an evaluation, information sharing by the health care professional is most useful. Often relatives are unfamiliar with the medical intervention and treatment options available to them or their children. Families are often comforted by learning that fra(X) syndrome is a common disorder that may cause only minimal problems in one individual but more serious problems in another. Letters may sensitively address these and other issues. Literature written by fra(X) families, as well as other lay literature, can be sent to those at risk. Contacting relatives by telephone may also provide a less threatening environment in which questions can be answered and specific concerns raised. Ideally, through education and understanding, a trusting relationship can be built between the professional and the patient.

Another interesting observation is the reaction of grandparents of the fra(X) diagnosis. Meryash and Abuelo (1988) noted that women were more concerned with the risk of having an affected grandchild than with the risk of having another affected child of their own. They postulated that these families, when surveyed, had already received adequate genetic counseling regarding their recurrence risks and therefore that this question no longer held importance. Nonetheless, the idea that one grandparent may have passed the gene to their grandchild seems to be an especially sensitive issue. In our experience, it is not infrequent that a child's parent is protective of her parents' feelings, concerned that they would be unable to cope if they heard this news. Overwhelming depression, sadness, and guilt in grandparents coping with the news that they are carriers is not uncommon.

Many and certainly the majority of families cooperate and share information willingly. Further studies of fra(X) family attitudes and needs is important if we are to consider this information in genetic counseling.

Counseling Needs of Fra(X) Families

Helping families adjust to and cope with the stresses of having a fra(X) child is an important role of the genetic counselor. This can be accomplished in a variety of ways and includes presenting pertinent medical information about diagnosis and prognosis, reviewing the inheritance and recurrence risks, discussing available testing and family planning options, and, as already discussed, assisting families in identifying and addressing the underlying psychosocial issues. Combining education with emotional support ideally helps prepare families to make informed decisions regarding treatment, management, and testing (Fraser 1974; Kessler 1979; Sorensen et al. 1981; Reif and Baitsch 1985).

Attaining these goals when counseling fra(X) families is a challenge. As already discussed, the inheritance pattern is still unclear and risks are not straightforward. The uncertainties and limitations in testing can lead to further confusion and in fact may raise anxiety. If genetic counselors are perplexed, imagine how the families feel. Thus, the challenge is to untangle all the facts and figures and simplify the information so that the families truly understand their options.

Appreciating a patient's prior knowledge, experiences, expectations, and apprehensions about fra(X) can provide insight into how to approach the counseling session. The most commonly asked question concerns treatment for the affected child and how to optimize his outcome. Families are seeking information that will help them explore what life in the future would be like if they had a fra(X) child, what they can expect for their child, and what they can hope for (Lipperman-Hand and Fraser 1979).

The role of the genetic counselor, therefore, moves beyond providing recurrence risks and available testing (Beeson and Golbus 1985). Genetic counselors must educate themselves about medical management and educational intervention available to families. When counseling fra(X) families, genetic counselors should have a general understanding of sensory integration therapy, be aware of the speech language needs of fra(X) children, and understand the benefits and drawbacks of mainstreaming. Medication is a key issue for many families. Certainly, genetic counselors are not expected to be experts in all of these areas. However, with few health care providers and educators experienced in fra(X) syndrome, genetic counselors must be prepared to answer general questions regarding long-term management and, importantly, must know where to refer families.

Because so few people are knowledgeable about fra(X) syndrome, parents will find themselves advocating time and time again for their child and fra(X) individuals in general. A variety of support groups exist for families with a disabled child. Because so many issues overlap, fra(X) families may also benefit from contact with other fra(X) parents who share similar experiences and who may be better suited to provide emotional support.

The National Fragile X Foundation is an international organization whose purpose is education and research regarding fra(X) syndrome and other forms of X-linked mental retardation. Genetic counselors and other health care providers are encouraged to refer all fra(X) families and concerned professionals to this organization for support, ongoing information, and resource centers in their area. Their address is 1441 York Street, Suite 215, Denver, Colorado 80206, and their telephone number is 800-688-8765 or 303-333-6155.

Conclusion

The genetic counselor plays a crucial role in the multidisciplinary approach to the fra(X) family. Assessing and addressing the counseling needs of each family is paramount. Explaining complex medical and genetic information in a manageable and meaningful way is a challenge that demands time, consideration, and practice. Each family will bring into the counseling session their own unique set of experiences, personal attitudes, and philosophical beliefs. It is the goal of the genetic counselor to help families adjust to and cope with unexpected circumstances. Families grappling to understand and confused by feelings of anger, guilt, or disappointment may be helped by the information shared by the genetic counselor. Through emotional support and understanding, moreover, families can once again feel in control and, ideally, regain hope in the future.

References

Beeson, D., and M. S. Golbus. 1985. Decision making: Whether or not to have prenatal diagnosis and abortion for X-linked conditions. *Am. J. Med. Genet.* 20:107–114.

Brondum-Nielsen, K., N. Tommerup, H. Poulsen, P. Jacobsen, and M. Mikkelsen. 1981. A pedigree showing transmission by apparently unaffected males and partial expression in female carriers. *Hum. Genet.* 59:23–25.

Brown, W. T., E. C. Jenkins, A. C. Gross, C. B. Chan, M. S. Krawczun, M. L. Alonso, E. S. Cantú, J. G. Davis, R. J. Hagerman, R. Laxova, M. Liebowitz, V. B. Penchaszadeh, S. Thibodeau, A. M. Willey, M. K. Williams, J. P. Willner, and N. J. Zellers. 1987a. Clinical use of DNA markers in the fragile(X) syndrome for carrier detection and prenatal diagnosis. In A. M. Willey (ed.), *Nucleic acid probes in diagnosis of human genetic diseases.* New York: Alan R. Liss, pp. 11–34.

Brown, W. T., E. C. Jenkins, A. C. Gross, C. B. Chan, K. Wisniewski, I. L. Cohen, and C. M. Miezejeski. 1987b. Genetics and expression of the fragile X syndrome. *Ups. J. Med. Sci. (Suppl.)* 44:137–154.

Brown, W. T., E. C. Jenkins, A. C. Gross, C. B. Chan, M. S. Krawczun, C. J. Duncan, S. L. Sklower, and G. S. Fisch. 1987c. Further evidence for genetic heterogeneity in the fragile X syndrome. *Hum. Genet.* 75:311–321.

Brown, W. T., A. Gross, C. Chan, E. C. Jenkins, J. L. Mandel, I. Oberlé, B. Arveiler, G. Novelli, S. Thibodeau, R. Hagerman, K. Summers, G. Turner, B. N. White, L. Mullegan, C. Forster-Gibson, J. J. A. Holden, B. Zoll, M. Krawczun, P. Goonewardena, K. H. Gustavson, U. Pettersson, G. Holmgren, C. Schwartz, P. N. Howard-Peebles, P. Murphy, W. R. Breg, H. Veenema, and N. J. Carpenter. 1988. Multilocus analysis of the fragile X syndrome. *Hum. Genet.* 78:201–205.

Butler, M. G., G. D. Vaithilingam, J. E. Ulm, D. Shah, P. Wilmot, and L. Shapiro. 1988. The use of early simultaneous percutaneous umbilical blood sampling (PUBS) and amniocentesis for prenatal fragile X chromosome analysis. *Am. J. Med. Genet.* 31:775–778.

Camerino, G., M. G. Mattei, J. F. Mattei, M. Jaye, and J. L. Mandel. 1983. Close linkage of fragile X-mental retardation syndrome to haemophilia B and transmission through a normal male. *Nature* 306:701–704.

Carr, J. 1970. Mongolism: Telling the parents. *Dev. Med. Child Neurol.* 12:213–221.

Cronister, A., S. N. Thibodeau, J. Jirikowic, and R. J. Hagerman. 1990. The usefulness of cytogenetic and DNA linkage analysis in counseling families with fragile X syndrome. *Birth Defects* 26:238–253.

Cronister, A., R. Schreiner, M. Wittenberger, K. Amiri, K. Harris, and R. J. Hagerman. 1991a. The heterozygous fragile X female: Historical, physical, cognitive and cytogenetic features. *Am. J. Med. Genet.* 38:269–274.

Cronister, A., R. J. Hagerman, M. Wittenberger, and K. Amiri. 1991b. Mental impairment in cytogenetically positive fragile X females. *Am. J. Med. Genet.* 38:503–504.

Davies, K. E., M. G. Mattei, J. F. Mattei, H. Veenema, S. McGlade, K. Harper, N. Tommerup, K. B. Nielsen, M. Mikkelsen, P. Beighton, D. Drayna, R. White, and M. E. Pembrey. 1985. Linkage studies of X-linked mental retardation: High frequency of recombination in the telomeric region of the human X chromosome. *Hum. Genet.* 70:249–255.

Drillien, C. M., and E. M. Wilkenson. 1964. Mongolism: When should parents be told? *Br. Med. J.* 5420:1306–1307.

Drotar, D., A. Baskiewicz, N. Irvin, J. H. Kennell, and M. H. Klaus. 1975. The adaption of parents to the birth of an infant with a congenital malformation: A hypothetical model. *Pediatrics* 56:710–717.

Emde, R. N., and C. Brown. 1978. Adaption to the birth of a Down syndrome infant. *J. Am. Acad. Child Psychiatry* 17:299–323.

Evans, M. I., A. Drugan, F. C. Koppitch, I. E. Zador, A. J. Sacks, and R. J. Sokol. 1989. Genetic diagnosis in the first trimester: The norm for the 1990's. *Am. J. Obstet. Gynecol.* 160:1332–1339.

Falek, A. 1984. Sequential aspects of coping and other issues in decision making in genetic counseling. In A. E. H. Emery and I. Pellen (eds.), *Psychological aspects of genetic counselling.* London: Academic Press, pp. 23–36.

Filippi, G., A. Rinaldi, N. Archidiacono, M. Rocchi, I. Balazs, and M. Siniscalco. 1983. Linkage between G6PD and fragile-X syndrome. *Am. J. Med. Genet.* 15:113–119.

Filippi, G., V. Pecile, A. Rinaldi, and M. Siniscalo. 1988. Fragile-X mutation and Klinefelter syndrome: A reappraisal. *Am. J. Med. Genet.* 30:99–107.

Forster-Gibson, C. J., L. M. Mulligan, N. E. Simpson, B. N. White, and J. A. Holden. 1986. An assessment of the use of flanking DNA markers for fra(X) syndrome carrier detection and prenatal diagnosis. *Am. J. Med. Genet.* 23:665–683.

Fraser, F. C. 1974. Genetic counseling. *Am. J. Med. Genet.* 26:636–659.

Friedman, J. M., and P. N. Howard-Peebles. 1986. Inheritance of fragile-X syndrome: An hypothesis. *Am. J. Med. Genet.* 23:701–713.

Froster-Iskenius, U., E. Schwinger, M. Weigert, and C. Fonatsch. 1982. Replication pattern in XXY cells with fra(X). *Hum. Genet.* 60:278–280.

Froster-Iskenius, U., B. C. McGillivray, F. J. Dill, J. G. Hall, and D. S. Herbst. 1986. Normal male carriers in the fragile(X) form of X-linked mental retardation (Martin-Bell syndrome). *Am. J. Med. Genet.* 23:619–631.

Fryns, J. P. 1986. The female and the fragile X: A study of 144 obligate female carriers. *Am. J. Med. Genet.* 23:157–169.

Fryns, J. P., and H. Van den Berghe. 1982. Transmission of fragile (X)(q27) from normal male(s). *Hum. Genet.* 61:262–263.

———. 1988. The concurrence of Klinefelter's syndrome and fragile X syndrome. *Am. J. Med. Genet.* 30:109–113.

Fryns, J. P., A. Kleczkowska, E. Kubien, P. Petit, M. Haspeslagh, I. Lindemans, and H. Van de Berghe. 1983. XY/XXY mosaicism and fragile X syndrome. *Am. Genet.* 26:251–253.

Fryns, J. P., A. Klexzkowska, I. Wolfs, and H. Van den Berghe. 1984. Klinefelter syndrome and two fragile X chromosomes. *Clin. Genet.* 26:445–447.

Gath, A. 1972. The effect of mental subnormality on the family. *Br. J. Hosp. Med.* 8:147–150.

———. 1977. The impact of an abnormal child upon the parents. *Br. J. Psychiatry* 130:405–410.

Hagerman, R. J., and W. E. Sobesky. 1989. Psychopathology in fragile X syndrome. *Am. J. Orthopsychiatry* 59:142–152.

Hofker, M. H., A. A. B. Bergin, M. I. Skraastad, N. J. Carpenter, H. Veneema, J. Connor, E. Bakker, G. J. B. van Ommen, and P. L. Pearson. 1987. Efficient isolation of X chromosome-specific single-copy probes from a cosmic library of a human X/hamster hybrid cell line: Mapping of new probes close to the locus for mental retardation. *Am. J. Med. Genet.* 40:312–328.

Israel, M. 1987. Autosomal suppressor gene for fragile-X: An hypothesis. *Am. J. Med. Genet.* 26:19–31.

Jacobs, P. A., T. W. Glover, M. Mayer, P. Fox, J. W. Gerrard, H. G. Dunn, and D. S. Herbst. 1980. X-linked mental retardation: A study of 7 families. *Am. J. Med. Genet.* 7:471–489.

Jenkins, E. C., W. T. Brown, J. Brooks, C. J. Duncan, M. M. Sanz, W. P. Silverman, K. P. Lele, A. Masia, E. Katz, R. A. Lubin, and S. L. Nolin. 1986. Low frequencies of apparently fragile X chromosomes in normal control cultures: A possible explanation. *Exp. Cell Biol.* 54:40–48.

Jenkins, E. C., W. T. Brown, M. S. Krawczun, C. J. Duncan, K. P. Lele, E. S. Cantú, S. Schonberg, M. S. Golbus, G. S. Sekhon, S. Stark, S. Kunaporn, and W. P. Silverman. 1988. Recent experience in prenatal fra(X) detection. *Am. J. Med. Genet.* 30:329–336.

Jenkins, E. C., M. S. Krawczun, S. L. Stark-Houck, C. J. Duncan, S. Kuraporn, H. Gu, C. Schwartz-Richstein, P. N. Howard-Peebles, A. Gross, S. L. Sherman, and W. T. Brown. 1991. Improved prenatal detection of fra(X) (q27.3): Methods for prevention of false negatives in chorionic villus and amniotic fluid cell cultures. *Am. J. Med. Genet.* 38:447–452.

Kelly, T. E. 1976. *Clinical genetics and genetic counseling.* Chicago: Yearbook Medical Publishers, pp. 343–364.

Kemper, M. B., R. J. Hagerman, R. S. Ahmad, and R. Mariner. 1986. Cognitive profiles and the spectrum of clinical manifestations in heterozygous fra(X) females. *Am. J. Med. Genet.* 23:139–156.

Kennerknecht, I., G. Barbi, N. Dahl, and P. Steinbach. 1991. How can the frequency of false-negative findings in prenatal diagnoses of fra(X) be reduced? Experience with first trimester chorionic villi sampling. *Am. J. Med. Genet.* 38:467–475.

Kessler, S. 1979. The psychological foundations of genetic counseling. In S. Kessler (ed.), *Genetic counseling: Psychological dimensions.* New York: Academic Press, pp. 17–33.

Kiely, L., R. Sterne, and C. J. Witkop. 1976. Psychological factors in low-incidence genetic disease: The case of osteogenesis imperfecta. *Soc. Work Health Care* 1:409–420.

Kupke, K. G., A. L. Soreng, and U. Müller. 1991. Origin of the supernumerary X chromosome in a patient with fragile X and Klinefelter syndrome. *Am. J. Med. Genet.* 38:440–446.

Laird, C. D. 1987. Proposed mechanism of inheritance and expression of the human fragile-X syndrome of mental retardation. *Genetics* 117:587–599.

———. 1991. Possible erasure of the imprint on a fragile-X chromosome when transmitted through a male. *Am. J. Med. Genet.* 38:391–395.

Lipperman-Hand, A., and F. C. Fraser. 1979. Genetic counseling: Parent's responses to uncertainty. *Birth Defects* 15:325–339.

Loesch, D. Z., and D. A. Hay. 1988. Clinical features and reproductive patterns in fragile X female heterozygotes. *J. Med. Genet.* 25:407–414.

Martin, J. P., and J. Bell. 1943. A pedigree of mental defect showing sex-linkage. *J. Neurol. Neurosurg. Psychiatry* 6:154–157.

McKinley, M. J., L. V. Kearney, K. H. Nicolaides, C. M. Gosden, T. P. Webb, and J. P. Fryns. 1988. Prenatal diagnosis of fragile X syndrome by placental (chorionic villi) biopsy culture. *Am. J. Med. Genet.* 30:355–368.

Mercer, R. T. 1974. Mothers' response to their infants with defects. *Nurs. Res.* 23:133–137.

Meryash, D. L. 1989. Perception of burden among at risk women of raising a child with fragile X syndrome. *Clin. Genet.* 36:15–24.

Meryash, D. L., and D. Abuelo. 1988. Counseling needs and attitudes toward prenatal diagnosis and abortion in fragile-X families. *Clin. Genet.* 33:349–355.

Miezejeski, C. M., E. C. Jenkins, A. L. Hill, K. Wisniewski, J. H. French, and W. T. Brown. 1986. A profile of cognitive deficit in females from fragile X families. *Neuropsychologia* 24:405–409.

Moric-Petrovic, S., and Z. Laca. 1983. A father and daughter with fragile X chromosome. *J. Med. Genet.* 20:476–478.

Mulley, J. C., and G. R. Sutherland. 1987. Letter to the editor: Fragile X transmission and the determination of carrier probabilities for genetic counseling. *Am. J. Med. Genet.* 26:987–990.

Navajas, L., C. Rosenberg, and A. M. Vianna-Morgante. 1987. Genetic counseling in Martin-Bell syndrome. *Rev. Bras. Genet.* 10:333–340.

Nihira, K., C. E. Meyers, and I. T. Mink. 1980. Home environment, family adjustment and the development of mentally retarded children. *Appl. Res. Ment. Retard.* 1:5–24.

Nussbaum, R. L., S. D. Airhart, and D. H. Ledbetter. 1986. Recombination and amplification of pyrimidine-rich sequences may be responsible for initiation and progression of the Xq27 fragile site: An hypothesis. *Am. J. Med. Genet.* 23:715–722.

Oberlé, I., J. L. Mandel, J. Bone, M. G. Mattei, and J. F. Mattei. 1985. Polymorphic DNA markers in prenatal diagnosis of fragile X syndrome. *Lancet* 1:871.

Oberlé, I., G. Camerino, K. Wrogemann, B. Arveiler, A. Hanauer, E. Raimondi, and J. L. Mandel. 1987. Multipoint genetic mapping of the Xq26–28 region in families with fragile X mental retardation and in normal families reveals tight linkage of markers in Xq26–27. *Hum. Genet.* 77: 60–65.

O'Brien, M. M., T. Padre-Mendoza, and S. M. Pueschel. 1982. Maternal nondysjunction of fragile X chromosome resulting in Klinefelter syndrome. *Am. J. Hum. Genet.* 35:146A.

Opitz, J. M. 1986. On the gates of hell and a most unusual gene. Editorial comment. *Am. J. Med. Genet.* 23:1–10.

Pearn, J. H. 1973. Patients' subjective interpretation of risks offered in genetic counseling. *J. Med. Genet.* 10:129–134.

Pembrey, M. E., R. Winter, and K. Davies. 1985. A premutation that generates a defect at crossing over explains the inheritance of fragile-X mental retardation. *Am. J. Med. Genet.* 21:709–717.

Purvis-Smith, S. G., S. Laing, G. R. Sutherland, and E. Baker. 1988. Prenatal diagnosis of the fragile X: The Australian experience. *Am. J. Med. Genet.* 30:337–345.

Raeburn, J. A. 1989. Mental handicap. In A. E. H. Emery and I. Pullen (eds.), *Psychological aspects of genetic counseling.* London: Academic Press, pp. 95–105.

Reif, M., and H. Baitsch. 1985. Psychological issues in genetic counseling. *Hum. Genet.* 70:193–199.

Rhoads, G. G., L. G. Jackson, S. E. Schlesselman, F. F. de la Cruz, R. J. Desnick, M. S. Golbus, D. H. Ledbetter, H. A. Lubs, M. J. Mahoney, E. Pergament, J. L. Simpson, N. J. Carpenter, S. Elias, N. A. Ginsberg, J. D. Goldberg, J. C. Hobbins, L. Lynch, P. Shiono, R. J. Wapner, and J. M. Zachary. 1989. The safety and efficacy of chorionic villus sampling for early prenatal diagnosis of cytogenetic abnormalities. *N. Engl. J. Med.* 320:609–616.

Rocchi, M., V. Pecile, N. Archidiacono, G. Monni, Y. Dumey, and G. Filippi. 1985. Prenatal diagnosis of the fragile-X in male monozygotic twins: Discordant expression of the fragile site in amniocytes. *Prenat. Diagn.* 5:229–231.

Schild, S. 1981. Social and psychological issues in genetic counseling. In S. R. Applewhite, D. C. Busbie, and D. H. Borgaonkar (eds.), *Genetic screening and counseling: A multidisciplinary perspective.* Springfield, Ill.: Charles C Thomas, pp. 104–133.

Schild, S., and R. B. Black. 1984. *Social work and genetics: A guide for practice.* New York: Haworth Press, pp. 49–70.

Schnur, R. E., D. H. Ledbetter, and R. L. Nussbaum. 1986. A family with a 47,XXY plus fragile X at Xq27.3 due to paternal nondisjunction. *Am. J. Hum. Genet. (Suppl.)* 39:A100.

Shapiro, L. R., P. Wilmot, P. Brenholz, A. Leff, M. Martino, G. Harris, M. Mahoney, and J. C. Hobbins. 1982. Prenatal diagnosis of fragile X chromosome. *Lancet* 1:99–100.

Shapiro, L. R., P. L. Wilmot, P. D. Murphy, and W. G. Breg. 1988. Experience with multiple approaches to the prenatal diagnosis of the fragile-X syndrome: Amniotic fluid, chorionic villi, fetal blood and molecular methods. *Am. J. Med. Genet.* 30:347–354.

Shapiro, L. R., P. L. Wilmot, and P. D. Murphy. 1991. Prenatal diagnosis of the fragile X syndrome: Possible end of the experimental phase for omniotic fluid. *Am. J. Med. Genet.* 38:453–455.

Sherman, S. L., N. E. Morton, P. A. Jacobs, and G. Turner. 1984. The marker (X) syndrome: A cytogenetic and genetic analysis. *Ann. Hum. Genet.* 48:21–37.

Sherman, S. L., P. A. Jacobs, N. E. Morton, U. Froster-Iskenius, P. N. Howard-Peebles, K. B. Nielsen, M. W. Partington, G. R. Sutherland, G. Turner, and M. Watson. 1985. Further segregation analysis of the fragile X syndrome with special reference to transmitting males. *Hum. Genet.* 69:289–299.

Sherman, S. L., A. Rogatko, and G. Turner. 1988a. Recurrence risks for relatives in families with an isolated case of the fragile X syndrome. *Am. J. Med. Genet.* 31:753–765.

Sherman, S. L., G. Turner, L. Sheffield, S. Laing, and H. Robinson. 1988b. Investigation of the twinning rate in families with the fragile X syndrome. *Am. J. Med. Genet.* 30:625–631.

Shore, M. F. 1975. Psychological issues in counseling the genetically handicapped. In C. Birch and P. Albrecht (eds.), *Genetics and the quality of life.* New York: Pergamon Press.

Sorensen, J. R., J. P. Swazey, and N. A. Scotch. 1981. *Reproductive pasts, reproductive futures: Genetic counseling and its effectivenes.* New York: Alan R. Liss.

Steinbach, P. 1986. Mental impairment in Martin-Bell syndrome is probably determined by interaction of several genes: Simple explanation of phenotypic differences between unaffected and affected males with the same chromosome. *Hum. Genet.* 72:248–252.

Sutherland, G. 1985. The enigma of the fragile-X chromosome. *Trends Genet.* 1:108–112.

Sved, J. A., and C. D. Laird. 1990. Population genetic consequences of the fragile-X syndrome based on the X-inactivation imprinting model. *Am. J. Hum. Genet.* 46:443–451.

Tabor, A., J. Philip, M. Madsen, J. Bang, E. D. Obel, and B. Norgaard-Pederson. 1986. Randomised control trial of genetic amniocentesis in 4604 low risk women. *Lancet* 2:1287–1293.

Thibodeau, S. N., H. R. Dorkins, K. R. Faulk, R. Berry, A. C. M. Smith, R. Hagerman, A. King, and K. E. Davies. 1988. Linkage analysis using multiple DNA polymorphic markers in normal families and in families with fragile X syndrome. *Hum. Genet.* 79:219–227.

Tommerup, N., F. Sondergaard, T. Tonnessen, M. Kristensen, B. Arveiler, and A. Schinzel. 1985. First trimester prenatal diagnosis of a male fetus with fragile X. *Lancet* 1:870.

Tommerup, N., P. Aula, B. Gustavii, A. Heiberg, G. Holmgren, H. von Koskull, J. Leisti, M. Mikkelsen, F. Mitelman, K. B. Nielsen, P. Steinbach, S. Stengel-Rutkowski, J. Wahlstrom, K. Zang, and M. Zanke. 1986. Second trimester prenatal diagnosis of the fragile X. *Am. J. Med. Genet.* 23:313–324.
Turner, G., and M. W. Partington. 1988. Fragile X expression, age and the degree of mental handicap in the male. *Am. J. Med. Genet.* 30:423–428.
Turner, G., A. Daniel, and M. Frost. 1980. X-linked mental retardation macroorchidism, and the Xq27 fragile site. *J. Pediatr.* 96:837–841.
Turner, G., J. M. Opitz, W. T. Brown, K. E. Davies, P. A. Jacobs, E. C. Jenkins, M. Mikkelsen, M. W. Partington, and G. R. Sutherland. 1986. Conference report: Second International Workshop on the Fragile X and on X-linked Mental Retardation. *Am. J. Med. Genet.* 23:11–67.
Veenema, H., N. J. Carpenter, E. Bakker, M. H. Hofker, A. Millington-Ward, and P. L. Pearson. 1987. The fragile X syndrome in a large family. III. Investigations on linkage of flanking DNA markers with the fragile X site Xq27. *J. Med. Genet.* 24:101–106.
Watkins, C., A. Lazzarini, M. K. McCormack, and C. S. Reis. 1989. Genetic counseling for the mildly mentally retarded client. In N. J. Zellers (ed.), *Strategies in genetic counseling.* New York: Human Sciences Press, pp. 219–234.
Watson, M. S., W. W. Breg, D. Pauls, W. T. Brown, A. J. Carroll, P. N. Howard-Peebles, D. Meryash, and L. R. Shapiro. 1988. Aneuploidy and fragile X syndrome. *Am. J. Med. Genet.* 30:115–121.
Weaver, D. D., and S. L. Sherman. 1987. A counseling guide to the Martin-Bell syndrome. Letter to the editor. *Am. J. Med. Genet.* 26:39–44.
Webb, T. P., C. H. Rodeck, K. H. Nicolaides, and C. M. Gooden. 1987. Prenatal diagnosis of the fragile X syndrome using fetal blood and amniotic fluid. *Prenat. Diagn.* 7:203–214.
Webb, T. P., S. Bundey, and M. McKinley. 1989. Missed prenatal diagnosis of fragile-X syndrome. *Prenat. Diagn.* 9:777–781.
Wertz, D. C., J. R. Sorenson, and T. C. Heeren. 1984. Genetic counseling and reproductive uncertainty. *Am. J. Med. Genet.* 18:79–88.
Wikler, L., M. Wasow, and E. Hatfield. 1981. Chronic sorrow revistied: Parent vs. professional depiction of the adjustment of parents of mentally retarded children. *Am. J. Orthopsychiatry* 51:63–70.
Wilmot, P. L., and L. R. Shapiro. 1986. The value of folate sensitive fragile sites in detecting false negative fragile X prenatal cytogenetic results in amniotic fluid cell cultures. *Am. J. Hum. Genet.* 39:A269.
Wilmot, P. L., L. R. Shapiro, and P. A. Duncan. 1980. The Xq27 fragile site and 47,XXY. *Am. J. Hum. Genet.* 32:94A.
Wolff, P. H., J. Gardner, J. Lappen, J. Paccia, and D. Meryash. 1988. Variable expression of the fragile X syndrome in heterozygous females of normal intelligence. *Am. J. Med. Genet.* 30:213–225.

CHAPTER 9

Medical Follow-up
and Pharmacotherapy

Randi Jenssen Hagerman, M.D.

The physician who follows children and adults with fragile X syndrome must be familiar with the physical and behavioral problems associated with this disorder to provide optimal treatment and intervention. Although a cure does not presently exist, a variety of effective interventions are available. Special education and individual therapy in speech and language, motor, and sensory integration, as discussed in chapter 11, are essential for children with fra(X) syndrome. Also helpful are counseling and behavior therapy for children, adults, and the family, as discussed in chapter 10. The most optimal intervention, however, is a multiprofessional approach that also includes the physician's input in health maintenance and, when necessary, pharmacotherapy, particularly for behavior problems. Usually, counseling, special education, individual therapy, and medication work synergistically to allow fra(X) children to achieve their highest potential. Treatment must be individualized, however, because the severity of the problems may vary. Similar problems are present in the majority of fra(X) males and significantly affected females, such that a preventive approach to medical complications is possible. The first section of this chapter focuses on medical complications and their treatment. This section is divided into ages, with an emphasis on what the physician should assess at each age. The second section concerns the pharmacotherapy of behavior problems.

Medical Follow-up

Infancy

Fra(X) infants are usually identified after an older relative, such as a brother or first cousin, is identified as fra(X) positive. Genetic counseling for extended family members should begin at the time of diagnosis and may also involve prenatal diagnosis for future pregnancies (chapter 8).

The newly diagnosed infant should be examined with a close look for possible connective tissue abnormalities (chapter 1). Fragile X infants are at increased risk for cleft palate, clubfoot, congenital hip dislocation, and hernias, perhaps all related to loose connective tissue. Fryns et al. (1988) also reported an increased incidence of sudden infant death syndrome (SIDS), so episodes of apnea, obstructive breathing, or possible seizures require a detailed work-up and subsequent careful monitoring.

Many fra(X) babies have been described as stiff, unable to cuddle, irritable, and poor feeders. We have noted several cases of failure to thrive related to difficulties in sucking, tactile defensiveness, aversion to food textures, and frequent infections. If feeding difficulties are a problem, particularly with sucking or later tolerance of foods, consultation with an occupational therapist and subsequent work on oral stimulation and oral motor coordination can be helpful. Significant hypotonia or motor delays also require therapy from an occupational therapist (OT) and/or physical therapist during the first year. This can be obtained through an infant stimulation program, which should also include a language therapist. Such programs also work with the parents to teach them how to stimulate the baby optimally at home. If the mother herself is severely learning disabled or retarded because of fra(X) syndrome, such intervention is essential to teach appropriate parenting skills and to provide ongoing guidance.

The Toddler Period

Beginning in the first year of life, frequent otitis media (middle ear) infections are a problem for approximately 60% of fra(X) boys (Hagerman et al. 1987). As discussed in chapter 1, this problem requires vigorous therapy to avoid a fluctuating hearing loss that may further compromise language development. If a conductive hearing loss is persistent after acute antibiotic treatment, the physician should consider the insertion of polyethylene (PE) tubes through the tympanic membrane to normalize hearing. Prophylactic antibiotics may also be helpful to decrease the incidence of recurrent otitis media.

Language development is often delayed in normal milestones, which include six words by 16 months, two word phrases by 18 months, and three word phrases by 24 months (Hagerman 1990). If language delays, articulation problems, or unusual characteristics such as cluttering, echolalia, stuttering, or perseveration develop, referral to a speech and language pathologist for a thorough evaluation and individual therapy is appropriate. The therapist can also develop a home program to enhance language stimulation.

Formal developmental tests, such as the Bayley Scales of Infant Development, allow the physician to monitor progress and focus on areas of delay. Motor problems and hypotonia are common among fra(X) children; therefore, continued therapy with an OT is recommended during childhood (chapter 11).

Behavioral difficulties often noted in the second year include excessive tantrums, eating problems, and sleeping difficulties. Maintaining consistency in routines, facilitating transitions, avoiding circumstances that are overwhelming in sensory input, and helping a child with calming techniques are outlined in chapters 10 and 11. Basic principles of child-rearing and discipline, such as reinforcing good behavior and ignoring or timing out negative behavior, can be discussed in detail with parents. Often negative behavior cycles develop at home, which involve negative attention for bad behavior and no reinforcement for appropriate behavior, both of which are counterproductive. If problems develop, early referral to therapists who can teach appropriate behavior modification techniques to the parents is essential. Pharmacotherapy, such as methylphenidate, is typically most helpful for the school-aged child, not the toddler, and it is used for impulsivity and attentional problems and not primarily for behavioral control. However, many families have associated folic acid therapy with improvement in attention, language development, and mood lability during early childhood, as reviewed below. Folic acid therapy may be started during infancy, unlike stimulants.

Preschool

The physician must continue to be supportive in ordering sensory-motor integration therapy, by an OT, to improve motor planning, motor coordination, joint stability, and coordination of visual, auditory, and tactile information into a motor output. The OT can be particularly helpful in teaching calming techniques to the parents, which may control tantrums. Continued language therapy to enhance pragmatic, attention, and problem-solving skills is beneficial for affected boys and girls. Regular preschool experience with normal children, when possible, is helpful in providing normal role models for the child (chapter 11).

The physician must be vigilant about taking a history for possible seizures, which occur in approximately 20% of fra(X) children. The type of seizure is variable; there may be staring spells or focal motor, grand mal, or psychomotor seizures, as described in chapter 1. If such a history is obtained, an electroencephalogram (EEG) that includes the waking and sleeping state should be done. Pharmacotherapy for seizures is described below.

An ophthalmologic examination should be carried out by four years of age because strabismus or other difficulties including ptosis, nystagmus, and myopia occur in over 50% of fra(X) children (chapter 1).

School-age

The physician can ensure that appropriate special education is provided for the school-aged child, including speech and language therapy and OT. As described in chapter 11, such support continues to be essential for sensory integration and cognitive development. If this therapy is not provided through the school, the family may need guidance in providing private therapy. When possible, mainstreaming for nonacademic areas is recommended so that the child will have models of normal behavior and will learn appropriate social skills.

The assessment and treatment of attentional problems and hyperactivity are important in the young school-aged child. Successful treatment is multimodal, including behavior management, special education, and individual therapies (Kendall and Braswell 1986). In addition, medication to improve attention and reduce impulsivity and hyperactivity is often helpful, as described below. For evaluation of possible attention deficit hyperactivity disorder (ADHD), a detailed history should be taken and questionnaires, such as the Conners (Conners 1973), can be given to the parent and teacher. In the clinical assessment, behavior can be monitored during play and during an examination that includes tasks that require concentration (Hagerman 1984).

Further signs of connective tissue dysplasia may be evident at this age, including scoliosis, flat feet, hernias, and a cardiac murmur. Mitral valve prolapse (MVP) may be manifested by a click or an early systolic murmur and occurs in approximately 50% of fra(X) males, although it is more common as the patient ages (chapter 1). On rare occasions, the MVP may be severe and a holosystolic murmur secondary to mitral regurgitation is heard. If evidence of MVP is detected on physical examination, further evaluation by a cardiologist, including an echocardiogram, is necessary. If the MVP is confirmed, prophylaxis for subacute bacterial endocarditis (SBE) is recommended for dental procedures or surgery that may be contaminated by endogenous bacteria. If scoliosis is present, baseline spinal films should be performed with careful follow-up. Referral to an orthopedist is important because progression of the scoliosis may require treatment such as bracing well before puberty.

Families who have ongoing difficulties with behavior in their child should be referred to a therapist who can provide ongoing support with behavior modification and counseling for the family and child (chapter 10).

Early Adolescence

Often hyperactivity decreases before or during puberty, but attention problems usually persist. Aggressive behavior may be a problem for some boys, and episodic violent outbursts are particularly problematic during and after puberty.

Treatment involves many of the same interventions mentioned at earlier ages, including calming techniques and individual counseling, as well as behavior management. Monitoring the environment to avoid overwhelming stimuli and facilitating transitions is also helpful (chapters 10 and 11). Medical intervention with pharmacotherapy (as described below) may work synergistically with these other interventions.

Testicular volume normally increases during the early stages of puberty, but in fra(X) boys this increase is usually quite dramatic, leading to macroorchidism, or a testicular volume of >30 ml bilaterally. These changes are typical for the syndrome, and they do not require intervention.

The physician may be consulted by a teacher or psychologist concerning an IQ decrease in the early adolescent fra(X) boy. This is common in fra(X) boys, and it does not represent neurologic deterioration (chapters 1 and 5). Therefore, a more detailed neurologic work-up is usually not indicated. Problems that may interfere with learning, however, such as subtle seizures, absence episodes, significant attentional problems, and emotional or behavioral difficulties, must be identified and treated to optimize the cognitive development of fra(X) children.

Late Adolescence

The problems at this stage are an extension of many issues discussed in the previous sections. The transition to adulthood is difficult for all individuals but particularly so for severely learning-disabled or retarded individuals. The cognitive abilities may prevent independent living, and varying degrees of supervision are necessary. Vocational training options are usually the primary focus throughout high school. The physician can provide ongoing support for programming in this area, which is usually developed by the educational system. The stresses of the transition from childhood to adulthood often intensify emotional or behavioral problems in fra(X) males. Individual counseling can be very helpful to the adolescent or young adult, particularly with sexuality issues and problems associated with separation from family (chapter 10).

Aggressive behavior is a common problem in adolescence and adulthood, and it requires a thorough medical and environmental assessment. Medical problems, such as psychomotor seizures, may precipitate aggressive behavior and require anticonvulsant therapy, as described below. Various environmental stressors may also precipitate an outburst, including overstimulating situations, crowding, transitions, physical discomfort, staff changes, and family conflict. Possible problems must be assessed and changes made to create an appropriate environment. Often a workplace without excessive stimuli and distractions or a living situation without disruptive roommates makes a significant difference in the frequency of aggressive outbursts. Additionally, a program of behavior management that may include tokens for good behavior and calming techniques can be helpful (chapter 11). Medications, as described below, can work synergistically with behavior and environmental management to help patients control aggressive behavior (Stewart et al. 1990).

Periodic physical examinations to monitor cardiovascular parameters including blood pressure, weight changes, and neurologic findings that may be influenced by medication are recommended. Health maintenance also includes an ongoing vigilance for connective tissue problems such as hernias, joint dislocations, scoliosis, and MVP.

Pharmacotherapy

The Treatment of Seizures

Approximately 20% of fra(X) males have well-documented seizures; therefore, the medical history should always include questions concerning possible seizures. Although many seizures are grand mal, other episodes may be partial complex seizures with subtle jerking of the face or hand associated with staring, sensory sensations, and guttural sounds. These episodes may be difficult to recognize as seizures, and careful questioning is necessary. Abruptly violent episodes that are not precipitated by environmental stimuli may be temporal lobe seizures. Violent outbursts may also be related to a lack of appropriate inhibition in the central nervous system (CNS), which may also give rise to frequent spike discharges on the EEG. Musumeci et al. (1991) found a correlation between violent outbursts and spikes in the EEGs of fra(X) males. If there are clinical questions about the possibility of seizures, an EEG is warranted.

The majority of fra(X) males with seizures have a benign variety with rolandic spikes that respond well to anticonvulsants, as previously described (Wisniewski et al. 1991). Carbamazepine (Tegretol) is most commonly used. It is an iminostilbine with a tricyclic structure unique among anticonvulsants (fig. 9.1). It is the drug of choice for partial motor, partial complex, and secondary generalized tonic-clonic seizures. It is usually well tolerated, but up to 30% of individuals may experience sedation, which is usually transient. The dosage is gradually increased from a starting dosage of 10 mg/kg/day to a maintenance dosage of 20–40 mg/kg/day, and serum levels should be checked before the morning dose to determine whether the patient is in the therapeutic range of 7 to 12 μg/ml. The dose is usually given two or three times a day, and side effects may rarely include a rash, hyponatremia, hematopoietic alterations, and liver toxicity. A benign transient neutropenia occurs in up to 20%, but it rarely requires discontinuation of the medication (Dodson 1989). Serious severe hematologic problems such as agranulocytosis are very rare (Pellock 1987). An

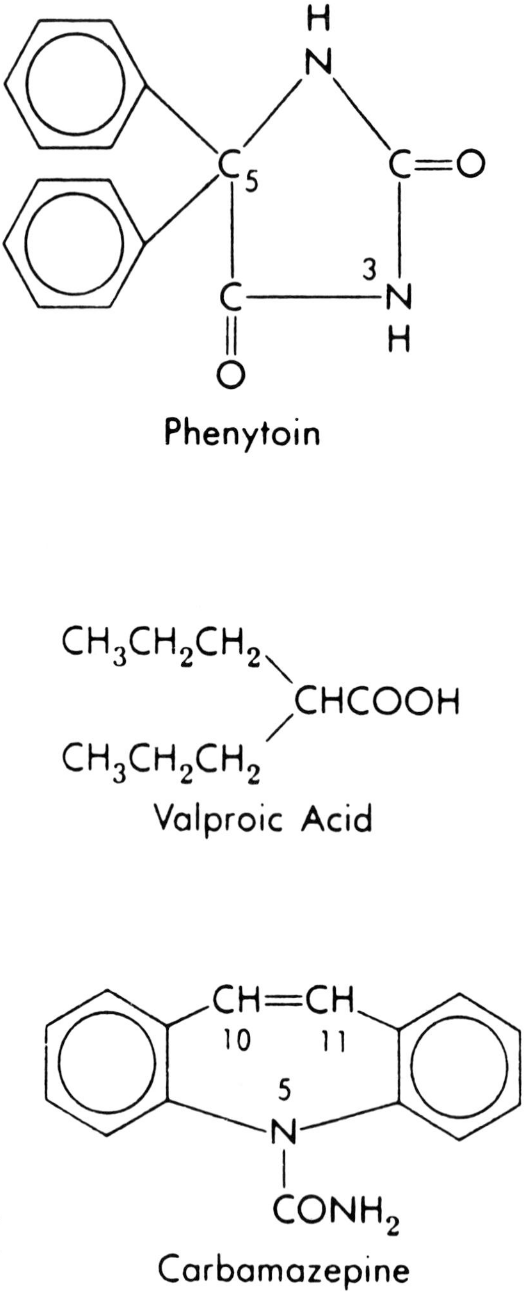

Phenytoin

Valproic Acid

Carbamazepine

Figure 9.1 The chemical structures of phenytoin, valproic acid, and carbamazepine.

occasional patient will develop behavioral problems such as hyperactivity, and this seems to be related to a metabolite, an epoxide of carbamazepine which can be assayed. Concurrent treatment with macrolide antibiotics (including erythromycin), cimetidine, propoxyphene, and isoniazid can interfere with the metabolism of carbamazepine with a subsequent increase in the levels and development of symptoms of toxicity, including nausea, vomiting, ataxia, lethargy, and diplopia (Pippenger 1987).

Carbamazepine is helpful for behavioral and psychiatric disorders in both retarded and nonretarded patients (Evans and Gualtieri 1985; Berkheimer et al. 1985). Problems including episodic dyscontrol, violent outbursts, hyperactivity, and self-injurious behavior may respond to carbamazepine in those with or without EEG abnormalities or seizures (Reid et al. 1981; Langee 1989). Although some patients may respond to the anticonvulsant effect, (i.e., the EEG abnormalities that may have precipitated the outburst are improved), there may also be a direct effect on behavior. No studies of the effect of carbamazepine on behavior problems in fra(X) patients have yet been done. A study by Langee (1989) showed improvement in 39% of 76 mentally retarded institutionalized males with behavior problems (usually aggression or episodic dyscontrol) when treated with carbamazepine. This is a medication, therefore, that should be considered in violent or significantly aggressive fra(X) males, particularly those with EEG findings of spike wave discharges.

Of the anticonvulsants presently available, phenobarbital has been used the longest, and it is effective for controlling seizures. However, it commonly increases hyperactivity and may exacerbate ADHD in fra(X) patients. It is, therefore, not recommended for routine use in fra(X) syndrome; however, it may be necessary for a poorly controlled seizure disorder that does not respond to other anticonvulsants. Primidone (mysoline) may also exacerbate hyperactivity because it is metabolized to phenobarbital.

Phenytoin (Dilantin) is very effective for all types of partial seizures, generalized tonic clonic seizures, and status epilepticus. It is commonly used in fra(X) patients with good results. Its side effects include gingival hyperplasia, hirsutism, acute cerebellar ataxia, and idiosyncratic allergic reactions. It can also lower serum folic acid levels, which is of concern in fra(X) patients because behavioral improvements can be seen with high serum folic acid levels (Hagerman et al. 1986). There is animal evidence that long-term use of phenytoin is associated with cerebellar atrophy, and it has the most significant cognitive effects, including memory and performance deficits, of the commonly used anticonvulsants (Trimble 1987). It is, therefore, not the drug of choice for seizures, but it is certainly an effective alternative drug if carbamazepine is not beneficial. If possible, serum folic acid levels should be brought to the normal range in individuals treated with phenytoin to avoid possible deleterious long-term effects of a lowered folic acid level in fra(X).

Valproic acid (Depakene) is an effective anticonvulsant for absence episodes and major motor seizures, and it is probably effective for partial motor seizures. It may be particularly effective when bilateral and multifocal spikes are present in the EEG. Its mechanism of action is through stimulation of gamma-aminobutyric acid (GABA) neurotransmission, and it has the fewest cognitive or behavioral side effects when compared to other anticonvulsants (Trimble 1987). Its side effects include appetite changes, usually with weight gain, and hair thinning. Stomachaches can be avoided by taking valproic acid after meals. The most serious side effect is hepatic toxicity and pancreatitis. Hepatic failure can occur, with the greatest risk (1 in 500) in young patients treated with multiple drugs (Dreifuss and Langer 1987).

The Treatment of Attention Deficit Hyperactivity Disorder

Attention deficits with or without hyperactivity are significant problems for almost all young fra(X) males and for many cognitively affected females (see chapter 1). Treatment for these problems includes special education with appropriate environmental structure and repetition, as well as individual therapies, such as language therapy and occupational therapy (see chapter 11). Medication, however, can significantly improve attention and concentration, although it is most effective in synergy with educational endeavors.

CNS Stimulants

Stimulants have been used to treat ADHD symptoms since Bradley's report of benzedrine's effectiveness in 1937. A dramatic increase in use occurred in the 1950s associated with the development of other psychotropic medications, including antipsychotics and antidepressants. Although stimulant medication is commonly used for intellectually normal children with ADHD, its use in retarded individuals has generated more caution. Attentional problems are frequent in the mentally retarded because of cognitive deficits (Karrer et al. 1979). Stimulant use is generally not considered helpful in the moderately or severely retarded individual (Aman 1982); however, several studies have demonstrated efficacy in the mildly retarded (Varley and Trupin 1982; Handen et al. 1990; Blacklidge and Ekblad 1971). Gadow and Poling (1988) reported that 7.5% of mildly retarded children are being treated with stimulant medication, which is similar to the rate in schoolchildren in the third grade in Baltimore City schools (Safer and Krager 1988).

The three stimulants that are most commonly used are methylphenidate (Ritalin), dextroamphetamine (Dexedrine), and pemoline (Cylert) (fig. 9.2). All three stimulants work by stimulating dopaminergic and norepinephrine pathways (Raskin et al. 1984). They seem to stimulate inhibitory systems, allowing children to inhibit their responses to extraneous stimuli and stay

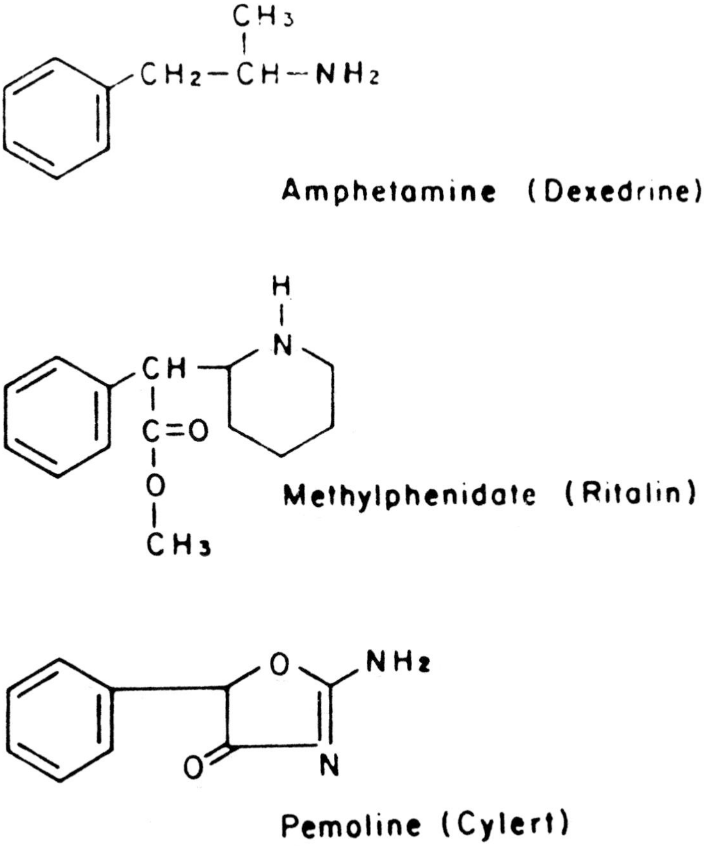

CH₃

Amphetamine (Dexedrine)

Methylphenidate (Ritalin)

Pemoline (Cylert)

Figure 9.2 The chemical structures of CNS stimulants: dextroamphetamine, methylphenidate, and pemoline.

focused on the tasks at hand (Barkley 1977). Improved inhibition can also decrease impulsivity and hyperactivity. The overall effect is a child who is in better control of attention, impulsivity, and hyperactivity. Auditory processing, reaction time, and even sensory integration and visual motor coordination are improved. Douglas et al. (1986) also showed academic improvements, particularly in the accuracy and efficiency of academic tests. The side effects include appetite suppression with possible weight loss which, when excessive, can decrease height growth. The cardiovascular system is also stimulated, including heart rate and blood pressure. Children on stimulant medication should be seen by their physicians at least every six months to monitor height, weight, and cardiovascular parameters. If weight is maintained at its appropriate percentile, height growth is not a problem. Allergic reactions are rare, although pemoline can occasionally cause a skin rash or liver irritation, requiring periodic monitoring of liver function studies. In approximately 10% of ADHD cases, stimulants may exacerbate an underlying tic disorder because of dopaminergic stimulation.

Stimulants are commonly used in young fra(X) boys before the diagnosis of fra(X) syndrome is made. In our clinical population, 38% of fra(X) boys under 13 years of age were treated with stimulants by their regular physicians (Hagerman 1987). A double-blind crossover trial of methylphenidate and dextroamphetamine compared to placebo was carried out in 15 prepubertal fra(X) boys (Hagerman et al. 1988). Ten were clinical responders to stimulants with improvements in attention span and socialization skills; 7 were improved on methylphenidate, and 2 were improved on dextroamphetamine. Dextroamphetamine was not the drug of choice for many because of an increased number of side effects, including mood lability and irritability. In general, fra(X) children are sensitive to stimulants and their mood often becomes brittle with an increase in outbursts at higher doses. For children up to five years old, a starting dose would be 2.5 mg of methylphenidate twice a day. For children older than five years, a methylphenidate dose of 0.2 to 0.3 mg/kg/dose is usually sufficient. An occasional fra(X) male may develop motor tics on stimulants, and then an alternative medication should be used.

In individuals with Tourette syndrome, which involves motor and vocal tics and is often associated with hyperactivity, the tic symptoms may worsen after treatment with stimulants in approximately 30 to 40% (reviewed by Shapiro et al. 1988). Therefore, in fra(X) patients who have motor or vocal tics, stimulants are not the first line treatment for ADHD symptoms.

Tricyclics

Both imipramine and desipramine are effective in the treatment of ADHD symptoms in childhood (Biederman et al. 1986; Pliszka 1987). Comparison studies, however, suggest that they are not as effective as stimulants for impulsivity and attentional problems (Rapoport et al. 1974; Pliszka 1987). Tricyclics are usually given only twice a day, in the morning and in the afternoon or evening. They have an easier dosage schedule and better coverage in the evenings, because of a longer half-life, than methylphenidate. They may also be more effective for the anxious or inhibited child with ADHD (Rapoport et al. 1974). This is important in fra(X) syndrome because anxiety is a significant problem in affected males and females. Very little work has been done in the treatment of retarded individuals with tricyclics (Gadow and Poling 1988); however, the study by Winsberg et al. (1972) is an exception. They evaluated 32 neuropsychiatrically impaired children with an IQ range of 40–113. Thirty-eight percent of this group responded to imipramine only, 13% responded to dextroamphetamine only, and 31% responded to both drugs.

No studies are available concerning the effectiveness of tricyclics in fra(X) patients. We have used tricyclics in fra(X) patients to treat ADHD symptoms when stimulants were unsuccessful. In approximately 50%, there was an increase in aggressive or outburst behavior, although 50% did well. An increase in aggressive behavior with imipramine was reported in nonfra(X) patients (Tec 1963), and such behavior may be exacerbated by the simultaneous use of stimulants.

Fra(X) children with enuresis and tics may benefit significantly from tricyclics. Imipramine has a long history of use for enuresis, and it is the most effective drug for this symptom (Blackwell and Currah 1973). Both imipramine and desipramine usually do not exacerbate tics when used in Tourette syndrome to improve ADHD symptoms (Dillon et al. 1985; Riddle et al. 1988; Hoge and Biederman 1986).

Imipramine has been used successfully in treating agoraphobic adults and in blocking panic attacks (Klein 1964), and it may, therefore, be helpful for heterozygous females who suffer from these problems, although other anxiolytic agents are also available. Imipramine's antianxiety effects have also been used in the treatment of school phobia in children (Gittelman-Klein and Klein 1971). Although tricyclics may lower the convulsive threshold, they usually do not exacerbate seizures and in some cases they have been used as an adjunct to other anticonvulsants.

The dosages used to treat ADHD symptoms, 1–3 mg/kg/day or 10–50 mg/day, are lower than the dosages used to treat depression, 3–5 mg/kg/day. Tricyclics stimulate norepinephrine transmission and may also potentiate serotonin transmission (Gualtieri 1977). They have anticholinergic side effects, including increased blood pressure, dry mouth, constipation, blurred vision, and appetite changes, although these are usually minor and transitory symptoms. A significant toxic effect, which includes prolongation of conduction time leading to arrhythmias, occurs in the myocardium. Regular monitoring with electrocardiograms (ECGs) is essential at higher doses, and safety precautions are important to avoid accidental overdoses. Serum levels of these medications should be followed.

Clonidine

Clonidine (Catapres) is an antihypertensive drug (Manheim et al. 1982) that is effective in the treatment of ADHD (Hunt et al. 1985). It has also been used to treat Tourette syndrome by reducing tics (Leckman et al. 1985). Clonidine is an alpha-adrenergic stimulating agent that acts on presynaptic alpha-neurons to inhibit norepinephrine activity (fig. 9.3). Norepinephrine mediates the expression of anxiety that occurs during phobic or panic states, and it also seems to mediate shifts in cognition, which are problematic in perseveration. Hunt et al.

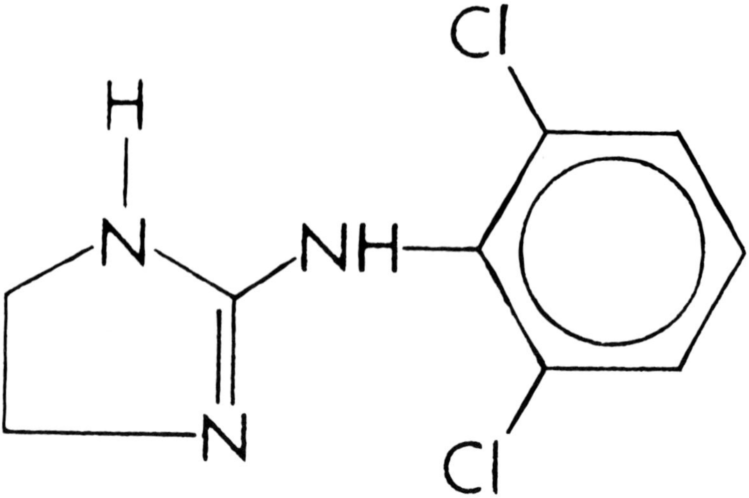

Figure 9.3 The chemical structure of clonidine

(1985) suggested that clonidine may be most beneficial in children with ADHD, who are easily emotionally overwhelmed, are anxious, and have a low frustration tolerance. Clonidine also stimulates growth hormone release (Leckman et al. 1984), so it may be helpful in treating the ADHD of fra(X) children with short stature. Leckman (1987) reported improved ADHD symptoms in three fra(X) males treated with clonidine. Three children completed a controlled trial comparing clonidine, methylphenidate, and placebo, and clonidine was the most effective medication in all three (F. Bregman, S. Ort, and J. F. Leckman, Controlled study of ritalin, clonidine and placebo, personal communication, 1989). In our experience with Tourette patients, clonidine was not as effective in improving attention span and concentration as was methylphenidate. However, in a young fra(X) boy, clonidine was used successfully in the afternoon, with methylphenidate in the morning and at lunchtime. Clonidine helped to alleviate mood lability in the late afternoon caused by stimulants, and it improved ADHD symptoms at home, where a lesser degree of concentration was demanded than at school.

The side effects of clonidine include sleepiness, which is dose dependent and usually subsides within three weeks after the medication is begun. The dose should be started low at 0.05 mg b.i.d. and gradually increased over two to three weeks to clinical effectiveness (approximately 4–5 µg/kg/day for school-aged children). Blood pressure and heart rate should be monitored and a follow-up ECG done because clonidine can also slow cardiac conduction time. Symptomatic hypotension rarely occurs in children. When clonidine is discontinued, the dose should be tapered gradually to avoid a significant increase in blood pressure and severe headaches, which may occur with abrupt withdrawal.

Folic Acid

Folic acid was the first medication reported to be beneficial for fra(X) individuals (Lejeune 1982). When added to tissue culture media, folate will decrease cytogenetic expression of the fragile site (see chapter 3). However, its mechanism of action in the central nervous system is probably unrelated to its cytogenetic effect. Preliminary reports from Lejeune (1982) and others (Harpey 1982; Lacassie et al. 1984; Lejeune et al. 1984) anecdotally demonstrated improvement in behavior and development in fra(X) males treated with folic acid. Subsequent controlled studies showed mixed results, with some reporting no benefit from folic acid (Rosenblatt et al. 1985; Froster-Iskenius et al. 1986; Madison et al. 1986; Brown et al. 1986; Fisch et al. 1988), whereas others demonstrated improvement with folic acid treatment (Carpenter et al. 1983; Brown et al. 1984; Gustavson et al. 1985; Gillberg et al. 1986; Hagerman et al. 1986; for review see Aman and Kern 1990).

Clearly, not all fra(X) patients respond to folic acid, but a significant number of prepubertal fra(X) boys are reported by their families to be less hyperactive and to have a better attention span. The cognitive improvements seen in young fra(X) boys by Hagerman et al. (1986) seem to be the result of improvement in attention span and concentration. The effect of folic acid is similar to the response noted with stimulant medication, although the latter usually causes a more dramatic improvement in attention. A rare patient will become more hyperactive on folate, and an occasional fra(X) adult will have more outbursts on folate. It is, therefore, not recommended for adult patients, who are less frequently plagued by hyperactivity.

Improvements in speech, language, and motor coordination are also occasionally reported by parents when their children are taking folic acid. The effectiveness of folic acid has been difficult to document in controlled studies; if a child responds to folate, however, parents insist on using it. As many parents are adamant about its effectiveness, perhaps future studies should focus on identifying the subgroup of fra(X) children who respond. There is no evidence for a metabolic defect in folate metabolism in fra(X) syndrome (Brondum-Nielsen et al. 1983; Wang and Erbe 1984). Its mechanism of action in the CNS is unknown, but it is probably not specific to fra(X) syndrome. There is one report of a fra(X) child who deteriorated behaviorally and developmentally after treatment with trimethoprim, an antibiotic that interferes with the metabolism of folic acid (Hecht and Glover 1983). Therefore, caution should be used in treating fra(X) patients with drugs that lower folate levels, including phenytoin.

Folate has been tolerated without significant side effects in dosages as high as 250 mg and 1000 mg/day (Brown et al. 1986; Zettner et al. 1981). However, Hunter et al. (1970) reported malaise, sleep problems, irritability, and an increased activity level when folate was given to normal, healthy volunteers. Folate has been reported to exacerbate the frequency of seizures in epilepsy (Reynolds 1967), but we have not experienced this problem in fra(X) patients with seizures. Folate treatment should be avoided, however, in patients with poorly controlled seizures. It may occasionally result in loose stools and can prolong diarrhea in children recovering from gastroenteritis. If diarrhea occurs, the dose of folate should be lowered or discontinued until the diarrhea resolves. We reported vitamin B_6 deficiency in fra(X) males taking 10 mg of folic acid per day (Hagerman et al. 1986). To avoid this problem, patients should take daily a multiple vitamin with B_6 while on folic acid therapy. Folate can also interfere with zinc absorption in the intestine, and serum levels should therefore be monitored once or twice a year (Milne et al. 1984).

Folic acid is manufactured only in 1-mg tablets in the United States; a liquid preparation of 5 mg/ml is more convenient and less expensive than the tablet form. Most patients who respond will demonstrate improvement on a dose of 10 to 50 mg/day. Many pharmacies will prepare the liquid preparation after a special request. Pharmacies can obtain folic acid powder U.S.P.-N.F through Tanabe U.S.A., Inc. (619-571-8410) or Apothecary Products, Inc. (1-800-328-2742). The following formula can be used to mix the folic acid solution to a dilution of 5 mg/ml (provided by Rob Rodgers, Pharm.D., at The Children's Hospital in Denver, Colorado): 10 g folic acid, 2000 ml H_2O (sterile), 15 ml NaOH 20%—add by titration until mixture clarifies in solution. Folic acid solution is sensitive to heat and photodegradation, and it must be refrigerated and protected from light in a covered or brown bottle. A syringe can be used to measure a typical dose of 5 mg or 1 ml twice a day. As folic acid is relatively tasteless, it can be squirted directly in the mouth or added to juice. The dose is usually given twice a day to avoid stomach irritation or diarrhea, which occasionally occurs.

The medical follow-up of patients treated with high dose folic acid includes a periodic physical and neurologic examination and at least annual blood work including a complete blood count (CBC); serum glutamic-oxaloacetic transaminase (SGOT); blood urea nitrogen (BUN); creatinine; urine analysis; serum levels of zinc, vitamin B_6, and folate; and red blood cell folate levels. A trial of folic acid therapy should last at least three months because improvements in behavior or attention may not begin until the second month. If folate is helpful, it should be continued, and it can be used together with stimulant medication. At least once every one to two years, the folic acid can be discontinued to assess whether it remains effective. There is some evidence to suggest a mild withdrawal effect in a limited number of patients, characterized by mood lability lasting one to two weeks. This is not uncommon in megavitamin therapy, and it has been described in pyridoxine and ascorbic acid therapy (American Psychiatric Association 1973; Gualtieri et al. 1987).

Fenfluramine

Fenfluramine (Pondimin), used to treat obesity, is an appetite suppressant. Its structure is similar to that of the amphetamines. Fenfluramine has also been reported to improve behavior in autistic patients, including hyperactivity, social awareness, and repetitive behaviors (Ritvo et al. 1986). However, multicenter trials have not shown consistent improvement with fenfluramine. A response rate as high as 33% has been reported, but some centers have shown no response (Ritvo et al. 1986). As with folic acid, there seems to be a subgroup of patients who respond to fenfluramine.

Reiss et al. (1988) treated seven autistic patients, one of whom was a seven-year-old fra(X) boy, with fenfluramine at a dose of 1.5 mg/kg/day in a double-blind fashion with placebo. There was a variable response to fenfluramine, and the fra(X) patient improved initially in social interactions, but this improvement was not sustained nor did hyperactivity improve. Further studies should be done before fenfluramine can be recommended.

The Treatment of Aggressive Behavior and Violent Outbursts

Beta-blockers

Propranolol (Inderal) is a beta-adrenergic blocking agent used primarily for treatment of cardiac disorders, including angina and hypertension (fig. 9.4). A number of studies have also shown propranolol to be effective in the treatment of aggressive behavior and intermittent explosive disorder (Williams et al. 1982; Ratey et al. 1983; Jenkins and Maruta 1987). The latter problem has also been termed *episodic dyscontrol* and is described as repeated discrete episodes of loss of control of aggression, disproportionate to the triggering event, with otherwise normal or nonaggressive behavior between episodes (Jenkins and Maruta 1987). Most patients with this symptom complex have some type of organic diagnosis, including traumatic brain damage, minimal brain dysfunction, or mental retardation. Approximately one-half to one-third have clinical seizures, and a decline in seizure frequency with propranolol has been reported (Williams et al. 1982). Intermittent explosive disorder is common in adult fra(X) men, as described in chapter 1. Episodic and unpredictable violence is a common reason for institutionalization of these men and, therefore, pharmacologic control is of critical importance. If there is an abnormal EEG with

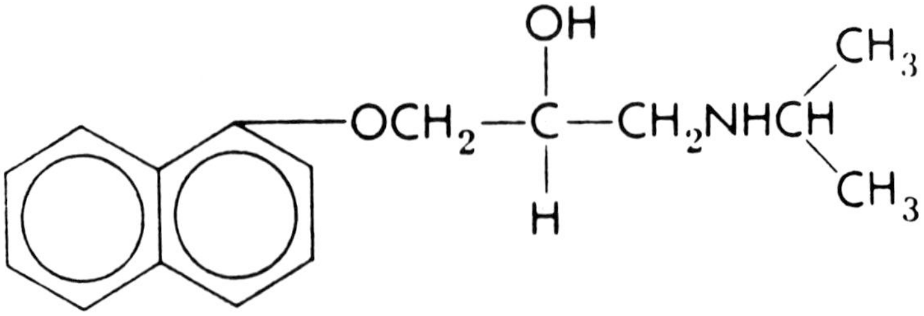

Propranolol

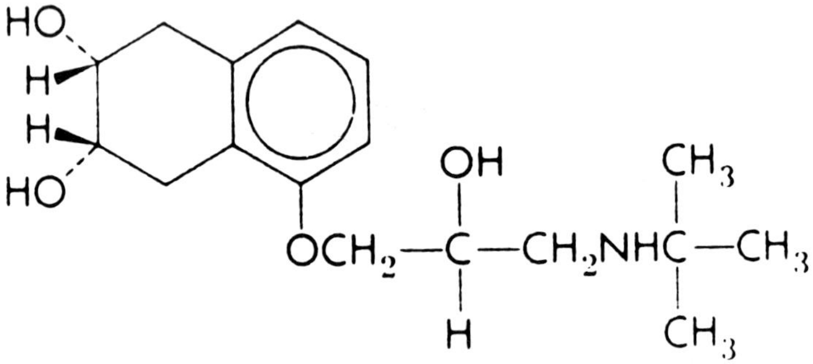

Nadolol

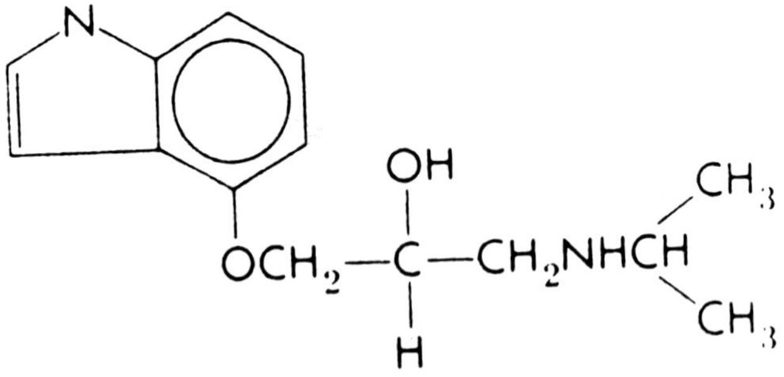

Pindolol

Figure 9.4 The chemical structures of beta-blockers: propranolol, nadolol, and pindolol.

spike/wave discharges, particularly in the temporal region, trial of an anticonvulsant such as carbamazepine is appropriate, as previously discussed. Propranolol is an additional option, although controlled studies have not been performed with fra(X) patients; however, significant experience with nonfra(X) patients has been reported.

Williams et al. (1982) studied one of the largest series of children, adolescents, and adults with violent behavior and found that 75% responded to propranolol in dosages of 50–1,600 mg/day (mean, 160 mg/day). Silver and Yudofsky (1985) outlined a treatment protocol that begins with 20 mg three times a day in adolescents and adults. The dose is gradually increased every other day until there is a beta-blocking response (pulse decrease below 55 beats/min or blood pressure less than 90/50) or improved behavior is achieved. If no response is achieved, a dosage of 640 mg/day in adults is maintained for four to six weeks. The response time may be two to six weeks before improvement is seen. Often a threshold level of propranolol is reached and a dramatic response is seen. Propranolol may interact with antipsychotic agents to increase their plasma levels. Thioridazine levels, in particular, may increase three to five times when propranolol is used simultaneously (Silver and Yudofsky 1985). Propranolol is contraindicated in patients with diabetes, asthma, or any other condition that is worsened with beta-blockers.

Newer generation beta-blockers, such as naldolol (Corgard) or pindolol, have also been effective in intermittent explosive disorder, with fewer side effects (Polakoff et al. 1986; Greendyke and Kanter 1986). Ratey et al. (1987) also showed that autistic patients may respond to propranolol or naldolol with an improvement in speech and communication abilities. They hypothesized that beta-blockers decrease hyperarousal and anxiety in these patients, allowing improved language and social behaviors.

Thioridazine

Thioridazine (Mellaril) is the neuroleptic medication most widely used in the mentally retarded. It is in the piperidine subclass of the phenothiazines, and it is most commonly used to treat aggressive behavior or hyperactivity (Gadow and Poling 1988; Aman and White 1988). The treatment for hyperactivity with neuroleptics is frequently associated with cognitive and academic impairment, unlike the treatment with stimulant medication. Therefore, thioridazine is not a first-line drug for ADHD symptoms; however, it has been shown to be beneficial in reducing stereotypies and self-injurious behavior (reviewed by Aman and Singh 1980).

No studies of the usefulness of thioridazine in fra(X) patients have been published, but in our experience it is commonly used for behavior problems in adults, particularly for aggression. It is probably chosen because it has a lower risk of extrapyramidal side effects compared to other neuroleptics. The extrapyramidal syndromes (EPSs), which are rarely seen with thioridazine, include akathisia or involuntary motor restlessness; tardive dyskinesia or rhythmic repetitive stereotypic movements, including sucking or smacking movements of the lips; parkinsonian syndrome or a decrease in spontaneous movements, mask-like facial expression, and tremor; and acute dystonic reactions including facial grimacing, torticollis, or oculogyric crisis (fixed upward gaze). With many neuroleptics, these findings can be seen in 20% of patients, and they are common with high dose, long-term use. Thioridazine has other side effects, including sedation, appetite enhancement, and anticholinergic effects, such as a dry mouth and orthostatic hypotension, which become more significant at higher doses.

Thioridazine has an antipsychotic effect in that delusions, hallucinations, loosening of associations, and inappropriate affect may also improve. Although psychosis or schizophrenia is not common in fra(X), it does occur and can be improved by antipsychotic medication (see chapter 1). A good response to low dose chlorpromazine was reported in a 15-year-old boy with fragile X who experienced a sudden onset of psychotic experiences including persecutory delusions, loosening of thought associations, and extreme anxiety in associa- tion with intercurrent stresses at home and school. Commencement of oral chlorpromazine (25 mg t.i.d.) led to entire symptom resolution within five days, with no significant side effects (J. Turk, personal communication, 1990). Further treatment trials of other neuroleptics are warranted when psychosis occurs.

A new atypical antipsychotic, clozapine (Clozaril), does not produce EPSs and, in fact, has been used to treat tardive dyskinesia. However, significant hematopoietic side effects occur, and 3% of patients can have a decrease in the white blood count. Clozapine is undergoing further studies in adults and has not yet been used with fragile X individuals, but it marks the beginning of an age of antipsychotics without EPS side effects. A further recent development in anti- psychotic medication is demonstrated by sulpiride, a substituted benzamide similar to metoclopramide. Specific dopamine-2 receptor activity allows for beneficial effects on abnormal beliefs and experiences while minimizing par- kinsonian side effects and sedation. Despite its relative expense, it has gained popularity in Europe because of its lack of adverse effects and its reported low incidence of tardive dyskinesia (J. Turk, personal communication, 1990).

Case History

RJ is one of twins delivered two months prematurely with a birth weight of $2\frac{1}{2}$ pounds. He required O_2 for the first few weeks of life, but he was never ventilated. He walked at 2 years and said words and phrases between 3 and 4 years. He received speech and language and occupational therapy in pre- school and special education programs throughout school. Fra(X) syndrome was diagnosed at 13 years of age when cytogenetic studies revealed 40% of 100 lymphocytes with the fra(X) chromosome.

Throughout childhood his speech was perseverative and he mumbled frequently. He was tactilely defensive, avoided cuddling, and intermittently bit his hand until 7 years of age. During childhood and adolescence he frequently demonstrated habits such as finger rubbing and more recently popping his jaw. Facial grimacing and inappropriate smiling also occurred throughout childhood. He was noted to have an occasional staring spell after 5 years of age. He was not hyperactive, but attention problems were an ongoing difficulty for him in school. In high school, he made progress in reading, but his math achievement was severely deficient.

At age 17, he was noted to have frequent episodes of prolonged staring, jerking of his left hand, and unusual facial expressions, including grimacing and smiling, lasting one minute or less but occurring several times a day. His mother also described him as "spacey" on frequent occasions during the day, as if he was in a world of his own and not in touch with reality. He would laugh inappropriately, have conversations with himself, and frequently appeared disoriented. His school progress deteriorated, as did his behavior.

On physical examination his height was at the twentieth percentile, weight was at the eighth percentile, and head circumference was at the sixtieth percentile for his age. His face was long and narrow, and his ears were mildly prominent. His palate was high, and cardiac examination demonstrated a systolic click without a murmur. Tanner stage III pubic hair development with a testicular volume of 25 ml bilaterally was seen. The extremities had hyperextensible finger joints with metacarpophalangeal (MP) extension to >90°. Muscle strength was normal, and deep tendon reflexes were 2+ in the upper and lower extremities. After the examination, while seated, RJ had an episode of tonic deviation of his head and left hand and left arm jerking lasting 10 seconds.

WAIS-R testing was notable for several episodes of staring followed by disorientation, inappropriate behavior, and unusual sensations, both visual and auditory. His verbal IQ was 60, performance IQ was 65, and full scale IQ was 62. His EEG was normal in the waking state, and a sleep record could not be obtained. A magnetic resonance imaging (MRI) scan demonstrated a small porencephalic cyst adjacent to the basal ganglia on the left, presumably secondary to an old ischemic event. Emotional evaluation documented hallucinations and an impending psychotic process complicated by probable seizures.

RJ was treated with carbamazepine (Tegretol) with a gradual increase in his dose until a therapeutic level was reached at 800 mg/day. He responded with a significant decrease in his partial motor seizures, but episodes of detachment from daily events continued. Thioridazine (Mellaril) was started at 25 mg twice a day, and his mother noted a remarkable improvement in reality orientation, socialization, and school work. He has continued to do well with only rare episodes of staring spells or daydreaming.

This case is unusual for fra(X) syndrome because the partial motor seizures worsened in adolescence and may have been associated with the anatomic abnormality of the porencephalic cyst. The ischemic brain damage probably occurred in utero or during the neonatal period. The psychotic behavior was associated with seizures but did not improve with anticonvulsants alone. The addition of thioridazine was associated with significant clinical improvement, even at a relatively low dose. The patient's clinical history also suggests motor tics including simple grimacing and more complex movements with his hands. His bursts of inappropriate laughter may be related to complex vocal tics or to the psychotic process, although such laughter is also seen in nonpsychotic patients.

Lithium

Lithium is used to treat both mood disorders and aggressive behavior in the mentally retarded (Gadow and Poling 1988). Although it has been used most effectively to treat manic depression in intellectually normal individuals, several studies have demonstrated its effectiveness in improving aggressive behavior or violent outbursts in mentally retarded individuals who do not suffer from depression or bipolar disease (Naylor et al. 1974; Dale 1980). It has also been used to reduce aggressive behavior in prisoners and delinquents who are not retarded (Sheard 1975; Sheard et al. 1976; Tupin et al. 1973).

Lithium carbonate is a salt whose exact mechanism of action is unknown. Its side effects involve the kidney, causing polyuria and electrolyte abnormalities because of diuresis. At higher levels (serum levels > 1.0 meq/L), sedation, ataxia, and a clouded sensorium occur. Serum levels must be monitored regularly to avoid toxicity. There is anecdotal evidence suggesting that maintenance at the low end of the therapeutic range may be sufficient to control aggressive behavior. Renal function studies (BUN, creatinine) and electrolytes should be monitored regularly. Long-term lithium treatment may also affect thyroid function, which should be monitored yearly.

Controlled studies have not been performed to evaluate lithium's effectiveness in fra(X) syndrome. However, anecdotal experience suggests that it is effective even at relatively low doses in the treatment of aggressive or violent behavior in fra(X) syndrome. We treated eight adult fra(X) men for these symptoms and found a beneficial effect beginning at serum levels of 0.4 meq/L in seven of these eight patients. The clinical effect is a decrease in anxiety and a decrease in the reactivity of the patient to stimuli that usually precipitate an outburst. Side effects are rare at low serum levels.

New Directions

The treatment of obsessive-compulsive disorder (OCD) has advanced significantly during the last few years, and new and effective medications, including
clomipramine (Anafranil), have moved from the experimental stage to clinical
availability. Clomipramine is a tricyclic, but it is relatively selective for serotonin pathways (Rapoport 1988). Many fra(X) individuals have significant problems with obsessive or compulsive behavior, although it may be difficult to
differentiate from perseverative behavior. Further work is needed to clarify
OCD symptoms in fra(X) and whether OCD medication would be helpful for
these symptoms.

No controlled studies of the pharmacologic therapy of depression or anxiety
in heterozygous females or affected males are yet available (chapter 1). Fluoxetine (Prozac), a relatively new antidepressant, causes fewer problems with
toxicity than do tricyclic antidepressants and is also helpful for mild OCD
symptoms that may complicate depression. Although anecdotal experience
suggests promise for its use in depressed heterozygotes, further studies are
required to clarify its efficacy. It may also turn out to be a helpful medication for
agitation and eating disorders in retarded patients, although it has been studied
only in dementia (Sabin 1989). If used in retarded individuals, it should be
started cautiously at a low dose, such as 20 mg every other day, to avoid
overstimulation initially (H. Crabbe, personal communication, 1990). Dr. An-
drew Levitas (personal communication, 1990) reported an adult fra(X) man
with depression who demonstrated remarkable improvement in his depression,
expressive language, and behavior on fluoxetine.

Anxiety is a problem for many cognitively normal heterozygotes and affected males. Further work is necessary to clarify the extent of this problem and
effective medications. Benzodiazepines, including alprazolam (Xanax) and
clonazepam (Klonopin), have been used frequently in adults, but the latter can
occasionally cause a paradoxical reaction with an increase in agitation. Both
drugs can block panic attacks, but they cause sedation and withdrawal effects.
A newer anxiolytic agent, buspirone (Buspar), does not cause physical dependence or sedation and is not related to benzodiazepines. It has affinity for
serotonin receptors, but it may take three to four weeks for maximal efficacy
and it does not block panic attacks (Jann 1988). Ratey et al. (1989) found that 9
of 14 individuals with a variety of developmental disabilities responded to
buspirone with reduction of anxiety and maladaptive behavior including aggression, hyperactivity, and self-injurious behavior. Information is not available concerning its efficacy in patients with fra(X) syndrome.

Treatment of self-injurious behavior (SIB) is difficult because no single
medication has been consistently effective. Naltrexone has had variable results
but has recently been reported to be most effective at lower doses in a group of

autistic children including one boy with fragile X syndrome (Leboyer 1990). Naltrexone deserves further study for SIB in fragile X patients.

Finally, an antiviral agent, amantadine (Symmetril), is also a dopaminergic agent that is proving to be helpful for aggressive behavior and agitation in individuals with developmental disabilities. However, formal studies have been performed only on head-injured patients (Gualtieri et al. 1989), and in hyperactive mentally retarded persons with a response rate of approximately 40% (Gualtieri 1990). One young fra(X) boy showed significant improvement in aggressive and oppositional behavior on amatidine (T. Gualtieri 1991, personal communication). These and other new medications hold promise for effective pharmacologic intervention in fra(X) syndrome.

Conclusions

The fra(X) patient usually presents with an array of physical and behavioral problems that require monitoring and treatment. Medical complications associated with the syndrome require detection and early treatment. Although no cure is available, several medication possibilities have been presented and can be used to treat specific behavior problems. Although some fra(X) patients have not required psychopharmacologic intervention, many have benefited from one or more of the medications discussed. If behavior problems exist, an appropriate medication trial should be considered in conjunction with additional intervention discussed in chapters 10 and 11. Further research is necessary to clarify the most effective medication options in children and adults with the fra(X) syndrome.

References

Aman, M. G. 1982. Stimulant drug effects in developmental disorders and hyperactivity: Toward a resolution of disparate findings. *J. Autism Dev. Disord.* 12:385–398.

Aman, M. G., and R. A. Kern. 1990. The efficacy of folic acid in the developmental disabilities. *J. Child. Adolesc. Pscyopharm.* In press.

Aman, M. G., and N. N. Singh. 1980. The usefulness of thioridazine for treating childhood disorders—fact or folklore? *Am. J. Ment. Defic.* 84:331–338.

Aman, M. G., and A. J. White. 1988. Thioridazine dose effects with reference to stereotypic behavior in mentally retarded residents. *J. Autism Dev. Disord.* 18:355–366.

American Psychiatric Association. 1973. *APA task force on vitamin therapy in psychiatry: Mega vitamin and ortho molecular therapy in psychiatry.* Washington, D.C.

Barkley, R. A. 1977. A review of stimulant drug research with hyperactive children. *J. Child Psychiatry* 18:137–165.

Berkheimer, J. L., J. L. Curtis, and M. W. Lann. 1985. Use of carbamazepine in psychiatric disorders. *Clin. Pharm.* 4:425–434.

Biederman, J., D. R. Gastfriend, and M. S. Jellinek. 1986. Desipramine in the treatment of children with attention deficit disorder. *J. Clin. Psychopharmacol.* 6:359–363.

Blacklidge, V., and R. L. Ekblad. 1971. The effectiveness of methylphenidate hydrochloride (Ritalin) on learning and behavior in public school educable mentally retarded children. *Pediatrics* 47:923–926.

Blackwell, B., and J. Currah. 1973. The psychopharmacology of nocturnal enuresis. In I. Kalvin, R. C. MacKeith, and S. R. Meadow (eds.), *Bladder control and enuresis.* London: Heinemann, pp. 231–257.

Bradley, C. 1937. The behavior of children receiving benzedrine. *Am. J. Psychiatry* 94:557–585.

Brondum-Nielsen, K., N. Tommerup, B. Frilis, K. Hjelt, and E. Hippe. 1983b. Folic acid metabolism in a patient with fragile X. *Clin. Genet.* 24:153–155.

Brown, W. T., E. C. Jenkins, E. Friedman, J. Brooks, I. L. Cohen, C. Duncan, A. L. Hill, M. N. Malik, V. Morris, E. Wolf, K. Wisniewski, and J. H. French. 1984. Folic acid therapy in the fragile X syndrome. *Am. J. Med. Genet.* 17:289–297.

Brown, W. T., I. L. Cohen, G. S. Fisch, E. Wolf, V. A. Jenkins, M. N. Milik, and E. C. Jenkins. 1986. High dose folic acid treatment of fragile(X) males. *Am. J. Med. Genet.* 23:263–271.

Carpenter, N. J., D. H. Barber, M. Jones, W. Lindley, and C. Carr. 1983. Controlled six-month study of oral folic acid therapy in boys with fragile X-linked mental retardation, abstract 243. *Am. J. Hum. Genet.* 35(suppl.):82A.

Conners, C. K. 1973. Rating scales for use in drug studies with children. *Psychopharmacol. Bull.* special issue, pp. 24–84, 219–222.

Dale, P. G. 1980. Lithium therapy in aggressive mentally subnormal patients. *Br. J. Psychiatry* 137:469–474.

Dillon, D. C., I. J. Salzman, and D. A. Schulsinger. 1985. The use of imipramine in Tourette's syndrome and attention deficit disorder: Case report. *J. Clin. Psychiatry* 46:348–349.

Dodson, E. W. 1989. Medical treatment and pharmacology of antiepileptic drugs. *Pediatr. Clin. North Am.* 36:421–433.

Douglas, V. I., R. G. Barr, M. E. O'Neill, and B. G. Britton. 1986. Short term effects of methylphenidate on the cognitive, learning and academic performance of children with attention deficit disorder in the laboratory and in the classroom. *J. Child Psychol. Psychiatry* 27:191–211.

Dreifuss, F. E., and D. H. Langer. 1987. Hepatic considerations in the use of antiepileptic drugs. *Epilepsia* 28(Suppl. 2):S23.

Evans, R. W., and C. T. Gualtieri. 1985. Carbamazepine neurophysiological and psychiatric profile. *Clin. Neuropharmacol.* 8:221–241.

Fisch, G. S., I. L. Cohen, A. C. Gross, V. Jenkins, E. C. Jenkins, and W. T. Brown. 1988. Folic acid treatment of fragile X males: A further study. *Am. J. Med. Genet.* 30:393–399.

Froster-Iskenius, U., K. Bodeker, T. Oepen, R. Matthes, U. Piper, and E. Schwinger.

1986. Folic acid treatment in males and females with fragile(X) syndrome. *Am. J. Med. Genet.* 23:273–289.

Fryns, J. P., P. Moerman, F. Gilis, L. d'Espallier, and H. Van den Berghe. 1988. Suggestively increased incidence of sudden death in children of fra(X) positive mothers. *Am. J. Med. Genet.* 30:73–75.

Gadow, K. D., and A. G. Poling. 1988. *Pharmacotherapy and mental retardation.* Boston: College Hill Press.

Gillberg, C., J. Wahlstrom, R. Johansson, M. Tornblom, and K. Albertsson-Wikland. 1986. Folic acid as an adjunct in the treatment of children with the autism fragile X syndrome (A FRA X). *Dev. Med. Child Neurol.* 28:624–627.

Gittelman-Klein, R., and D. F. Klein. 1971. Controlled imipramine treatment of school phobia. *Arch. Gen. Psychiatry* 25:204–207.

Greendyke, R. M., and D. R. Kanter. 1986. Therapeutic effects of pindolol on behavioral disturbances associated with organic brain disease: A double blind study. *J. Clin. Psychiatry* 47:423–426.

Gualtieri, C. T. 1977. Imipramine and children: A review and some speculations about the mechanism of drug action. *Dis. Nerv. Syst.* 38:368–375.

Gualtieri, C. T., R. W. Evans, and D. R. Patterson. 1987. The medical treatment of autistic people: Problems and side effects. In E. Shopler and G. Mesibov (eds.), *Neurobiological issues in autism.* New York: Plenum Publishing.

Gualtieri, C. T., M. Chandler, T. B. Coons, and L. T. Brown. 1989. Amantadine: A new clinical profile for traumatic brain injury. *Clin. Neuropharmacol.* 12:258–270.

Gualtieri, C. T. 1990. *Neuropsychiatry and behavioral pharmacology.* Berlin: Springer-Verlag.

Gustavson, K. H., K. Dahlblom, A. Flood, G. Holmgren, H. K. Blomquist, and G. Sanner. 1985. Effect of folic acid treatment in fragile X syndrome. *Clin. Genet.* 27:463–467.

Hagerman, R. J. 1984. Pediatric assessment of the learning disabled child. *J. Dev. Behav. Pediatr.* 5:274–284.

———. 1987. Fragile X syndrome. *Curr. Probl. Pediatr.* 11:627–674.

———. 1990. Growth and development. In W. Hathaway, J. R. Groothuis, W. Hay, J. Paisley (eds.), *Current pediatric diagnosis and treatment.* Hartford, Conn.: Appleton and Lange, pp. 8–28.

Hagerman, R. J., A. W. Jackson, A. Levitas, B. Rimland, and M. Braden. 1986. Oral folic acid versus placebo in the treatment of males with the fragile X syndrome. *Am. J. Med. Genet.* 23:241–262.

Hagerman, R. J., D. Altshul-Stark, and P. McBogg. 1987. Recurrent otitis media in boys with the fragile X syndrome. *Am. J. Dis. Child.* 141:184–187.

Hagerman, R. J., M. Murphy, and M. Wittenberger. 1988. A controlled trial of stimulant medication in children with fragile X syndrome. *Am. J. Med. Genet.* 30:377–392.

Harpey, J. P. 1982. Treatment of fragile X. Letter. *Pediatrics* 69:670.

Harden, B. L., A. M. Breaux, A. Gosling, D. L. Ploof, and H. Feldman. 1990. Efficacy of methylphemalate among mentally retarded children with attention deficit hyperactivity disorder. *Pediatrics* 86:922–930.

Hartman, N., R. Kramer, W. T. Brown, and R. B. Devereux. 1982. Panic disorder in patients with mitral valve prolapse. *Am. J. Psychiatry* 139:669–670.

Hecht, F., and T. W. Glover. 1983. Antibiotics containing trimethoprim and the fragile X chromosome. Letter. *N. Engl. J. Med.* 308:285.

Hoge, S. K., and J. Biederman. 1986. A case of Tourette's syndrome with symptoms of attention deficit disorder treated with desipramine. *J. Clin. Psychiatry* 47:478–479.

Hunt, R. D., R. B. Mindera, and D. J. Cohen. 1985. Clonidine benefits children with attentional deficit disorder and hyperactivity. *J. Am. Acad. Child Adolesc. Psychiatry* 24:617–629.

Hunter, R., J. Barnes, H. F. Oakeley, and D. M. Matthews. 1970. Toxicity of folic acid given in pharmacological doses to healthy volunteers. *Lancet* 1:61–63.

Jann, M. 1988. Buspirone: An update on a unique anxiolytic agent. *Pharmacotherapy* 8:100–116.

Jenkins, S. C., and T. Maruta. 1987. Therapeutic use of propranolol for intermittent explosive disorder. *Mayo Clin. Proc.* 62:204–214.

Karrer, R., M. Nelson, and G. C. Galbraith. 1979. Psychophysiological research with the mentally retarded. In N. R. Ellis (ed.), *Handbook of mental deficiency, psychological theory and research*, 2nd ed. Hillsdale, N J.: L. Erlbaum Associates, pp. 231–288.

Kendall, P. C., and J. Braswell. 1986. Medical applications of cognitive-behavioral interventions with children. *J. Dev. Behav. Pediatr.* 7:257–264.

Klein, D. F. 1964. Delineation of two drug responsive anxiety syndromes. *Psychopharmacology (Berlin)* 5:397–408.

Lacassie, Y., B. Curotto, M. A. Alliende, I. de Andraca, and A. Zavala. 1984. Evaluacion preliminar del tratamiento con acido folico en dos pacientes con retraso mental ligado al sexo y macroorquidismo. *Rev. Med. Chil.* 112:469–473.

Langee, H. R. 1989. A retrospective study of mentally retarded patients with behavior disorders who were treated with carbamazepine. *Am. J. Ment. Retard.* 93:640–643.

Leboyer, M. 1990. A double blind study of naltrexone in infantile autism. Presented at the Consensus Conference on Biological Basis & Clinical Perspective in Autism, Troina, La Citta dell'Oasi, Sicilia, October 19, 1990.

Leckman, J. F., D. J. Cohen, J. M. Dertner, S. Ort, and D. F. Harcherik. 1984. Growth hormone response to clonidine in children age 4–17: Tourette's syndrome vs. children with short stature. *J. Am. Acad. Child Psychiatry* 23:174–181.

Leckman, J. F. 1987. Medications in fragile X children. Presented at the 1st National Fragile X Conference, Denver, Colo., December 3–4.

Leckman, J. F., J. Detlor, D. F. Harcherik, S. Ort, B. A. Shaywitz, and D. J. Cohen. 1985. Short and long-term treatment of Tourette's syndrome with clonidine: A clinical perspective. *Neurology* 35:343–351.

Lejeune, J. 1982. Is the fragile X syndrome amenable to treatment? Letter. *Lancet* 1:273–274.

Lejeune, J., M.-O. Rethore, M. C. de Blois, and A. Ravel. 1984. Assay of folic acid treatment in fragile-X syndrome. *Ann. Genet.* 27:230–232.

Madison, L. S., T. E. Wells, T. E. Fristo, and C. G. Benesch. 1986. A controlled study of folic acid treatment in 3 fragile X syndrome males. *J. Dev. Behav. Pediatr.* 7:253–256.

Manheim, D., L. Paalzow, and B. Hokfelt. 1982. Plasma clonidine in relation to blood pressure, catecholamines, and renin activity during long-term treatment of hypertension. *Clin. Pharmacol. Ther.* 31:445–451.

Milne, D. B., W. K. Canfield, J. R. Mahalko, and H. H. Sandstead. 1984. Effect of oral folic acid supplements on zinc, copper and iron absorption and excretion. *Am. J. Clin. Nutr.* 39:535–539.

Musumeci, S. A., R. J. Hagerman, K. Amiri, and A. Cronister. 1991. Epilepsy, EEG findings and associated complaints in fragile X syndrome. Submitted for publication.

Naylor, G. T., J. M. Donald, D. Le Poidevin, and A. H. Reid. 1974. A double-blind trial of long-term lithium therapy in mental defectives. *Br. J. Psychiatry* 124:52–57.

Pellock, J. M. 1987. Carbamazepine side effects in children and adults. *Epilepsia* 28(Suppl. 3):S64-S70.

Pippenger, C. E. 1987. Clinically significant carbamazepine drug interactions: An overview. *Epilepsia* 28(Suppl. 3):S71-S76.

Pliszka, S. R. 1987. Tricyclic antidepressants in the treatment of children with attention deficit disorder. *J. Am. Acad. Child Adolesc. Psychiatry* 26:127–132.

Polakoff, S. A., P. J. Sorgi, and J. J. Ratey. 1986. The treatment of impulsive and aggressive behavior with nadolol. *J. Clin. Psychopharmacol.* 6:125–126.

Rapoport, J. L. 1988. The neurobiology of obsessive-compulsive disorder. *JAMA* 260:2888–2890.

Rapoport, J. L., D. O. Quinn, G. Bradbard, K. D. Riddle, and S. E. Brook. 1974. Imipramine and methylphenidate treatment of hyperactive boys. *Arch. Gen. Psychiatry* 30:789–793.

Raskin, L. A., S. E. Shaywitz, B. A. Shaywitz, G. M. Anderson, and D. J. Cohen. 1984. Neurochemical correlates of attention deficit disorder. *Pediatr. Clin. North Am.* 31:387–396.

Ratey, J. J., R. Morrill, and G. Oxenkrug. 1983. Use of propranolol for provoked and unprovoked episodes of rage. *Am. J. Psychiatry* 140:1356–1357.

Ratey, J. J., J. Bemporad, P. Sorgi, P. Bick, S. Polakoff, G. O'Driscoll, and E. Mikkelsen. 1987. Brief report: Open trial effects of beta blockers on speech and social behaviors in 8 autistic adults. *J. Autism Dev. Disord.* 17:439–446.

Ratey, J. J., K. Sovner, E. Mikkelsen, and H. E. Chmielinski. 1989. Buspirone therapy for maladaptive behavior and anxiety in developmentally disabled persons. *J. Clin. Psychiatry* 50:382–384.

Reid, A. H., G. T. Naylor, and D. S. G. Kay. 1981. A double blind placebo controlled crossover trial of carbamazepine in overactive severely mentally handicapped patients. *Psychol. Med.* 11:109–113.

Reiss, A. L., A. L. Egel, C. Feinstein, B. Goldsmith, and M. A. Caruso. 1988. Effects of fenfluramine on social behavior in autistic children. *J. Autism Dev. Disord.* 18:617.

Reynolds, E. H. 1967. Effects of folic acid on the mental state and fit frequency of drug treated epileptic patients. *Lancet* 1:1086–1088.

Riddle, M. A., M. T. Hardin, S. C. Cho, J. L. Woolston, and J. F. Leckman. 1988. Desipramine treatment of boys with attention deficit hyperactivity disorder and tics: Preliminary clinical experience. *J. Am. Acad. Child Adolesc. Psychiatry* 27:811–814.

Ritvo, E. R., B. J. Freeman, A. Yuwiler, E. Geller, P. Schroth, A. Yokota, A. Mason-Brothers, G. J. August, W. Klykylo, B. Leventhal, K. Lewis, L. Piggott, G. Realmuto, E. G. Stubbs, and R. Umansky. 1986. Fenfluramine treatment of autism: UCLA collaborative study of 81 patients at nine medical centers. *Psychopharmacol. Bull.* 22:133–140.

Rosenblatt, D. S., E. A. Duschenes, F. V. Hellstrom, M. S. Golick, M. J. Vekemans, S. F. Zeesman, and E. Andermann. 1985. Folic acid blinded trial in identical twins with fragile X syndrome. *Am. J. Hum. Genet.* 37:543–552.

Sabin, P. 1989. Fluoxetine in the treatment of agitated dementia. *Am. J. Psychiatry* 146:1636.

Safer, D. J., and J. M. Krager. 1988. A survey of medication treatment for hyperactive/inattentive students. *JAMA* 260:2256–2258.

Shapiro, A. K., E. S. Shapiro, J. G. Young, and T. E. Feinberg. 1988. *Gilles de la Tourette syndrome,* 2nd ed. New York: Raven Press, pp. 405–410.

Sheard, M. 1975. Lithium in the treatment of aggression. *J. Nerv. Ment. Dis.* 160:108–118.

Sheard, M., J. L. Marini, C. I. Bridges, and E. Wagner. 1976. The effect of lithium on impulsive aggressive behavior in man. *Am. J. Psychiatry* 133:1409–1412.

Silver, J. M., and S. C. Yudofsky. 1985. Propranolol for aggression: Literature review and clinical guidelines. *Int. Drug. Ther. News* 20:9–12.

Stewart J. T., W. C. Myers, R. C. Burket, and W. B. Lyles. 1990. A review of the pharmacotherapy of aggression in children and adolescents. *J. Am. Acad. Child Adolesc. Psychiatry* 29:269–277.

Tec, L. 1963. Unexpected effects in children treated with imipramine. *Am. J. Psychiatry* 12:603.

Trimble, M. R. 1987. Anticonvulsant drugs and cognitive function: A review of the literature. *Epilepsia* 28(Suppl. 3):S37-S45.

Tupin, J., D. B. Smith, T. L. Clanon, L. I. Kim, A. Nugent, and A. Groupe. 1973. The long-term use of lithium in aggressive prisoners. *Compr. Psychiatry* 14:311–317.

Varley, C. K., and E. W. Trupin. 1982. Double blind administration of methylphenidate to mentally retarded children with attention deficit disorder: A preliminary study. *Am. J. Ment. Defic.* 86:560–566.

Wang, J., and R. W. Erbe. 1984. Folate metabolism in cells from fragile X syndrome patients and carriers. *Am. J. Med. Genet.* 17:303–310.

Williams, D. T., R. Mehl, and S. Yudofsky. 1982. The effect of propanolol on uncontrolled rage outbursts in children and adolescents with organic brain dysfunction. *J. Am. Acad. Child Psychiatry* 21:129–135.

Winsberg, B. G., I. Bailer, S. Kupietz, and J. Tobias. 1972. Effects of imipramine and dextroamphetamine on behavior of neuropsychiatrically impaired children. *Am. J. Psychiatry* 128:1424–1431.

Wisniewski, K. E., S. M. Segan, C. M. Miezejeski, E. A. Sersen, and R. D. Rudelli. 1991. The fragile X syndrome: Neurological, electrophysiological, and neuropathological abnormalities. *Am. J. Med. Genet.* 38:476–480.

Zettner, A., G. Boss, and J. E. Seegmiller. 1981. A long-term study of the absorption of large doses of folic acid. *Ann. Clin. Lab. Sci.* 11:517–524.

CHAPTER 10

The Treatment of Behavioral
and Emotional Problems

John Brown, Ph.D., Marcia Braden, Ph.D.,
and William Sobesky, Ph.D.

This chapter provides three approaches to psychotherapeutic intervention with fragile X [fra(X)] individuals. Little has been written about psychotherapy with those affected by fra(X) syndrome. Hence, much of the content of this chapter is based upon the anecdotal experiences of the authors. In all three sections, the importance of considering the unique pattern of strengths and weaknesses characteristic of fra(X) when developing and implementing intervention programs is stressed. Progress in devising effective treatment programs will occur as we learn more about the nature of disabilities associated with fra(X) and become able to tailor interventions to meet the particular needs of individuals with fra(X).

The first part of the chapter focuses on the experiences of providing an eclectic psychotherapeutic approach to people with fra(X) retardation. In this section, some of the important issues of assessment are covered, especially in relation to the specific areas of thought and behavior associated genetically with fra(X). Some suggestions for capitalizing on strengths and addressing needs specifically in therapy are discussed.

The second section concentrates on behavior therapy from an operant perspective. Specific problems common to fra(X) males are reviewed, and intervention procedures are suggested. This section concentrates on the needs of children more than on those of adults.

The third section discusses the less studied area of working therapeutically with fra(X) females. This section concentrates on a life-span perspective, which is especially important considering the increased incidence of depression and anxiety-related disorders and the number of less-affected individuals who marry and raise children.

Overall, the authors try to convey the conviction that psychotherapy is a valuable and perhaps underutilized tool to offer affected individuals and their families.

Psychotherapy with Fragile X Males

Treatment of the fra(X) client continues to evolve as professionals learn more about the manner in which the syndrome manifests itself. Hagerman et al. (1983) noted that the most significant problem involving the fra(X) syndrome was the lack of education within the professional community about the syndrome. This statement is probably still true as it pertains to psychotherapy with fra(X) patients. Much of the information on psychotherapy with fra(X) patients comes from research and literature pertaining to psychotherapy with mentally retarded patients, with extrapolations and modifications as they are perceived to apply to fra(X) patients.

The efficacy and appropriateness of using psychotherapy with mentally retarded patients are controversial. Although there are differences of opinion, most studies conclude that psychotherapy can be useful with retarded individuals (Chess 1962; Bozarth and Roberts 1970; Silvestri 1977; Sinason 1989). Sigman (1985) noted that much of the reluctance to use psychotherapy with the retarded is a function of two misconceptions. One is the lack of recognition that emotional problems are often independent of cognitive deficits, and the other views psychotherapy as inappropriate because of its reliance on the patient's capacity to reflect on his or her own experience, a capacity that the retarded individual is considered to lack.

There are also different opinions regarding the retarded individual's capacity to experience emotional conflicts and the complexity and nature of the feelings that they have. Doll (1953) described the "clinically feebleminded" as socially incompetent, having relatively simple emotional lives with disturbances becoming apparent only in those suffering from psychosis or severe emotional trauma. Hirsch (1959), on the other hand, noted that "the knowledge that the intelligence is dulled seems to carry with it the false implication that the retarded are less sensitive to hurt, less responsive to disappointment and not in need of gratifications which come with the knowledge that one's efforts are appreciated." McLachlan (1955) stated that the correlation between emotional disturbance and intellectual deficiency is not invariable and suggested that the retarded may be more susceptible to emotional problems as a result of lower stress tolerance and inadequate integration. Sternlicht and Deutsch (1972) also emphasized the greater susceptibility of the retarded to emotional problems. Eaton and Menolascino (1982) do not align with either of these positions but point out that, in people with severe or profound retardation, symptoms of emotional disturbances tend to be highly individualistic and frequently are accompanied by demonstrable brain pathologic and other organic conditions. Current views reflect the observations of Eaton and Menolascino and those of Sternlicht and Deutsch with the assumption that, with proper handling, these problems can be alleviated. Appropriate handling would mean that the retarded would be protected from and prepared for those situations where demands may exceed their capabilities and be provided outlets for the effective release of emotional tensions. It is from this perspective that psychotherapy with the retarded in general and with fra(X) patients in particular is being approached. Some of the extrapolations are based on a trial and error approach of trying different techniques to determine the degree of effectiveness with which they can be applied. It is assumed that, as we acquire more information about fra(X) and various attempts to treat these clients, we will become more refined in the manner in which we provide psychotherapy.

Gearheart and Litton (1975) offered the following premises as a rationale for providing psychotherapy for the retarded:

- The mentally retarded have an active emotional life and normal reactions to a variety of situations.
- The personality stresses and maladjustments of the mentally retarded are similar to those of the nonretarded.
- Emotional disturbance is as frequent among the retarded as among the nonretarded.
- Severe personality stresses may depress an individual's mental functioning so as to be indicative of retardation.
- Mentally retarded persons must have the same right to any available service that may benefit their overall functioning as any other person.

The goal of psychotherapy is to facilitate the adjustment of an individual in such a way that it enhances the capacity of the individual to deal with new situations as they are encountered. Gearheart and Litton (1975) indicated that the goals of treating the retarded are no different and that specific objectives involve the development of self-confidence and a feeling of self-worth, the ability to express and clarify emotional reactions, the development of methods for achieving emotional control, the development of standards for acceptable conduct, and the ability to seek help when needed.

Insight is often cited as a major goal of psychotherapy. Because retarded persons may have limited capacity for insight (Sigman 1985), many professionals consider them inappropriate candidates for psychotherapy. However, Maslow (1954) indicated that progress in psychotherapy takes place in six main ways:

- by expression (act completion, release, catharsis);
- by basic gratification (giving support, reassurance, protection, love, respect);
- by removing threat (good social, political, and economic conditions);
- by suggestion or authority;

- by positive self-actualization, individualization, or growth; and
- by improved insight, knowledge, and understanding.

One implication of Maslow's observations is that it is the therapist's responsibility to adapt strategies and techniques to accommodate the characteristics and needs of the patient rather than requiring the patient to adapt to the approach utilized by the therapist. It follows, then, that the applicability of psychotherapy to retarded persons depends, in part, on the capacity of the therapist to analyze, conceptualize, and understand the patient's problems in ways that facilitate the development and implementation of strategies that are meaningful in helping to ameliorate the patient's difficulties.

A critical aspect of the psychotherapy process is the assessment phase (i.e., determining the nature of the problem to be treated). Several problems are encountered in assessing retarded patients. Jura and Sigman (1985) identified a major factor influencing the treatment of emotional disorders in retarded patients, noting that there is a tendency to attribute aberrant response patterns to cognitive deficits once the diagnosis of mental retardation has been made. Reiss et al. (1982) labeled this phenomenon *diagnostic overshadowing* and cited it as a major variable influencing the decision-making process regarding the nature of the treatment to be provided to a particular patient. However, problems remain even when one avoids diagnostic overshadowing. The dearth of assessment tools designed specifically to assess emotional problems in retarded persons is a major problem (Jura and Sigman 1985). Jura and Sigman responded to this deficiency by offering several suggestions regarding ways currently used projective tests may be modified to get a better understanding of the emotional issues confronting retarded patients. Jura and Sigman saw this as being particularly useful with adolescents and adults and noted that the examiner must be more active than usual in eliciting important thematic material and in supporting the productive efforts of the patient. Jura and Sigman further indicated that one must take into consideration the developmental level, manner of presenting, and history when interpreting projectives to avoid overestimating the degree of psychologic disruption.

History, in terms of significant changes and/or deterioration in levels of functioning and behavior, is especially important when trying to tease apart cognitive disability and emotional disturbance in the more severely retarded patient. As Eaton and Menolascino (1982) pointed out, in cases involving more severe retardation, symptoms of emotional disturbance are frequently accompanied by demonstrable brain abnormalities and other organic conditions. Therefore, the historical data provide some of the information necessary to make a differential diagnosis and thus provide appropriate treatment. Consequently, without adequate background information, less confidence can be placed in diagnosis.

Similar precautions must be taken when assessing fra(X) patients because they also manifest a variety of symptoms that are associated with the fra(X) syndrome as well as with other psychiatric disorders, such as autism and attention deficit hyperactivity disorder (ADHD). One could easily overestimate the level of pathology present if the only available data were how the person presented in one situation or performed in response to a test. This certainly would alter one's perspective regarding the nature of the treatment required and, possibly, the effectiveness with which one would be able to treat the patient.

Heber (1965) pointed out that the intellectual limitations of the retarded patient necessitate modifications in usual counseling techniques and require the use of a wider range of approaches. Sigman (1985) echoed Heber's point and elaborated on ways in which therapy may be modified. She noted that many mildly retarded adolescents and adults have the cognitive skills and experience necessary to understand social situations to a considerable degree and, there-fore, would be able to benefit from less directive, more traditional forms of therapy. The same logic would seem to apply to fra(X) adolescents and adults, with the additional caution that some fra(X) clients who seem to function at a lower cognitive level as a result of perceptual/motor and language difficulties may also have the capacity to engage in therapy. Fra(X) clients need repetition and time to process and use information because of attentional and auditory processing problems and they also need help refocusing on a task; thus, the therapist must be more active than usual. A distinction should be made, how-ever, between being active and being intrusive. The therapist needs to redirect the patient's behavior in a calm and supportive manner, lest the patient interpret the therapist's actions as being critical and rejecting.

Therapy can also vary in terms of the degree of focus on current situations versus more formative events in the patient's past history. With retarded pa-tients, this may require active participation of family members and/or other relevant individuals to provide the therapist with information regarding signifi-cant events that occur, especially if the patient does not provide adequate information. This can be a major problem with fra(X) patients because of their difficulties involving intersensory integration and language that may result in misinterpretations and/or idiosyncratic meanings being ascribed to their expe-riences. Therapy can also vary in terms of the frequency and length of sessions and the use of concrete activities or tasks to facilitate the process. Drawings, pictures, role-playing, etc., are all viable techniques.

Sigman (1985) noted that patients' developmental level, level of psycho-logic differentiation, and chronologic age are important for understanding how patients relate and the issues they present in therapy. Developmental level is most simply defined as mental age. Psychologic differentiation reflects the nature of the emotional and social concerns as well as the behavioral, adaptive, and social skills manifested by the person. Sigman sees the level of psychologic differentiation being determined by both developmental level and chronologic age. Environment should be added to the list, for it is clear that the level of psychologic differentiation varies according to the environmental support available to the individual as well as according to the individual's capacity to benefit from the support available.

It would be presumptuous to assume that a therapist using any one approach could be completely effective in treating the fra(X) patient. Because the deficits associated with the syndrome involve so many different disciplines, a therapist should consult a variety of professionals to treat the fra(X) patient effectively. These include speech/language clinicians regarding language difficulties and techniques that might be helpful in circumventing this problem in therapy, occupational therapists regarding intersensory integration and tactile defensiveness (chapter 11), and physicians/psychiatrists regarding medical issues and psychopharmacology for behavior problems (chapters 1 and 9).

The typical fra(X) adolescent or adult male patient is referred for treatment as a result of concerns about aggressive, impulsive, and occasionally self-injurious behavior or inappropriate sexual behavior. The concern of the referring agency is control of the behavior; however, the therapist must assume a larger role. The therapist must try to understand the significance of the patient's behavior in terms of what needs are involved. The therapist must assist the patient in understanding and expressing those needs in more adaptive ways by either working directly with the patient or consulting with those responsible for the patient. For example, many retarded individuals are not taught appropriate ways of expressing affect. Instead, they grow up having few words for feelings and even fewer adaptive ways of expressing them. To the extent possible, a significant part of the treatment would be helping the person label and understand feelings and adaptive ways of expressing them. Treatment would also involve educating significant others about the meaning of the person's behavior and trying to help them find ways of facilitating positive behavior. It is imperative that contact between the therapist and others who are actively involved in the patient's programming be maintained because, as in other situations, it is the coordination and consistency of the treatment that influences the degree of success in treatment. An effective therapist for fra(X) patients is likely to be one who can conceptualize and understand the psychodynamics of the person's behavior and translate this into cognitive-behavioral and/or behavioral strategies that are designed to facilitate more adaptive functioning.

Case History

Jim is a 22-year-old fra(X) man living in a quasi-supervised residential setting and involved in a vocational training program. In the past he has been tested and found to be functioning at the high moderate to low mild range cognitively, with a variety of perceptual processing difficulties. He was referred for periodic impulsive and aggressive outbursts and concerns about inappropriate sexual behavior. Previous attempts to manage these problems through behavioral techniques had resulted in only minimal success. Initially, Jim exhibited many schizoid features in the manner in which he related in therapy, but gradually he became more comfortable and was able to engage in sustained dialog regarding his problems. He was concerned about his maladaptive behavior but primarily because it made other significant adults (e.g., parents and staff) upset with him and he was afraid that they would not like him and would ultimately abandon him. His solution, therefore, was to avoid strong affect, especially anger. In other words, it was not okay to be angry. This was a direct translation of his early training, which emphasized the inappropriateness of anger and aggressiveness. It was noted that Jim had ambivalent feelings about living apart from his parents and that there were times when he would become reactive to what he perceived as people trying to tell him what to do.

Exploring issues involving sexuality revealed a rather curious but naive person whose knowledge and information about sexuality were very limited. Jim had received no formal or informal training about sexuality at home or anywhere else. The picture that developed was that of a young man who was conflicted about his own drive for greater autonomy/independence, need to conform to please others, and fear of abandonment. Add to this picture a growing interest in and awareness of sexuality and you have a person who is chronologically an adult but developmentally dealing with issues similar to those of young adolescents. Processing difficulties associated with language problems complicated matters and made it necessary to teach Jim how to inhibit impulsive responding and be certain of what was said before he reacted. For example, he was taught to ask people to repeat what they had said or to say "I didn't understand that; could you explain it again?" Beyond empathetic listening and supportive techniques designed to foster a treatment alliance, early treatment involved teaching Jim how to recognize when he was beginning to get upset and how to use relaxation techniques to maintain control and enhance his sense of efficacy. Cognitive-behavioral strategies were also used to enhance his sense of self-control. As therapy progressed, the emphasis was placed on helping Jim to explore issues related to autonomy and independence as they related to anger and his concerns about abandonment.

He was quite resistant to exploring issues about anger, especially in terms of it being acceptable. Techniques including pictures depicting various emotional states, drawings, and audio- and videotaped parts of sessions were utilized, in addition to traditional therapy, to help him explore this issue. As he became more comfortable with this issue, other concerns emerged, especially those related to being on his own and fears of being abandoned by his family. Issues involving sexuality are being dealt with in a group context and individually.

Behavioral Approaches

In contrast to dynamically oriented psychotherapy, behavior therapy represents a more symptom-oriented approach. It has experienced broad use in the field of mental retardation because more classic approaches to psychotherapy can be limited by cognitive deficits. For a review of the use of behavior therapy in individuals with mental retardation, see Matson and McCartney (1981) and Whitman and Johnston (1987). At present, there are no studies concerning the use of behavior therapy in fra(X) patients and there are no "foolproof" behavioral treatment packages. Additionally, the type of therapeutic intervention may vary according to the level of affectedness in each patient.

The less-affected fra(X) patient, for example, may benefit greatly from cognitive behavioral interventions (Ellis 1962; Beck 1970, 1976; Turk and Francis 1990). These methods of intervention stress beliefs and thoughts as an integral part of emotion and how that effects behavior. They differ from the psychodynamic model, which concentrates on relieving internal conflicts and focuses less on behavioral change.

The cognitive-behavioral model can be applied to fra(X) patients who are able to generalize behaviors across environments and conditions. The therapist would teach strategies that are appropriate to assist in a behavioral adjustment. For example, if the fra(X) patient became aroused and excited every time a routine was changed, the therapist would shape and reinforce a desired behavior to be substituted for the excitability. As the process continued, the therapist would teach the patient to mediate or "think" through the adjustment so that it became an automatic, inherent treatment agent.

Another offshoot of this treatment model is that of self-instruction. Vygotsky (1962) and Luria (1959, 1961) posited a relationship between behavior and internalization of verbal commands. This theory has particular application for fra(X) patients. Fra(X) males have been observed repeating a sequence of instruction that was used in another setting for controlling behavior. The behavior might be regarded as a delayed echolalic speech pattern but, unlike echolalia, it often appropriately relates to the current situation. Therefore, the verbalization of an adult cue may become a mechanism by which the fra(X) patient gains internal control. This verbal cuing, which often occurs naturally without intervention, can be encouraged and modeled as a therapeutic means of controlling difficult behavior. It has been used in conjunction with calming techniques (chapter 11) to aid the patient in replacing a maladaptive physical reaction with a self-directed verbal control.

The research using this intervention was mainly documented with children of normal intelligence. There is strong support for this method in dealing with anxiety related to fear (Kanfer et al. 1975) and hyperactive/disruptive behavior (Goodwin and Mahoney 1975). Neilans and Israel (1981) conducted a comparison study with children from a residential treatment center which compared a token economy system (giving or removing tokens when on or off task) to a self-instruction system. The results indicated that the self-instruction, self-regulated program maintained the appropriate behavior longer than that of the token economy system which failed when the tokens were withdrawn. With some fra(X) patients who demonstrate more significant cognitive deficits and lack the language necessary to self-instruct, this would not be the method of choice. The lower-cognitive-functioning individual may require behavior modification techniques that are more concrete and may always require some system of external monitoring.

The most important aspect of a behavior modification program is the consistency of delivery. The child must be able to anticipate the outcome based on the choice of behavior. This encourages independence and ultimately self-monitoring. Operant conditioning and behavioral procedures have been successfully used with other handicapping conditions to decrease aggressive behavior (Brown et al. 1969), increase social interactions (Koegel et al. 1974; Strain et al. 1979), reduce self-injurious behavior (Repp and Dietz 1974; Tate and Baroff 1966), and manage other behavioral excesses (Ando 1977; Simpson 1977). Based on the success of these approaches with other populations, the principles have been used with fra(X) patients. Unfortunately, there has been no controlled research on the application and efficacy of behavioral techniques with the fra(X) patient.

Operant conditioning as espoused by Skinner (1953, 1958), a change in behavior through small approximations elicited and then reinforced, has been successfully used in treating self-stimulatory and aggressive behavior in the fra(X) population. The idea is to shape more appropriate behavior through an association with a positive condition or reinforcement. For example, a fra(X) patient who demonstrates destructive behavior (tearing up materials, pushing over tables, throwing work material) may be physically guided to indicate frustration through a communication board and then be removed from the work environment and placed in a time-out area, void of external distracters and environmental noises, to calm down. This program can then be modified to begin to shape the behavior of asking for assistance when frustrated. The maladaptive destructive behavior is gradually replaced by a conditioned response of indicating a need to calm down or leave the area when overstimulated. As the process progresses, the need for break time can then be included, with support from staff to assist in scheduling. This approach can help the individual to replace a maladaptive behavior that escalates feelings of failure and fear of one's own behavior. Demonstration of self-calming is more socially acceptable and will evoke positive reinforcement in the environment.

For responsible promotion of behavior modification interventions, it is essential to consider if the behavior significantly interferes with the fra(X) individual's performance. If there is a definite connection between the behavior and an interruption of cognitive/social functioning, then an intervention is warranted. Equally as important is the connection between the inappropriate behavior and social interaction. Often, behavioral excesses (hand flapping, hand biting, gaze avoidance, and perseverative speech patterns) set the fra(X) individual apart from normal peers. This deviance can create negative attention and often precludes the fra(X) individual from fully integrating into the mainstream, making educators and therapists realize the need to develop strategies to enhance social interactions using behavior modification.

In establishing a method of behavioral intervention, it can be helpful to explore behavioral features that seem to be consistent in this population and, to some extent, unique. Developmental histories provided by parents can help the therapist identify certain symptoms that can be addressed through the use of behavior modification techniques. The therapist can assist the parent in developing home programs and provide consultation to school/vocational staff.

Behavioral problems that appear commonly in this population were extracted from a compilation of over 50 developmental history interviews of parents with fra(X) children by one of the authors (M. B.). These situations were often cited by parents of fra(X) children as causing significant problems at home and in school/public environments: eating, mouthing objects, sleeping, atypical speech patterns, grooming, toileting, and eye gaze avoidance. These behaviors not only create extreme challenges in early development but often in later years may become an issue when other situational stresses occur. For example, a fra(X) adolescent may respond to the stress of beginning junior high by developing sleeping or eating problems previously experienced in early childhood.

Historically, a wide array of problems associated with eating emerge in infancy. Fra(X) babies usually have difficulty drinking from a bottle and are slow to develop food tolerance. This often results in poor eating habits. Parents who are concerned about nutrition may be tempted to give in to food idiosyncrasies and supplement the diet with protein drink. Eating can bring on tantrumming and noncompliance because of the stress it creates in fra(X) patients. Often children gag or eat sloppily, using both hands to push food into the mouth. Because fra(X) children need more tactile stimulation to interpret incoming tactile input, they may use their fingers to smear food over the face and cheeks. The therapist can assist in developing food tolerance programs to gradually incorporate less well liked foods into the diet.

Sleeping also causes great difficulty for families. Sleeping problems often relate to hyperactivity, infrequent naps, and an inability to self-calm so that, when a child awakens at night, crying occurs instead of falling back to sleep. In addition, these children are often light sleepers because of a hypersensitive response to noise in their environment. The therapist might suggest that the parents run fans or humidifiers to filter out extraneous sounds and consult a pediatrician familiar with fra(X) for medical assistance with the hyperactivity. Putting a child to bed while awake in infancy helps a child learn self-calming techniques, which allows them to fall asleep initially and subsequently when they awake in the middle of the night.

Speech development is clearly delayed and is often characterized by initial throaty or squealing sounds. As speech develops, it becomes repetitive and dysfluent—lacking organization (chapters 5 and 11). An unusual quality is the enjoyment of certain environmental sounds such as machinery running, washer/dryer sounds, car engines, and vacuum cleaners. These sounds are reported to be somewhat calming and enjoyable. The therapist and parent may utilize these sounds to assist in the development of a program to calm the patient.

Grooming presents a difficult dilemma because of the extreme sensitivity of the head and facial area. The fra(X) patient often dislikes haircuts, hair washing, hair brushing, or combing of hair and usually dislikes wearing hats. Sensory deficits contribute to the negative reaction elicited by certain clothing or materials. For example, many fra(X) patients dislike the feel of certain fabrics, turtle-necked shirts, or short pants. Usually, sensory integrative therapy is recommended to help the patient become desensitized to certain clothing textures, thus reducing the negative reaction (chapter 11).

The fra(X) patient usually prefers to avoid eye contact and often squints or turns his head downward when socializing (Cohen et al. 1988). Lack of eye contact can preclude successful social interaction and will often bring on a negative reaction from the environment. It is important to understand that the fra(X) patient is hypersensitive to social input and that direct attention, even when positive, may create a feeling of being "spotlighted" and overstimulated.

Even though these behavioral features may have resulted from sensory or speech deficits inherent in this population (chapters 1 and 11), the unusual responses may be reinforced by the environment. For example, one particular fra(X) patient will not eat anything but yogurt and pizza. His parents consistently deal with severe tantrums anytime a different food is introduced. The child continues the tantrums with higher frequency until the parents remove the different food and replace (reinforce) it with yogurt. These behaviors can be maintained or reduced simply by changing the responses from caretakers or other factors in the environment.

Case History (reported by Sonny Spielman and Diane Riggs, Cheyenne Village, Manitou Springs, Colorado)

CJ is a 26-year-old fra(X) man living in a four-bed residential cabin. He displays panic-related symptoms and aggressive behavior, which includes self-abuse, throwing of objects, property damage, and the hitting/kicking of others. The staff developed a behavioral plan to reduce the frequency, intensity, and duration of these aggressive events. Environmental controls were utilized to provide CJ with a dimmer-switch in his room to control lighting. To assure privacy, he did not share his room, and housemates have their own rooms as well. Window glass was replaced with clear lexan panels to avoid breakage. The general house activity level, including temperature, noise, resident interactions, and lighting, was monitored so as to minimize fra(X) hypersensitivity. New or unfamiliar people and events were previewed via video tape or photographs. Verbal and visual previewing was done at least four times a day so as to structure his vocational and residential day. CJ reviewed past, present, and future events in the morning after getting out of bed and during the transition from residential to vocational settings using a structured checklist. During the transition back to the residential setting from the vocational setting, the same checklist was used. In the evening, planning included a synopsis of the day as well as a preview of the following day.

CJ was involved in physical activity daily. A modified jacobsonian relaxation training and thought-stopping techniques were used via cassette tapes and verbal prompts to breathe deeply and "stop" in relation to thought perseveration and precursor behavior. Self-management behavior training was used whereby he learned to self-monitor his behavior, starting with easily identified behaviors and self-monitoring picture charts. Redirection was used whenever staff could foresee a potentially sensitive or overstimulating situation.

CJ responded best to the use of cue words to help him focus and redirect to positive and calming thoughts. Such words as "grumpy versus happy," "straight across versus rainbow talk," "peaceful stranger," "adding up (or down) the ladder," and similar simple cues or analogs were very helpful. Visual (hand motion) cues done in conjunction with verbal cues were often used.

Medical intervention included lithium and a beta-blocker, which helped in decreasing the number of outbursts (chapter 9). He attended both individual and group psychotherapy as well as a residential meeting to assist with internalizing the processes he learned. Physical management of aggressive behavior was used as a last resort by staff members who were adequately trained in the safe use of state-approved intervention techniques.

Treatment of Heterozygous Females

Although many heterozygotes may be unaffected by the fra(X) gene, others suffer from learning difficulties and emotional problems including shyness, anxiety, and depression (chapters 1 and 5). Hagerman and Sobesky (1989) suggested three foci for intervention around various problems of fra(X) females. As in the case with fra(X) males, there is no controlled research to verify the efficacy of these interventions with fra(X) females. The first focus is aimed at helping individuals to feel greater control over their internal world. Intervention such as biofeedback and various relaxation techniques may be helpful. Additionally, medication for attentional problems and impulsivity or to relieve depression might be of assistance. The second intervention consists of skill building. This can focus upon self-monitoring techniques that would help individuals learn to modulate their thinking, use anxiety as a signal rather than being overwhelmed by it, and develop the ability to observe their own behavior. The third focus of intervention is geared toward addressing self-esteem issues as well as addressing feelings of depression.

Our clinical experiences indicate that there is a need to adopt a life-span perspective in viewing the needs of fra(X) females. Different pressures in different phases of the life cycle may interact with various vulnerabilities to produce difficulties. These difficulties may tend to be more episodic than chronic; however, the quality of life of heterozygotes may be enhanced by appropriate, short-term interventions.

During school age, three sorts of problems tend to cause the greatest difficulty: shyness, learning problems, and attentional problems. In terms of shyness, we suggested that parents encourage their daughters to engage in activities outside the home. This is often painful for parents because their daughters initially are quite apprehensive and reluctant. However, our experience is that over time these daughters do adapt and actually enjoy their outside activities. Also, involvement in such activities may lead to less painful shyness during adolescence. In terms of attentional and learning problems, it is valuable for parents to be advocates for their children's needs in school settings. Special supportive services can be helpful in providing the requisite structure and learning enhancements to help these young women (chapter 11).

During adolescence several issues may become problematic. Many women, as adults, recall their adolescence as a very painful time. The pressures to socialize intensify during adolescence under the social demands of that developmental period. Given the shyness and social anxiety experienced by some fra(X) women, it may be very difficult for some fra(X) females to engage with their peers. Additionally, adolescents are beginning to look forward to adulthood. For fra(X) individuals this requires coming to terms with the meaning of their fra(X) diagnosis and the implications of this diagnosis in terms of marrying, having children, and selecting a career. Under such pressures there may be a tendency to withdraw from school and social activities. Individual counseling can help the fra(X) female come to terms with her diagnosis and to value her strengths. Additionally, family therapy may help all members of a family to gain an understanding of the meaning and implications of the fra(X) diagnosis. Therapy can also be a valuable resource in strengthening family support systems and can also help family members "let go" of one another as children become more independent.

Finally, during adulthood the pressures associated with child-rearing, especially of fra(X) children, are frequently a great stress. Additionally, there may be biologic stresses such as estrogen deficiency after pregnancy and during menopause, which may increase the heterozygote's vulnerability to depression and anxiety. Again, supportive treatment to help the individual understand what is happening biologically as well as support around the stresses of child-rearing can be of assistance.

These suggestions regarding interventions have not been substantiated by formal study. Indeed, various kinds of behavioral and psychologic interventions are probably underutilized by the fra(X) population as a whole. As we come to understand better the biologic side of fra(X) difficulties and their manifestations through the life-span, we should be more able to devise appropriate and effective intervention techniques, not only for daughters, but for affected mothers as well.

References

Ando, H. 1977. Training autistic children to urinate in the toilet through operant conditioning techniques. *J. Autism Child. Schizo.* 7:151–163.

Beck, A. T. 1970. Cognitive therapy: Nature and relation to behavior therapy. *Behav. Res. Ther.* 1:184–200.

———. 1976. *Cognitive therapy and the emotional disorders.* New York: International Universities Press.

Bozarth, J. D., and R. R. Roberts. 1970. Effectiveness of counselor-trainees with mentally retarded sheltered workshop clients. *Training School Bull.* 67:119–122.

Brown, R. A., L. S. Pace, and W. C. Becker. 1969. Out of the classroom: Treatment of extreme negativism and autistic behavior in a six-year-old boy. *Except. Child.* 36(2):115–122.

Chess, S. 1962. Psychiatric treatment of the mentally retarded child with behavior problems. *Am. J. Orthopsychiatry* 32:863–869.

Cohen, I. L., G. S. Fisch, E. G. Wolf-Schein, V. Sudhalter, D. Hanson, R. J. Hagerman, E. C. Jenkins, and W. T. Brown. 1988. Social avoidance and repetitive behavior in fragile X males: A controlled study. *Am. J. Ment. Retard.* 92:436–446.

Doll, E. A. 1953. Psychodynamics of the mentally retarded. *Am. Med. Assoc. Arch. Neurol. Psychiatry* 70:121.

Eaton, L. F., and F. J. Menolascino. 1982. Psychiatric disorders in the mentally retarded: Types, problems and challenges. *Am. J. Psychiatry* 139:1297–1303.

Ellis, A. 1962. *Reason and emotion in psychotherapy.* New York: L. Stuart.

Gearheart, B. R., and F. W. Litton. 1975. *The trainable retarded.* St. Louis: C. V.
Mosby.

Goodwin, S., and M. J. Mahoney. 1975. Modification of aggression through modeling:
An experimental probe. *J. Behav. Ther. Exp. Psychiatry* 6:200–202.

Hagerman, R. J., and W. E. Sobesky. 1989. Psychopathology in fragile X syndrome.
Am. J. Orthopsychiatry 59:142–152.

Hagerman, R. J., A. C. M. Smith, and R. Mariner. 1983. Clinical features of the fragile
X syndrome. In R. J. Hagerman and P. M. McBogg (eds.), *The fragile X syndrome.*
Dillon, Colo.: Spectra Publishing, pp 17–53.

Heber, R. 1965. *Vocational rehabilitation of the mentally retarded.* Rehab. Serv. Series
65–16. U. S. Department of Health, Education and Welfare, Washington, D. C.

Hirsch, E. 1959. The adaptive significance of commonly described behavior of the
mentally retarded. *Am. J. Ment. Defic.* 63:639–646.

Jura, M., and M. Sigman. 1985. Evaluation of emotional disorders using projective
techniques with mentally retarded children. In M. Sigman (ed.), *Children with
emotional disorders and developmental disabilities.* New York: Grune and Stratton,
pp. 229–248.

Kanfer, F. H., P. Karoly, and A. Newman. 1975. Reduction of children's fear of the dark
by competence-related and situational threat-related averbal cues. *J. Consult. Clin.
Psychol.* 43:251–258.

Koegel, R. L., P. B. Firestone, K. W. Kramme, and G. Dunlap. 1974. Increasing
spontaneous play by suppressing self-stimulation in the autistic child. *J. Appl. Behav. Anal.* 7:521–528.

Luria, A. R. 1959. The directive function of speech in development and dissolution.
Word 15:341–352.

———. 1961. *The role of speech in the regulation of normal and abnormal behaviors.*
New York: Liveright.

Maslow, A. H. 1954. *Motivation and personality.* New York: Harper and Row.

Matson, J. L., and J. R. McCartney. 1981. *Handbook of behavior modification with the
mentally retarded.* New York: Plenum Press.

McLachlan, D. H. 1955. Emotional aspects of the backward child. *Am. J. Ment. Defic.*
60:323–330.

Neilans, T. H., and A. C. Israel. 1981. Towards maintenance and generalization of
behavior change: Teaching children self-regulation and self-instructional skills. *Cognition Ther. Res.* 5:189–196.

Reiss, S., G. Levitan, and J. Szysko. 1982. Emotional disturbance and mental retardation: Diagnostic overshadowing. *Am. J. Ment. Defic.* 86:567–574.

Reiss, A. L., R. J. Hagerman, S. Vinogradov, M. Abrams, and R. J. King. 1988.
Psychiatric disability in female carriers of the fragile X chromosome. *Arch. Gen.
Psychiatry* 45:25–30.

Repp, A. C., and S. M. Deitz. 1974. Reducing aggressive and self-injurious behavior of
institutionalized retarded children through reinforcement of other behaviors. *J. Appl.
Behav. Anal.* 7:313–326.

Sigman, M. 1985. Individual and group psychotherapy with mentally retarded adolescents. In M. Sigman (ed.), *Children with emotional disorders and developmental disabilities*. New York: Grune and Stratton, pp. 259–276.

Silvestri, R. 1977. Implosive therapy treatment of emotionally disturbed retardates. *J. Consult. Clin. Psychol.* 45:14–22.

Simpson, R. L. 1977. Behavior modification with the severely emotionally disturbed. Working Paper 5, Severe Personal Adjustment Project, Bureau of Education for the Handicapped, United States Office of Education, Department of Health, Education and Welfare, Washington, D.C.

Sinason, V. 1989. Uncovering and responding to sexual abuse in psychotherapeutic settings. In H. Brown and A. Craft (eds.), *Thinking the unthinkable: Papers on sexual abuse and people with learning difficulties*. London: FPA Education Unit.

Skinner, B. F. 1953. *Science and human behavior.* New York: Macmillan.

———. 1958. Reinforcement today. *Am. Psychol.* 13:94–99.

Sternlicht, M., and M. R. Deutsch. 1972. *Personality development and social behavior in the mentally retarded.* Lexington, Mass.: D. C. Heath.

Strain, P. S., M. M. Kerr, and E. U. Ragland. 1979. Effects of peer-mediated social initiations and prompting/reinforcement procedures on the social behavior of autistic children. *J. Autism Dev. Disord.* 9(1):41–53.

Tate, B. G., and G. S. Baroff. 1966. Aversive control of self-injurious behavior in a psychotic boy. *Behav. Res. Ther.* 4(4):281.

Turk, M. V., and E. Francis. 1990. An anxiety management group: Strengths and pitfalls. *Ment. Handicap* 18:78–81.

Vygotsky, L. 1962. *Thought and language.* New York: Wiley.

Whitman, T. L., and M. B. Johnston. 1987. Mental retardation. In M. Hersen and V. B. Van Hasselt (eds.), *Behavior therapy with children and adolescents*. New York: Wiley, pp. 184–223.

CHAPTER 11

An Integrated Approach
to Intervention

Sarah Scharfenaker, M.A., C.C.C., Lois Hickman, M.S., O.T.R., and Marcia Braden, Ph.D.

Newly diagnosed families coming to a clinic for initial evaluation are there to gather information. For many families, an important question is what treatment is available to meet their children's special needs. Although there is no cure for fragile X syndrome, many intervention strategies are useful in managing the behavioral problems and learning difficulties so common among fra(X) children and adults. Because of the multifaceted needs of these patients, an integrated approach to special education which combines the expertise of the speech and language pathologist, occupational therapist, and teacher is most beneficial. In this chapter, we review the history and philosophy behind the concept of integrated services and discuss its implications for working with the fra(X) population. Specific strategies applicable within the academic, speech/language, and occupational therapy domains are presented for the infant-toddler, school-aged child, and late adolescent-adult. Although the emphasis of this chapter is on integrated services for the fra(X) male, the information can be extrapolated for use with the learning-disabled and mild to moderately impaired fra(X) female.

Most methods discussed in this chapter are based on clinical observation rather than controlled research because of the lack of studies in this area. Further research is necessary to improve our understanding of beneficial treatment techniques in all areas of education.

In the absence of research specific to fra(X) treatment, we attempted to cite applicable research studying other populations whose features are similar to those of the fra(X) population, while bearing in mind the unique cognitive, speech/language, and sensory deficits of fra(X) individuals.

Overview of Integrated Services

The concept of integrated services emerged when special education legislation was passed at the federal level in the mid-1970s (U.S. Congress 1975). PL 94-142 posited that all handicapped children were entitled to a free and appropriate education within the "least restrictive environment." The term *least restrictive environment* implies that handicapped children are entitled to the same education as their nonhandicapped peers and that the school experience should not be restricted to the programs already established within school districts.

When PL 94-142 was passed, the new objective was to identify individuals with multiple needs in the cognitive, behavioral, speech/language, and occupational therapy areas as "multiply handicapped." The development of a transdisciplinary team model evolved to accommodate the needs of these children within a public school setting (Hutchinson 1983). Within this model, each member of the team trains others, thus abandoning a traditional role and building competence in other disciplines to meet the complex needs of the student (Sternat et al. 1977).

In October 1986, another public law was passed, PL 99-457, which ensured that each handicapped infant and toddler and their families receive a written individualized family service plan (IFSP) (U.S. Congress 1986). This act further served to acknowledge the multidisciplinary team concept by including the parent or guardian as a member of the team and thus an active participant in the educational process.

PL 94-142 and PL 99-457 significantly changed the public school system. With this legislation, more multiply handicapped children moved from private and public institutions into the public school system. As a consequence, the growing need for normalization, mainstreaming, and providing the least restrictive environment was evident. These laws also caused changes in educational treatment, related services, and therapeutic intervention. It was no longer appropriate to educate a child in an isolated facility, with occupational therapy in a hospital and speech therapy in a rehabilitation center. Instead, there was a legal mandate to centralize services in the public school. Thus, the focus shifted from isolated delivery to a multidisciplinary approach. Input from speech pathologists, occupational and physical therapists, educators, psychologists, and other specialists provided an integrated framework from which a child's educational curriculum could evolve. The success of treatment was less contingent on the technique or philosophy of an individual therapist or educator and more dependent on the positive treatment effects of an integrated program. Only a few studies have evaluated the advantages of integrative therapy and the multidisciplinary model. Preliminary findings from several studies suggest that implementing therapy within a functional environment and context is more effective than teaching skills in isolated environments (Campbell et al. 1984; Giangreco 1986).

Fra(X) and Integrated Service Delivery

Although there is a dearth of research specific to fra(X) intervention, a great deal of knowledge can be gained by examining the related fields of autism, mental retardation, and learning disabilities. In addition, observations from trained professionals can provide insight into the special educational needs of fra(X) children.

The fra(X) individual has a number of complex needs which present the educator and therapist with a programming challenge (see chapters 1 and 5). These complex needs include

- a hypersensitivity to visual, auditory, olfactory, and tactile stimuli;
- difficulty with motor planning and sequencing;
- attentional difficulties, hyperactivity, and impulsivity;
- difficulty making physical transitions;
- difficulties with social interaction;
- communication difficulties, including phrase, sentence, and topical perseverations; and
- cognitive deficits ranging from learning disabilities to severe retardation.

These cognitive, communicative, and sensory difficulties preclude learning through a traditional classroom model. With the fra(X) individual, integrated services involving the occupational therapist and speech/language pathologist are often critical to a successful educational program. The cognitive and speech/language skills, as well as the sensory-motor skills addressed by occupational therapy, vary significantly in the fra(X) population. What may benefit a severely handicapped fra(X) individual is inappropriate for a high-functioning child. Thus, the educational and therapeutic needs of each fra(X) child must be assessed on an individual basis. The programming goals of an integrated education plan are listed in table 11.1.

The decisions for classroom placement must be based on individual needs and ability (Baroff 1986). Although PL 94-142 has been misinterpreted by some to be a mandate that all special education students should be mainstreamed into regular classrooms, the public law does not require mainstreaming. Instead, an appropriate education must be provided with specific procedures defined to protect that right. Mainstreaming can be a positive educational practice if the regular classroom teacher has had special education training or experience (Walker et al. 1989). Modifications of the mainstreaming

Table 11.1

Programming Goals for an Individualized Educational Plan

1. Sensory integrative therapy to:
    a. Decrease hypersensitivity to tactile, visual, olfactory, gustatory, and auditory stimuli
    b. Increase tolerance of change in routine and environment
    c. Decrease mouthing, hand biting, chewing on clothing
    d. Decrease ritualistic behaviors
    e. Improve gross and fine motor skills
    f. Improve motor planning skills
2. Speech/language therapy to:
    a. Increase receptive and expressive language levels
    b. Increase mean length of utterance
    c. Increase problem-solving skills
    d. Increase play skill competency
    e. Increase use of a variety of speech acts
    f. Decrease verbal perseverations
    g. Increase frequency of spontaneously initiated verbalizations
    h. Decrease fast rate and oral and speech dyspraxia
3. Combined sensory integration and speech/language therapy to apply basic sensorimotor strategies into developing speech, language, and pragmatic skills
4. Educational intervention to:
    a. Increase attending behaviors in all situations
    b. Increase compliance to direct cues
    c. Increase independent toileting
    d. Decrease person/environment specific behaviors
    e. Decrease tantruming
    f. Increase play skill competencies
    g. Increase mainstreaming with normal age-appropriate peers

experience can also be helpful. One example is reverse mainstreaming, in which a small number of normal-functioning peers attend the special education classroom. A variety of structured play and leisure activities can help the handicapped and normal children accept each other and learn together.

Higher-functioning fra(X) children may also do well in the regular classroom for nonacademic periods and in some cases for limited academic subjects, such as reading [an academic strength for some fra(X) children]. Fra(X) children demonstrate strong verbal and behavioral imitation skills. Because of this, placement in a regular classroom, where development of normal socialization skills can be encouraged, is desirable.

Sensory Integration Therapy and Fra(X)

To understand and in turn work effectively with fra(X) individuals, one must recognize any underlying deficits in sensory integrative function. Sensory integration dysfunction is commonly seen in the fra(X) population, although the degree of deficit in each individual may vary.

The central nervous system (CNS) has evolved with complex interrelationships of the sensory modalities (Sarnat and Netsky 1981; Marks 1978; Nobak 1975; Smith 1985). Ayres (1965) recognized this principle and investigated the importance of its application in the study and treatment of children with a variety of central nervous system disorders. This research indicated that dysfunction in the proprioceptive, vestibular, tactile, and visual systems could adversely affect the development of higher level functions (Ayres 1972, 1978). Ayres postulated that treatment enhancing basic sensory integration would have a positive influence on motoric, tactile, emotional, and cognitive functions.

Remediation using a sensory integrative approach has been an effective form of intervention for certain diagnostic groups. Importantly, some populations previously studied display behaviors similar to those seen in the fra(X) population. Among these are autistic children, who are hypersensitive to touch (Ayres and Tickle 1980), individuals with stereotypic rocking behavior (Bonadonna 1981), and children who display self-stimulatory or self-injurious behavior (Storey et al. 1984; Bright et al. 1981). There is also evidence that sensory integrative therapy can facilitate the development of language skills in mentally retarded, developmentally delayed, learning-disabled, and autistic children (Densom et al. 1989; Kantner et al. 1982; Kawar 1973; Meegrum et al. 1981; Reilly et al. 1983). Table 11.2 summarizes seven sensory integration efficacy studies and provides comparative data on subjects, treatment design, research parameters, and findings (Parham 1988).

The quality of higher level functioning in the CNS may depend on the integrity of more basic integration, with the individual's behavior often a clue as to this integrity (Ayres 1979). For example, if there has been inadequate vestibular and proprioceptive integration, individuals may be fearful when their feet are off the ground. Others may be unable to tolerate vigorous movement. On the other hand, a visual fascination with spinning tops or other toys, watching water twirling out of a faucet or flushing down a toilet, or ritualistic movements may be used to satisfy a need for movement in the head or body. It has been postulated that this type of self-stimulation may be an attempt to stimulate the vestibular system (Ayres 1979).

Another basic system involves tactile perception. If dysfunction of this system is manifested by hypersensitivity to touch, persons may prefer wearing long-sleeved clothing or avoiding light touch while craving being held tightly. They may even bite or hit themselves when overly excited in an attempt at self-

Table 11.2

Sensory Integration Studies

Reference	Diagnosis	Age	No.	Design	Procedure	Duration	Parameter	Findings
Arnold et al. (1985)	Attention deficit disorder w/hyperactivity	Kindergarten to 9 yr	37	Split sample Latin square crossover	Control, then combined visual & vestibular, then vestibular alone or total control, then combined visual & vestibular, then visual alone.	2 sessions/wk; 4 wk each condition, 12 wk	Hyperactivity, behavior ratings	Significant improvement in hyperactivity particularly with solitary vestibular stimulation ($P < .05$); effects still significant at 1 yr follow-up.
Ayres and Mailloux (1981)	Aphasia	4–5 yr	4	Single case	Sensory integration	2 sessions/wk, 1 yr	Language	Children with depressed postrotary nystagmus showed improved rate of language development
Ayres and Tickle (1980)	Autism	3 yr 6 mo to 13 yr 2 mo	10	Quasi-experimental	Sensory integration	2 sessions/wk, 1 yr	Reaction to sensory input, language, awareness of environment, purposeful activity, self-stimulation, social and emotional behavior	Sensory integration procedures more effective w/hyperreactive than hyporeactive children
Bonadomma (1981)	Mental retardation	13–22 yr	3	Single-case multiple	Vestibular stimulation	10 min/d, 5 d/wk, 3 wk	Stereotypic rocking	Stereotypic rocking reduced & re-

332

Study	Population	Age	N	Design	Intervention	Duration	Outcome	Results
				baseline				mained low 6 d after program end
Magun et al. (1981)	Mental retardation	3–10 yr	10	Treatment baseline reversal	Vestibular stimulation	10 min/d for 5 d	Spontaneous verbalizations	Significant relationship between vestibular stimulation & spontaneous verbalization
McKibben (1973)	Developmental apraxia & poor tactile perception	5–10 yr	27	Experimental w/controls	Gross motor or tactile stimulation or eye-hand coordination activities	1-hr sessions 3/wk, 16 wk	Motor planning & tactile perception	Motor planning & tactile perception showed significant improvement in all groups ($P <$ .01). Gains were maintained. Group receiving additional tactile stimulation did not show significantly greater improvement ($P >$ .10).
Ottenbacher (1982)	Severely or profoundly retarded	39–97 mo	14	Experimental (pre-post), with controls	Vestibular stimulation	30–40 min, 3–4 sessions/wk for 13 wk	Seizures	No significant differences in the control of seizures between groups

inhibition through input to deep proprioceptors (Ayres 1979).

Olfactory stimuli, which input at the cortical rather than the brain stem level (Scott 1986) and which influence the limbic system and memory (Gustavson et al. 1987; Nobak 1975), may cause primitive defensive or nondiscriminatory behavior. One study demonstrated that fra(X) children initially perceive non-aversive scents as either noxious or undifferentiated (Burns and Hickman 1989). This response to olfactory stimuli is yet another example of disorganized sensory processing. Improvements in sensory processing at all levels may be reflected in improved sensory integration and subsequent output, both motor and vocal (Windeck and Laurel 1989; Bellman and Goldberg 1984; Clark and Steingold 1982; de Quiros and Schrager 1978; de Quiros 1976; Zivin 1979; Luria 1976).

Early learning occurs through the child's basic sensory experiences with people and with the environment. For meaningful interaction to occur, a child must be at a normal level of arousal (Windeck and Laurel 1989). Inadequate early sensory experiences resulting from decreased central nervous system organization may lead to poor environmental and social interaction and delays in language development. Tactile defensiveness in infants and young children, for example, may lead to decreased interactions with care givers and other children, disrupting the natural development of social interaction (Wilbarger and Wilbarger 1988; Short-DeGraff 1988).

The goal of therapy is to help the person develop more adaptive responses in a developmentally appropriate sequence. Vestibular, proprioceptive, and tactile systems underlie and contribute to later skills in visual, auditory, and language areas.

A sensory integrative problem involving poor sensory inhibition may include general hypersensitivity and hyperactivity. The individual with this problem is unable to screen important from unimportant environmental information and must be helped to develop appropriate inhibitory and discriminatory, rather than global or stereotypic, reactions.

Throughout testing and therapy sessions, appropriate principles, activities, and environment should be provided. The therapist must also respond to the complex behavioral needs of the fra(X) individual. This is accomplished by understanding the stereotypic behavior and then responding with appropriate intervention. The therapist may respond with a reassuring touch, a quieter voice, a slower rate of speech, or singing rather than speaking directions. A therapist should acknowledge the agitation a person may feel and perhaps help with verbalization or expression of the person's emotional state. Expressing the reasons for the stereotypic behavior used to control his emotion can also be helpful. Once discussed, alternative behaviors can be suggested and demonstrated. For example, the person may bite his hand when stressed by testing procedures. The therapist may say, "It is uncomfortable to be tested. Biting your hand helps you to calm down. Here's another way to feel better." Techniques that can be used by the person, either alone or with the assistance of family or staff, are listed in table 11.3.

As previously mentioned, the fra(X) individual with disordered central nervous system function may be sensitive to environmental stimuli. General principles that may be applied to maintain a more normal level of arousal during testing or therapy or at home include the

- use of natural lighting;
- use of clothing made of natural fibers that do not irritate;
- avoidance of foods that may worsen behavior problems, such as hyperactivity;
- awareness of the effect of color and olfactory stimuli on emotional state.

It is also critical for therapists and educators working with fra(X) individuals to understand that many behavioral problems result from sensory integrative deficits and are not intentional acts on the part of the child. The underlying cause of behavioral problems in this population must be examined as it will have a significant effect on the type of therapy used to change undesirable behaviors. A strict behavior modification program may not be appropriate if behaviors are resulting from sensory integrative deficits.

Speech and Language Therapy and Fra(X)

No research on specific speech and language treatment regimes with fra(X) individuals has been reported. However, because the fra(X) population is similar in many ways to the learning-disabled, mentally retarded and autistic populations, intervention strategies found useful with those individuals can be utilized with fra(X) individuals.

Professionals often hunt for cookbook techniques for therapy. Because of the wide variation in skill levels of fra(X) individuals, this approach is not feasible. Instead, therapy goals for each child should be determined by his or her specific strengths, weaknesses, and skills in a variety of areas. Sensory integrative dysfunction and cognitive and attentional deficits will significantly affect speech/language development and learning. Therefore, before speech and language therapy is initiated, these areas of difficulty must be addressed (see chapter 5). Assessment of the sensory integration, cognitive, and attentional domains is vital. To establish a strong foundation for future learning, the therapeutic principles of each area must be applied.

General guidelines in planning programming for speech and language therapy have been compiled in table 11.4. Many of the suggestions are based on

Table 11.3
Integrative Therapy Model

	Intervention Strategies
Disorganization in basic systems . . .	
Tactile	Deep pressure
Hypersensitivity	Joint compression
	Vibration
	Brushing (Wilbarger and Wilbarger [1988])
(As additional systems and interventions are added, previous ones are incorporated.)	
Vestibular-proprioceptive	"Heavy work" activities—in quadruped
(Movement-weight bearing)	Gradual introduction of rhythmic movement
Fear of being off the ground	with tactile, weight-bearing activities
Stereotypical movements	
Poor postural control & balance	
Poor antigravity postures	
Auditory	Calming music
Aversion or sensitivity to sounds	"Mantra" sounds such as mm,
	Headphones to dampen environmental sounds
Visual-spatial	Experiences in going "through," "around,"
Fascination with primitive visual	"over" objects
stimuli	Combining tactile, vestibular-
Visual distractibility	proprioceptive, and focused visual input
Poor spatial orientation	
. . . leads to disorganization in progressively "higher level" systems	
Motor planning and sequencing	Weight shifting
Poor trunk flexion	Weight bearing and movement combined
Poor trunk rotation	with activities requiring trunk flexion and
Poor crossing midline skills	rotation
Poor left/right orientation	Music (singing), rhyming, poems, limer-
Oral and verbal dyspraxia	icks; slow, whispered speech
Fast rate	
Social interaction play	
Aggression or withdrawal	Calming activities
Stereotypical motor responses	Modeling alternative responses
Poor eye contact	Use of language to prepare for upcoming transition
Difficulty with transitions	Use of music to signal transition
Attending skills	
Hypersensitivity to sensory input	Calming, focusing techniques
Inability to attend to specific meaning and discriminate	Use of interest areas in teaching

Table 11.3 (*Continued*)

	Intervention Strategies
Auditory memory deficits	Auditory memory and sequencing
	Short, simple instructions
	Several short sessions rather than one long one
	Decrease auditory and visual distractions
Speech & language	
Pragmatic deficits	Provide appropriate external speech
	Model and expand desired utterances
	Provide opportunity for communicative interactions in child-centered, naturalistic setting
Learning	Use any of the above techniques as needed
	Use strength in visual area when teaching
	Combine visual and tactile with auditory input
	Utilize interest areas
	Computers
	Peer tutoring
	Mainstreaming or
	Reverse mainstreaming

clinical experience and our understanding of the specific learning style of fra(X) individuals.

Fra(X) individuals usually exhibit difficulties with topic maintenance, tangential comments, initiation of conversation, short-term memory, cluttering, verbal and motor dyspraxia, abstract reasoning, perseveration (repetition of words, phrases, sentences, or topics), and eye gaze (see chapter 5). Many of these deficits relate to a disorder of pragmatics. Pragmatics is the study of the conversational act and its components. The purpose of conversation is to control or influence a listener's thoughts, beliefs, actions, and attitudes (Lucas 1980). Conversation may serve a variety of communicative functions: labeling, denying, requesting, or stating information, among others. For individuals to be proficient in pragmatic or conversational skills, they must have developed a repertoire of socially acceptable rules and strategies for influencing their listener. They must be able to utilize the correct linguistic structures as well as nonverbal cues (eye contact, gestures, body posture) to get their message across effectively. Children with pragmatic difficulties may not have developed the linguistic knowledge necessary to communicate effectively or may not use

Table 11.4

Speech/Language Deficits and Intervention Strategies

Deficit Areas	*Intervention Strategies*
Attention	Utilize child's interest areas
	Supplement auditory with visual input, including photographs
	Keep auditory and visual distractions at a minimum
	Work in small, partitioned area
	Use headphones to dampen sound
	Have the occupational therapist provide calming activities
	Work for several short periods
Delayed onset of expressive speech	Utilize a total communication approach—fade out signs as verbalizations increase
	Reinforce any attempts at speech, shape responses by modeling correct utterances
Rate, rhythm, "cluttering"	Model correct rate/rhythm
	Perform melodic intonation therapy (Sparks et al. [1987]; Sparks and Holland [1976])
	Increase self-monitoring
	Use voice synthesizer for auditory and visual feedback
Oral and verbal dyspraxia	Use music, singing, and movement
	Integrate therapy with occupational therapist (Windeck and Laurel [1989])
Memory	Elicit attention before task
	Pair auditory information with visual cue
	Practice rhythm and music to cue recall
	Use short instructions intrinsic to task
Abstract reasoning, problem-solving skills	Utilize realistic, meaningful materials of interest to the child
	Begin at the level of the concrete and systematically increase the level of abstraction
	Use a microcomputer/game format, *Think Aloud Program* (Camp and Bash [1981])
Verbal perseveration, tangential comments, topic maintenance	Allow increased processing time
	Model desired utterances
	Reduce complexity of utterances to child's level
	Monitor anxiety level and adapt accordingly (calming and focusing activities)

Table 11.4 (*Continued*)

Deficit Areas	Intervention Strategies
	Provide opportunities to practice a variety of speech acts
	Redirect the child verbally
	Have the child reauditorize to help process
	Emphasize "topic" through use of high interest materials

General Strategies:

Because imitative skills are often strong in fra(X) individuals, small groups consisting of higher-functioning children should be utilized to augment individual therapy.

Maintain close coordination of goals among all those working with the child. Encourage the parents to follow through on home programs.

Evaluate the need for combined speech/language and occupational therapies.

conversational rules and strategies appropriately. In addition, they may not be able to correctly interpret verbal and nonverbal messages from others. Difficulties with conversational rules and strategies are common within the fra(X) population; examples of typical pragmatic difficulties are outlined in table 11.5.

One of the more distinctive pragmatic features of the fra(X) syndrome is the use of perseveration. As with repetitive self-stimulatory behaviors (such as hand biting and rocking), perseveration may reflect the fra(X) individual's difficulty with inhibition of responses. Perseveration may also be an anxiety-based response to excessive language demands. For example, increased receptive and expressive as well as pragmatic demands may cause the fra(X) individual to become anxious, resulting in increased use of perseveration. Anxiety is often experienced during formal assessments. As the assessment demands become more complex, perseveration is more frequent. For the fra(X) individual, perseveration may provide a conversational time filler as well as increased time for processing information, as has been documented in non-fra(X) aphasics (Arwood 1984; Travis 1971). By providing more time for processing, the therapist is more apt to elicit an appropriate response and conversation may be facilitated.

Because there is such variability of speech and language deficits in the fra(X) individual, a thorough assessment of pragmatic skills is necessary. Although formal assessment tools are available through publishers, many therapist-made tools are equally sensitive. Suggestions for developing specific pragmatic treatment programs for fra(X) individuals can be drawn from the related fields of autism and developmental disabilities. Pragmatic skill programs that take ad-

Table 11.5

Examples of Pragmatic Deficits Seen in Fra(X) Individuals

Off-Target Responses

Therapist:	Eli, tell me about your day.
Patient:	I like Hawaii, I like the hula.
Therapist:	Eli, how was your day? Tell me about it.
Patient:	It was okay; Luis, you're looking skinny.

Tangential Comments

Patient:	I really loved the movie "Tootsie."
Therapist:	Yeah, it was funny.
Patient:	You know, Tootsie's wig was all poofed up; she was a scream.
Therapist:	Yeah, she was great.
Patient:	You know you look like Julie Andrews, did I ever tell you that?

Perseveration

Patient:	These transformers are hard to take apart. Where'd you buy them?
Therapist:	At the department store.
Patient:	Can I try the white one?
Therapist:	Sure; it's pretty hard.
Patient:	That weather's really bad out today, really bad.
Therapist:	Is that white one hard to take apart?
Patient:	That weather's bad, really windy. Don't you think the weather's bad?
Therapist:	Jimmy, please pass the apples.
Patient:	They're in the chocolate milk, in the milk.
Therapist:	I need the apples, please pass the apples.
Patient:	Chocolate milk, where's chocolate milk?

Topic Closure

Therapist:	I'm rolling my play dough with a rolling pin.
Patient:	A rolling pin! A rolling pin! Roll it out, Molly, very good, very good! I like play dough, I do! Let's use a star cookie cutter, here it is, Molly. The star is very pretty, very nice. Push down hard. It's a Christmas star.

Nonverbal Difficulties

Poor eye contact

Perseverative rocking, head nodding, swaying

Exaggerated gestures

---

vantage of naturally occurring events in the child's environment, facilitate the spontaneous use of communication, and encourage a wide generalization of learning are best (Stokes and Bauer 1977). Conversely, a dogmatic, therapist-centered approach to teaching pragmatics may inhibit or disrupt social interaction and communication (Wetherby 1986) and is not desirable.

Fra(X) individuals demonstrate strong verbal and social imitative skills, and they should be placed with others functioning at the same or a slightly higher language level. Many of the suggestions listed in table 11.3 are applicable in a group setting. These include using the group's interest areas, utilizing visual cues, and allowing extra response time. Modeling of correct utterances (reducing the complexity of therapist verbalizations), expansion (expanding the child's utterance with one or two words), and parallel talk (verbalizing what the patient is doing or thinking) are useful in improving pragmatics (Koegel et al. 1987) and, more specifically, perseveration. Modeling and expansion are also used to target the growth of specific linguistic structures. These techniques have been used successfully with the autistic population (Scherer and Olswang 1989; Schwartz and Leonard 1985). A fast rate of speech, oral and verbal dyspraxia, and difficulties with auditory memory and abstract reasoning skills also require remediation. Although specific therapeutic techniques for these deficits can be found in the general speech and language literature, some adaptations should be made in structure and presentation when working with the fra(X) population. Suggestions for adaptations in the therapy setting are found in table 11.3, and other specific strategies may be found in table 11.4.

The nonverbal fra(X) individual presents a particular challenge to the speech/language pathologist. A total communication approach (the use of sign in combination with verbal output) has been useful in stimulating language growth. Therapists have noted that, as the fra(X) child's spontaneous verbalizations increased, the use of sign language decreased and gradually faded out (Scharfenaker and Hickman 1989). General motor skills, including motor planning and sequencing skills, should be assessed before the use of sign language. The *Assessment, Behavior Management & Communication Training Program* by Krug et al. (1980) was used successfully with several moderately handicapped, nonverbal fra(X) children. Sign language and speech imitation are taught independently and then combined into total communication when the student initiates vocalizations while signing. As speech production increases, the use of signs fades. The curriculum is centered on the child's interests and desires. Programming is presented through a hierarchical series of structured cues and responses, allowing quick and easy assessment of progress and areas of need.

The technology in the area of augmentative and alternative communication is expanding rapidly. If total communication or sign language is not helpful to a specific child, alternative communication systems must be evaluated. The decision to use a specific communication device or computer is based upon evaluation of the child's motor, cognitive, perceptual, social, and communicative skills and needs. Montgomery (1980), Musselwhite and St. Louis (1982), Silverman (1982), Yoder (1982), and Schiefelbush (1980) provided information useful in evaluating appropriate alternative communication choices for children.

Integrating Occupational and Speech Therapies: A Rationale

The combined therapy approach, in a small group setting, can facilitate integration of sensory, language, and cognitive skills for the fra(X) individual. The calming and centering provided by the occupational therapist, using sensory integrative techniques, enable the fra(X) person to focus on more cognitive and language-related activities. The problems of oral and verbal dyspraxia also lend themselves well to the combined approach (Windeck and Laurel 1989). Use of movement, rhythm, music, singing, and limericks can facilitate and enhance motor planning and sequencing (Sparks et al. 1974; Sparks and Holland 1976).

Table 11.3 represents the developmental, integrative model, illustrating the concept that higher skills are built upon more basic sensory modalities. Techniques or activities are given for each area of need in each of the three disciplines of occupational therapy, speech therapy, and educational intervention. These are only examples and cannot substitute for individual treatment planning. Children and adults diagnosed as having fra(X) syndrome have common behavioral characteristics, but they also have significant individual differences, strengths, and weaknesses. Even though a treatment session is planned to follow a certain sequence, the reciprocal therapeutic interactions between therapists and clients must reflect the client's and the group's immediate and evolving needs.

Education and Fra(X)

Curricular needs vary based on the functioning level of the fra(X) individual. In any instructional setting, materials should be age and IQ appropriate. In general, it is best to utilize functional or real life materials whenever possible. Simulated or representational materials are often too abstract for the fra(X) individual because of language and cognitive difficulties. Concrete, realistic, and familiar materials seem to stimulate learning. This allows the learner to organize the incoming information into an already familiar schema.

Observation indicates that these patients learn through associations made in a particular context, as opposed to normal learning, which involves the acquisition of a concept with subsequent generalization into other contexts until the concept is widely known and readily accessed. The concept is accessed in the context in which it was initially learned or within an association. Often the fra(X) learner seems to be confused or disassociated from the material presented because it is not being presented or associated within the context in which it was learned. This hypothesis is further validated by performance on the Kaufman Assessment Battery for Children (K-ABC) (Kemper et al. 1988; Leckman et al. 1989). On this assessment, the fra(X) patient typically performs better using simultaneous processing rather than sequential processing. The fra(X) patient demonstrates more success when asked to access information presented in a global manner (e.g., visual closure, identifying an object whole that is presented with missing components). The fra(X) patient demonstrates more difficulty with the reverse, the formulation of a whole from individual parts presented in order.

The educational challenge with this population is to adapt teaching materials that promote success through familiar contexts. The phenomenon of incidental learning is also important and is reflected in the high score usually obtained by fra(X) boys on the faces and places subtest of the K-ABC (Kemper et al. 1988). Abilities or skills may be acquired by fra(X) patients in a subtle, nontraditional method. Again, this seems to be related to interest areas as well as associated contexts. The fra(X) patient may produce information in a rather nonchalant manner to the surprise of parents and/or educators. The acquired information is often unrelated to the designated curricular focus and seems to be acquired incidentally or without formal teaching.

When establishing an appropriate curriculum, integrating the child's incidentally acquired knowledge is important. For example, when teaching numbers, a clock, microwave touch plate, computer keyboard, or license plates may be used in preference to flashcards, workbooks, or number lines. Flags, cars, or product labels may be used when teaching reading or vocabulary. Also important is the identification and use of high interest materials to reduce student resistance and distractibility. An assessment of interests can be helpful when creating curricular content and strategies (table 11.6).

Educators often fail to recognize the influence of the environment on learning. Fra(X) children performed better at tasks that accessed information learned through a familiar environment than at tasks that accessed information learned from novel situations (Kemper et al. 1988). Classroom noise, teacher/peer interactions, lighting, and curricular materials will significantly affect the learning environment of the fra(X) individual. As these variables are addressed, modifications can be made to facilitate learning. Tables 11.3 and 11.4 present some useful suggestions for altering the environment and programs to fit the fra(X) individual's need.

Some areas of visual perception seem to be a strength for many fra(X) boys. Utilizing this strength (e.g., when giving instructions and drawing or acting out stories) is often more useful than limiting the presentation to auditorily presented instruction.

Often fra(X) individuals experience motor deficits manifested in poor eye-hand coordination and motor dyspraxia (Levitas et al. 1983). This has implications for academic expectations related to writing. Even though the individual often demonstrates motivation to draw or write, the task becomes so difficult that often inappropriate behavioral responses emerge. Wide margin paper or

Table 11.6
Interest Inventory

FAVORITE PEOPLE	FAVORITE TV SHOWS
1. _____	1. _____
2. _____	2. _____
3. _____	3. _____
4. _____	4. _____
5. _____	5. _____
FAVORITE PLACES	FAVORITE SUBJECTS
1. _____	1. _____
2. _____	2. _____
3. _____	3. _____
4. _____	4. _____
5. _____	5. _____

FAVORITE ACTIVITIES (even those that are perseverative and seem to be nonproductive)

1. _____

2. _____

3. _____

4. _____

5. _____

Source: © Copyright 1988 Marcia L. Braden, Ph.D.

paper with nubbed lines to guide motor output through tactile input can be beneficial. Adaptive devices, such as a pencil grip, primary-sized pencils, or markers may provide more tactile input and promote better production. Templates or fine motor tracing devices have also been useful in providing structure and boundaries when the individual is first learning to draw or write. Storytelling while the individual is moving the pencil from left to right can provide motivation to comply. For example, a child might be given a picture of a car on the left margin, a copy of a logo from a favorite fast food chain on the right margin, and a line between. A student could be asked to "drive his car to McDonald's," staying on the "road" as he "drives."

Integrated Service Approach: Infants and Toddlers

The benefit of early education intervention programs has long been debated (Caldwell and Stedman 1977). One of the earlier surveys commissioned by Elliott Richardson, Secretary of Health, Education and Welfare, indicated that educational programs for preschool handicapped children, whether infants or five-year-olds, could significantly improve the quality of the children's lives. Of particular interest was the finding that the effects of early intervention were most salient when they occurred during the period of rapid development. In addition, if access to the child could be gained in the early years (one to two years of age) when language was emerging, the programs were even more effective than if begun later. This intervention contributed to the child's social and intellectual development. Several preschool programs have been successful with autistic children with pervasive developmental delays. The approach is usually developmental with an emphasis on language and affect development within an integrated setting (Rogers and Lewis 1989; Rogers et al. 1986; Strain 1987).

A plateau and then decline in IQ score is typically seen in the majority of fra(X) males (chapter 5). This seems to be related to deficits in abstract reasoning that are emphasized in cognitive testing during middle and later childhood. Consequently, the learning potential may be greatest during preschool and early school years (Paul et al. 1987). Early sensory integration and attentional deficits often contribute to difficulty in learning for the fra(X) child. Hypersensitivity to sounds, sights, and touch makes normal interactions with one's environment difficult at best and interferes with social, motor, play, and emotional development (Scharfenaker and Schreiner 1989). Therefore, the need for a multidisciplinary and integrated approach at this age level is critical for the fra(X) child.

Occupational Therapy and Sensory Integration

Several early warning signs have been observed clinically and have been described as indicators of an infant's or child's need for therapeutic intervention. These warning signs are outlined in table 11.7. Some of these behaviors have been observed in infants and young children with fra(X) syndrome and reflect difficulty in processing environmental stimuli and difficulty with interpersonal interactions.

Table 11.7

Warning Signs for Developmental Delay, Deficits in Sensory Integration, or Language Problems

---

Behavior that may be present from infancy
- Inability to calm
- Arrhythmic movements; not in synchrony with speech or with music
- Fear of new activities, especially off the ground (i.e., being held up in the air, playing on slides, swings, merry go rounds)
- Aversion to new textures on body or to new textures or tastes in mouth
- Passive, nonexpressive facial features
- Difficulty with transitions
  1. Leaving caregiver
  2. Going from one activity to another
- Late-developing babbling

Problems that may become more obvious in the toddler or older child
- Poor posture: may be lordotic (swayed lower back) or kyphotic (rounded upper back) with stiff, perhaps broad-based walk, with little or no trunk rotation
- May walk on toes
- Lack of grading of movements: may be jerky or exaggerated, without smoothness or subtlety
- Aversion or hypersensitivity to smells, with possible lack of differentiation among odors
- Clumsy, with poor balance
- Overly aggressive or passive
- Hurrying from one activity to another and unable to stay with one activity more than momentarily
- Trouble with motor planning, whether imitating others' movements, figuring out how to climb, or maneuvering around objects; may be able to do an activity one day, but unable to the next
- Poor social interaction with peers
- Difficult to understand after age 3
- Late in developing first words and phrases

Because the young fra(X) child often has difficulty cooperating or performing on standardized tests, plans for therapeutic intervention can be made based on observed behaviors. The therapist should attempt to administer developmental assessments or standardized tests to observe the child's responses to a variety of sensory, motor, and visual tasks. In addition, intervention strategies that may help the child calm or focus on an activity can be explored. Whether or not standardized scores are obtainable, the observations made in a testing session are invaluable in planning subsequent treatment. Parents can provide the most pertinent and reliable information regarding the child's preferences and patterns in movement, response to touch and visual stimulation, responses to transitions, and other stresses in his or her life. They can also describe ways the child interacts with toys, objects, and people and the degree of independence in self-care activities.

Many children with fra(X) syndrome are extremely sensitive to environmental stimuli, especially to touch and movement. As a result, there may be difficulty modulating behavior, and they may exhibit hostility or aggressiveness or may simply withdraw to avoid being overwhelmed by the environment. For these children, individual occupational therapy may be preferred, with sensory integrative treatment structured to reduce these hypersensitive responses. The therapist may work with the child in a dimly lit room and use only essential play equipment. Additional structure and calming may be provided by using taped environmental sounds or music with a strong underlying beat. Initially, transitions may be facilitated by holding the child firmly and carrying him in a prone position from one activity to the next. Additional techniques are suggested in table 11.8.

Speech and Language

The relationship between functional and symbolic play and language acquisition is well established (Bates 1979; McCune-Nicolich 1981; Ungerer and Sigman 1985). An early intervention program must be based on interactive play in a natural setting through which communication can evolve. Play provides children with an opportunity for observation and imitation of others, which are basic prerequisites for language and learning (Bloom and Lahey 1978).

The role of speech/language pathologists in early intervention is multidimensional. Therapists must provide direct or consultative services within the classroom as part of the multidisciplinary team. They must provide parents with ongoing suggestions on how they can apply speech/language intervention techniques at home. In addition, therapists must integrate intervention techniques from other disciplines into the therapy program.

For this age level, the therapy techniques of imitation, modeling, and expansion are most beneficial. Facilitating imitation of environmental and animal sounds may be the starting point of therapy for very young children. Modeling and expansion can then be utilized as receptive and expressive vocabulary increases.

Educational Components

Social and behavioral skills are important preacademic aspects of an early intervention program for the fra(X) child. Infant training programs should focus on attending behaviors, tolerating change in routine, and social awareness of the environment. The fostering of consistency and predictability of a

Table 11.8

Calming Activities

Activity	Appropriate for:		
	Infants/Toddlers	*Children*	*Adolescents/Adults*
Brushing: Using a surgical scrub brush, vigorously brush person's back, arms, hands, legs. (Avoid stomach and face.) Follow with joint compression through elbow to shoulder, wrist to elbow, fingers and thumb. Then apply pressure downward through shoulders and head.	X	X	X
Quieting sounds such as environmental sounds, imagery, music	X	X	X
Chewing crushed ice or "slushy"		X	X
Slow stroking on the back: Light stroking with your fingers beginning at the nape of the neck and stopping at the top of the hips. Do this no more than 3 min for children, 5 min for adults.	X	X	X
Joint compression: Push-ups or pushing against wall		X	X
Quadruped activities	X	X	
Creeping through tunnels	X	X	
Deep pressure: Swaddling or wrapping in blankets	X		
Wearing ace wraps on legs, arms, trunk, even around head (if person wants it)		X	X
Holding child so his back is against your chest, press down lightly on his head; provides neutral warmth and rhythmic pressure	X	X	
Lying on mat, apply firm pressure on gymnastic ball as it is rolled over person's legs, back.		X	X
Kneading bread dough		X	X

Table 11.8   (*Continued*)

Activity	Appropriate for:		
	Infants/Toddlers	*Children*	*Adolescents/Adults*
Wedging into barrel with pillows	X	X	X
Wedging into "squeeze machine" (Grandin and Scariano 1988) or crawling through short, tight, foam-lined tunnel.		X	X
Wearing inflatable vest to provide constant comforting pressure	X	X	X
Wearing headphones: pressure to head and dampening of environmental "noise"		X	X
Vibration:			
Vibrating pillow, activated with pressure	X	X	X
Electric toothbrush		X	X
Vibrating or "Mantra" sounds such as "mm" or "zz"	X	X	X
Feeling vibration of music on tape deck, on feet, hands	X	X	
Yoga and deep breathing (Uma et al. 1989)		X	X
Aerobics, exercise programs, jogging, swimming		X	X
Massage	X	X	X
Animal therapy: petting, caring for		X	X

Source: Data from Birren (1979); Farber (1982); Grandin and Scariano (1988); Huss (1976); Kawar (1973); and Wilbarger and Wilbarger (1988).

schedule allows the child to trust the environment. This may reduce anxiety and in turn maladaptive behaviors that may result from anxiety.

A daily routine can be established by training the child to anticipate particular activities (bath, breakfast, dressing, play, lunch, bedtime, etc.). As the process evolves, the child will become familiar with the schedule and then can be cued to anticipate a change of activity using a bell, timer, or music.

Behavior in the fra(X) patient will vary with each individual. For example, a child may eat for his mother but not for his father, or he will only allow his father to bathe him. To ensure generalization of behaviors, one must rotate caretaker interaction with the child in the home and in other settings.

The shaping of appropriate behavioral responses through imitation and modeling is an important programming need for the infant/toddler. Toddlers may jump or hand flap when they become excited or overstimulated while watching television, looking at books, hearing music, or observing movement. The hand flapping behavior can be shaped into a behavior that is more socially acceptable through modeling something like hand clapping and then reinforcing the child whenever he or she substitutes that more adaptive behavior.

Again, it is important to explore interests at this age and to expand upon a variety of materials that are motivating and promote self-initiation. With early programming, these individuals more easily integrate into the structure of a school placement.

Case History

CA, aged four, attends a small private preschool, receiving combined occupational and speech therapy three times a week in a classroom setting. Educational intervention is provided by the speech therapist. In addition, a music therapist and a physical therapist join the staff for weekly integrated sessions. Parents are involved in monthly informational and emotional support groups and are encouraged to have daily classroom contact. CA demonstrated difficulty with motor planning and defensiveness to touch. His speech was characterized by a fast rate, perseveration, and consistent off-topic utterances. His speech did not exhibit boundaries such as pauses or topic closure, which resulted in an excessive and constant stream of verbalizations. He resisted sitting for long periods as it was difficult to inhibit motor behavior. This was also evident in his difficulty inhibiting excessive verbalizations. In each therapy session, the occupational therapist provided activities to focus and calm him. He was not responsive to bouncing a ball or being brushed. Parallel talk and modeling of correct and slow utterances were used in conjunction with the occupational therapist's calming and focusing suggestions at home and at school. These techniques were useful in reducing the perseveration, slowing his rate of speech, and providing him with a model for conversational boundaries.

The School-aged Child

Occupational Therapy and Sensory Integration

Fra(X) teenagers usually have not developed the normal skills that would enable them to cope with the complicated adjustments involved in development through childhood. The physical, emotional, and intellectual changes common to adolescent development intensify the problems. The ability to screen out environmental stimuli, a sense of competence and self-reliance, and tolerance for change may not develop. At a time when peer acceptance is gaining importance, fra(X) children are apt to exhibit behaviors that alienate them from group interaction. A clinical study with a group of learning-disabled non-fra(X) teenagers (Jones et al. 1986) demonstrated that learning style, communication, and pragmatic areas were affected by sensory integration difficulties. Underlying all of these dysfunctional areas was the complication of a poor self-image.

Emotional complications such as depression, anger, and rebellion may emerge and must be dealt with. Treatment in a group setting to address all areas of need with occupational and speech therapies and educational and emotional support is critical. Tables 11.3 and 11.8 offer specific suggestions for this age group.

Speech and Language

A thorough assessment of speech/language, occupational therapy, and academic needs will help direct the focus of speech therapy and determine the frequency of intervention. In general, small group speech/language therapy is beneficial, yet individual therapy offers one-on-one therapist-student interaction and decreased distractions. A combination of group and individual therapy therefore is optimal.

During the school years, peer modeling should play an important role in fra(X) speech/language therapy. Small groups are best in teaching pragmatic skills through role playing, modeling, and problem solving (Lucas 1980). Typical experiences and topical interests of the group can further be used to increase motivation and ultimately increase generalization of learned skills. The input of an occupational therapist is important in providing calming and focusing strategies for the group.

Peer tutoring is a useful strategy when working with fra(X) individuals in a variety of educational and therapeutic settings. Tutoring provides the student with more individualized teaching and with repetition and practice. Tutoring within the classroom, rather than having a child removed from the room, is preferable. In addition, this technique encourages and gives the student a chance to practice social and pragmatic skills (Jenkins and Jenkins 1981).

The benefits of computers in regular and special education classrooms have been documented (Mokros and Russell 1986; Maddux 1984). Microcomputers have been used successfully with fra(X) children in both the academic and therapy settings. The visual presentation of microcomputers capitalizes on the strong visual skills of fra(X) children. A computer allows the child to learn independently of the teacher and also gives an important sense of control over learning (Ellis and Sabornie 1986). The colorful nature of many programs helps to focus a child's attention, which is usually a problem in fra(X) syndrome. However, many microcomputers lie idle in classrooms or are used primarily as reinforcing games for classwork finished early. Regular and special education teachers should be encouraged and instructed in how to use microcomputers effectively in the classroom.

The National Special Educator's Alliance, a program of Apple Computer, Inc., has several member centers across the United States. These centers provide information and programs for children with disabilities, their families, and professionals working with them. The centers emphasize the use of specially adapted computers to reinforce learning and play skills and guide parents and professionals in choosing developmentally appropriate software for their children and students. A list of these centers and of major publishers of software for the speech/language profession may be found in appendix 11.1.

Many types of software are available for a variety of topics in special education. Programs that teach the basic skill of cause-effect are available, as are programs in problem solving skills for the higher-functioning child. Special concerns in evaluating software for the fra(X) child include the auditory and visual distractibility of the program and its complexity. Placing the keyboard on the floor with the child lying in front of it or having the child sit in a bean bag chair with the keyboard in his lap may be more beneficial than using traditional seating. Similarly, special adaptations for keyboards are available. A child's cognitive level and visual-spatial, memory, motor, and language skills must be evaluated so that appropriate software can be matched to the student. The input of the occupational therapist in assessing perceptual-motor abilities, recommending optimal seating, and suggesting approaches to help the child focus attention is also beneficial.

Educational Components

Parents and clinicians report that fra(X) children have an ability to identify missing items and recall specific visual detail in their environment. This is considered a cognitive strength, and a mode of intervention using visual gestalt (presenting information within a visual context that is familiar to the child) seems to be successful. The use of photographs has been effective in providing familiar visual stimuli that can be used to develop basic concepts. For example, color naming in isolation is often difficult, but if pictures of familiar automobiles are associated with a specific color the accuracy improves. When a numeral is associated with a photograph of a familiar license plate, it is more easily retained within that context. Other academic materials found useful with this population are described in appendix 11.2.

A pictorial, visual cuing technique can also be applied to behavior management. A pictorial approach showing a more appropriate behavioral response is reinforced by using a routine bedtime story with pictures of the child in his or her own home environment. For many fra(X) children, independent grooming before bed (showers or baths, hair washing, teeth brushing, toileting, or dressing) may provoke extreme resistance. A picture album of the child going through the behavioral sequence at home with captions that reflect the child's own language can be read before beginning the bedtime ritual. This process seems to give the child additional information that may have more meaningful or concrete application.

Fra (X) patients exhibit great difficulty with basic math concepts and numeric calculation (Kemper et al. 1988; Hagerman 1987). Given the nature of their learning style, it follows that sequential calculation processes present great difficulty. In addition, language deficits may further complicate math delays. For example, basic concepts of more/less, big/little, half/whole, long/short are related to mathematic operations. Even if the student is able to master basic level computations through rote memory or practice, progress becomes increasingly difficult when abstractions, formulas, and representational symbols are required.

Because numbers represent a value concept, numbers will most likely hold little meaning for the fra(X) student (McEvoy and McConkey 1986). To provide meaning, one must tie the number of something concrete to something the student already understands. Counting and number use must have direct value to the student. There must be a reason for the student to use numbers or counting—a means to an end. Board games can assist in counting and numeracy. Because the fra(X) student is directly involved in the game, counting dice and moving a game piece the designated number can produce a favorable outcome with less resistance. The game-playing paradigm also diffuses the confrontational nature of direct teaching and may encourage spontaneous responses that are more likely to be accurate (McEvoy and McConkey 1986).

Again, the success of this approach is contingent upon basic interest. Some therapists have designed board games that revolve around the child's interests and include favorite pictures, logos, or object obsessions. The game can be as simple as marking spaces with the throw of a die to get to a designated picture. Functional use of mathematical concepts is again the focus. The fra(X) patient will be far more motivated to learn to use measuring to make a favorite food than to complete a work page with fractions. Ultimately, the use of a small hand calculator will be helpful once number concepts are understood.

For a non–special education classroom teacher to be effective with fra(X) children in a mainstreaming experience, it is critical to understand possible interfering behaviors associated with the syndrome: strong reaction to change, overstimulation, poor verbal output on command, hypotonia, difficulty with fine motor tasks, and academic deficits. It is also important to be aware of the events that may exacerbate levels of anxiety, especially when in a large group with a variety of distractions. For instance, confrontation, loud yelling, and inflexibility often lead to further stimulation and eventual outbursts of behavior.

Case History

ND is a nine-year-old fra(X) male. ND was diagnosed five years ago and was immediately referred into a specialized classroom for autistic and fra(X) students. The program was highly specialized to include a 2:1 teaching ratio, a full time speech/language therapist, educational and psychologic consultation, and an occupational therapist. The program effectively followed the interdisciplinary model, with all professionals interacting to provide a consistent, integrated approach.

Initially, ND had great difficulty complying with entry level behaviors (giving eye contact when spoken to, sitting at a table, attending to cues, making the transition from one trainer to another). He exhibited little language, few preacademic skills, and poor social relatedness. ND demonstrated extreme deficits in sensory motor integration and was tactilely defensive. He felt discomfort wearing certain textures of clothing and never wanted his skin exposed. For example, if he wore short pants, he would pull at his socks until they covered his knees. He disliked short-sleeved shirts for the same reason and constantly pulled at this clothing. In the early stages, he lacked the language to communicate basic needs; thus, his frustration often manifested in explosive behavioral outbursts.

A systematic daily schedule involved ND in 30-minute training sessions rotated on a half-day school placement with speech, occupational therapy, and educational intervention. All of his programs were presented using a direct 1:1 teaching format, which forced interaction at an accelerated frequency. If a response was requested and not given, the trainer modeled a correct response and repeated the cue.

Eventually, ND looked forward to the structure of the program and began to anticipate the next activity. At this point, he was ready to experience gradual routing changes and to begin integration into the mainstream of the regular school setting. At age nine, he is mainstreamed for approximately one-third of his school day and is a school messenger, taking routine packages to the school office. He has made friends in the mainstream and models their more appropriate social responses.

He is currently learning to read using the Logo Reading System (Braden 1989), which utilizes logos from fast food and grocery store chains to encourage word recognition. Assistance from the occupational therapist has enabled ND to benefit from fine motor programs. Collaboration from the speech/language therapist, occupational therapist, and teaching staff has promoted individualized instruction and optimal learning strategies based on specific interests.

ND experiences great difficulty with writing. He has a strong desire to learn to write his name so that he can put it on his papers and sign his name. He is currently involved in a program where he writes his name on a copied blank check and exchanges it for money in the school office. This has provided him with the motivation to reproduce his name carefully.

His success has related directly to integrated services and an individualized curriculum based on his interests.

Late Adolescence through Adulthood

As the fra(X) child progresses through the junior high and high school years, the emphasis for many will shift to prevocational and vocational training. Although there is no research available on vocational training for the fra(X) population, information can be drawn from the literature that describes vocational training for handicapped students in general (Wehman and Hill 1981, 1982; Mithaug and Hagmeier 1978; Levy 1983; Wehman et al. 1985). Many investigators think that vocational training begins too late in the school experience and that comprehensive training, including training in social and pragmatic competence, should occur at all levels of schooling (Brown et al. 1979; Hamre-Nietupski et al. 1982; Wimmer 1981; Hayes 1987).

Important information pertinent to job training and placement can be derived from the general behavioral and cognitive features of the fra(X) population. For example, an adult who has difficulty screening out visual and auditory stimuli would not be a good candidate for sacking groceries at a supermarket. Because of the excellent imitative skills of most fra(X) individuals, placement with more severely handicapped or emotionally/behaviorally disturbed adults would not be desirable as maladaptive behaviors would most likely be imitated. Other general considerations when placing fra(X) individuals in a vocational setting are listed in table 11.9.

In developing the vocational experience for the fra(X) individual, environmental limitations are as critical as cognitive and behavioral ones. The occupational therapist, then, plays an important part in vocational planning. Coping with the challenges of late adolescence and adulthood can be especially stressful for individuals with fra(X) syndrome and their families. All of the expected maturation issues common to a normal individual can be compounded by the sensory integrative problems and behavioral anomalies with which the fra(X) person has dealt since infancy. Behavioral responses to sensory sensitivity or defensiveness are often maladaptive and may include ritualistic movements, self-abuse (i.e., biting the back of the hand), aggression, and withdrawal.

The beneficial effect of sensory integrative methods, including vibratory and vestibular stimulation, with retarded adults has been documented (Ottenbacher

Table 11.9
Considerations in Vocational Planning

Client Considerations	Employer Considerations

Environment
  Overall noise level
  Level of auditory, visual, olfactory, tactile distractions; degree of sensitivity to various stimuli
  Physical proximity of other employees
  Number of other employees
Basic Skills
  Verbal and motor imitation
  Visual discrimination and memory
  Auditory memory and sequencing
  Complexity of receptive and expressive language
  Complexity of motor skills
  Ability to generalize
  Client's interests
Social and Work Skills
  Personal grooming
  Social language
  Ability to interact appropriately with other employees and public
  Degree of independence in using transportation
  Physical strength and stamina
	Understanding employee's needs, strengths, and deficits
	Willingness to modify work setting to encourage optimal performance
	Length of work day
	Willingness to provide rest periods for needed calming or exercise; flexibility in providing time off for scheduled therapies
	Assess safety of employee and other workers
	  Environmental hazards
	  Possible emotional or physical outbursts
	Expectations for appropriate social interaction

and Altman 1984; Clark and Miller 1978). Vigorous physical activity, which would naturally include vestibular and proprioceptive input, has also been reported to have a calming influence (Autism Research Review 1989). Exercise tapes may be used to augment a treatment program for fra(X) individuals. The ability to mimic behaviors, love of imitation of movement, a fascination with visual stimuli, and interest in music could make this approach useful. Because of the importance of fostering social interaction, it is advisable to have this type of exercise program incorporated into a group setting.

Techniques to decrease auditory, visual, and tactile sensitivity should be incorporated into work and living situations, as well as into therapy sessions. The fra(X) adult should be encouraged to assume increasing responsibility for self-calming and organization. Individual psychotherapy may also be helpful in teaching calming techniques and control of anger and frustration (see chapter

10). The following case studies demonstrate how two fra(X) adults have discovered ways of coping with their "uncomfortable" environment and sensory integrative dysfunctions.

Case History

TO, a mildly mentally retarded 26-year-old fra(X) man, was extremely sensitive to light touch and to sound. Although he actively sought socialization, he had difficulty grading his approach to others. His discomfort in social situations could rapidly develop into aggressive behavior. When confronted with novel or perhaps mildly threatening situations, he would spontaneously use "mm" or "zz" sounds, seemingly in an effort to calm himself. If a cognitive task became overly challenging, he often attempted to direct himself verbally. His relatively good development of basic muscle tone and balance contrasted with deficits in more complex motor patterns requiring trunk rotation and crossing midline skills. TO had received intervention but without specific sensory integrative or combined occupational and speech therapy approaches. After his evaluation, he began to attend a combined speech and language and occupational therapy group, where his individual sensory integrative and pragmatic problems could be addressed. It was not long before a dramatic occurrence presented itself and gave a definite focus for therapy.

As stated above, TO's volatile temper often got him into trouble. In one incident, while waiting at a bus stop to go by himself to an amusement park, he exchanged insults with a mentally retarded woman acquaintance, ended up physically fighting, and was subsequently jailed.

This experience was the main topic of conversation at the next therapy session. TO was very upset and asked for help in controlling his temper so he would not get into trouble again. After a group discussion, a few calming techniques he could use by himself were developed, and he agreed to do them religiously. (1) He would brush four times a day with a surgical scrub brush. (2) About a half hour before he would be going on an outing by himself or before an activity he knew would stir up aggressive emotions, he would brush again. (3) If he felt himself becoming even slightly upset, he would count to 20 and press his hands together or push down hard on the top of his head with both hands. (4) It was also pointed out to TO that his habit of humming an "mm" sound when he was nervous was a good technique.

The next therapy session provided a perfect chance to try the techniques in a real life situation. TO, another fra(X) man and the occupational therapist walked six blocks to a supermarket in the heart of the city to buy snacks for that day's session. How would TO handle the crowd, the noise, the decision making? (To complicate matters, the therapist had taken very little money, which would force the two men to negotiate their purchases.)

Before leaving the clinic, TO used the brushing technique. Then, before going into the store, TO stopped, counted softly to 20, pushed hard on his head, and hummed briefly. Once in the store, the two men came close to a heated argument about what snacks to buy but were able to come to agreement.

The walk back to the hospital was uneventful but, while sitting at a picnic table outside the clinic, the group was approached by two suspicious-looking men who were later found to be wanted by the police. Both fra(X) men were able to stay calm, with TO, after a glance at the therapist, pressing his hands together and humming softly. In a later therapy session, on the way to visit his fellow group member's home, TO repeatedly asked, "Tell me again what to do if I'm upset?" The speech and occupational therapists helped him review all of the techniques discussed previously, but he was finally told, "We've gone over all these ideas many times. You've tried them. They work. I can't tell you anymore. It's your life and your decision and you have to do it for yourself."

Previous reports suggested that hyperactivity or extreme behavioral reactions to stimulation seem to decrease with age (Fryns 1985). In this case, TO had been able to restrict his hyperactivity and emotional lability some of the time but always felt "on the edge." He showed indications of residual sensory integrative problems from early childhood. Perhaps with early intervention these problems would be less severe. The low muscle tone that is more obvious in young children can evolve into a relatively flexed posture, with shoulders forward and hips slightly flexed in adulthood. Even in adults with relatively erect posture, full extension to prone is difficult because of the influence of tightness from habitual hip flexion used as a compensatory strategy to deal with hypotonia. The ability to rotate the trunk and cross the midline of the body, which is made possible by maturation of the balance between flexion and extension and by the ability to shift weight from side to side, is usually poor.

The speech/language pathologist can also provide needed support in vocational planning. Specific vocabulary and social skills necessary for the job and a more independent lifestyle should be emphasized. These can be taught most effectively through the use of small groups in a real life experiential setting. Social skill development is equally important as it is necessary to understand and relate to others in the work environment. Social communication skills such as greetings, making requests, and turn taking should be incorporated into the communication and academic curriculum. Verbalization of emotions must be taught as an alternative to violent behavioral outbursts, which often occur when a patient is overwhelmed by stimuli. Problem-solving skills around conflict resolution are essential for the fra(X) individual in any work setting.

Facilitating the transition from school to work is the ultimate goal of public education. To encourage the vocational training and placement process, one should address several areas in an academic setting. Dalrymple (1986) provided a model for transition that was suggested for the autistic population. Based on behavioral and language similarities, this model can also be addressed in the adolescent fra(X) individual. Overall competency, self-care, and language, social, academic, and prevocational skill development is recommended. Dalrymple (1986) suggested that basic academic skill building will further assist in an effective transition. Within the fra(X) population, basic attending and listening skills are critical. These skills can be trained by involving the adolescent in a listening program that will require attending for a sustained period and by having the individual follow oral directions of increasing length and difficulty. Pharmacologic intervention may also improve attention during the adolescent period, as in earlier childhood (chapter 9). Taking advantage of the fra(X) individual's visual strengths, one can provide a sequence of tasks in a visual format that will cue the adolescent/adult to the next step of the sequence in the workplace.

Academic emphasis in vocational training should be presented in a functional format (real coins versus plastic coins, real job applications, actual work objects from the real work environment, etc.). Training in identifying coins, making the correct change, budgeting, endorsing paychecks and making deposits should be a part of the instructional program. Functional sight vocabulary or comprehension of basic instruction should also be the focus of the reading curriculum at this level.

Success in the workplace is dependent upon a developed ability to make transitions and adjust to new environments and routines. The importance of training these skills early in the academic environment cannot be overemphasized. If the strong reaction to change is gradually desensitized during school placement, it will not be a problem when the workplace is entered.

Appropriate behavior in the work environment is essential for compliance and success. Hyperactivity in the fra(X) population can interfere with maintaining a job station and properly caring for work-related materials. Appropriate behavior should be trained by beginning with short work periods and extending them, with more work materials and distractors gradually introduced. This will build tolerance and reduce the likelihood of overstimulation in the workplace.

Case History

EG, a 22-year-old man, was mildly mentally retarded. The occupational therapist identified low muscle tone, difficulties with balance, mild sensitivity to touch, and distractibility. He sometimes used hand biting when overstimulated. Visual and tactile perception (in combination rather than as isolated sensory perceptions) and imitation motor tasks were strengths for him, as was visual memory.

EG's speech and language was characterized primarily by developmentally appropriate utterances. His verbal and behavioral imitative skills were areas of strength. Social interaction was extremely difficult for him, and he often avoided interactions with his peers by physically leaving any situation requiring direct verbal interchange, eye contact, or touch. When over-stimulated by sensory input, particularly during social interactions, his speech became perseverative and at times echolalic.

The combined occupational/speech therapy group that EG attended incorporated calming techniques, music, cooperative games, and vigorous physical activity with the communication techniques of modeling, self-talk, and parallel talk. Treatment in the clinical setting expanded to include hikes, shopping excursions, and visits to other group members' homes.

Close communication among EG's parents, therapists, and vocational guidance counselors was critical in developing an optimal vocational site. EG's primary responsibilities in filing and computer processing utilized his strengths in visual memory and sequencing. At his job, he was not required to interact with many people. He did, however, enjoy his responsibility of answering phones. This allowed him to practice his social language skills without the difficulty of interacting with people on a personal basis. His employer was surprised and pleased at EG's ability to learn the names of his 15 co-workers within 30 minutes. His employer also provided EG with several short periods during the day for calming activities.

Integrated Services and the Affected Fra(X) Female

Cognitive functioning in fra(X) females ranges from normal to severely retarded (Hagerman and Smith 1983; Kemper et al. 1986; Webb et al. 1982; Cronister et al. 1991). Importantly, one-third to one-half of fra(X) females exhibit mild to moderate learning disabilities or mild mental retardation (chapters 1 and 5). Affected females may exhibit behavioral problems similar to those of fra(X) males but usually less severe. Poor eye contact, impulsivity, and attending problems, as well as difficulties with shyness, anxiety, and depression, may be present (Hagerman and Sobesky 1989).

Deficits in math, especially with math reasoning and conceptual skills, have been reported (Kemper et al. 1986; Miezejeski et al. 1986; Theobald et al. 1987). Often females have difficulty generalizing math concepts into a variety of situations for future problem solving. Algebraic formulas, symbolic associations that include missing elements, and the computation of word problems often cause great difficulty in this population. A curriculum that utilizes concrete and manipulative materials to introduce basic mathematic operations should be considered. Teaching methods should include patterns and visual gestalt whenever possible to reinforce complex mathematic processes. Suggested materials are listed in appendix 11.2.

Table 11.10

Intervention Strategies Suggested for Affected Heterozygous Females

Math deficits
    Use concrete manipulative materials to teach concepts and mathematical operations
    Use visual cues whenever possible to reinforce mathematical operations
    Allow additional time to reduce the possibility of provoking performance anxiety
    Minimize auditory distractions during time periods when concentration is required (computation, problem solving)
    Use diagrams, illustrations and visual patterns whenever teaching a new concept
    Use repetition and patterning whenever rote memory tasks are required

Auditory memory and attentional problems
    Give specific instruction in a slow, simple, and concrete manner
    Place the student in close proximity of the instruction to ensure attention and concentration
    Structure the environment to be void of auditory distractions (earphones, carrels, or seating arrangements)
    Vary presentation to include frequent breaks to avoid attentional difficulties and lack of concentration

Visual Disorganization
    Limit amount to be copied from printed or written materials
    Simplify visually presented materials to eliminate a cluttered or excessively stimulating format
    Provide visual cues, such as color coding, numbering, and arrows, to organize written tasks
    Give specific concrete cues when giving oral directions that require an organized format
    Additional time may be required for written assignments

In the language area, problems with distractibility, inattentiveness, abstract reasoning, pragmatic language, topic maintenance, and a run-on narrative style have been reported (Madison et al. 1986; Hagerman 1987; see chapter 1). The pragmatic language deficits may be related to a "tangential" and impulsive thought process that affects reasoning and problem-solving skills (Hagerman and Sobesky 1989). These problems should be the focus of language therapy (chapter 5).

Therapists have noted various sensory integration problems within the female population. As in males, defensiveness to touch, low tone, and a lack of trunk rotation, which results in difficulty with praxis and subsequent inability to cross the midline, can be seen. The defensiveness to touch and shy, withdrawn behavior may contribute to poor interactional skills and may result in decreased pragmatic skills.

Intervention strategies for the female population can be drawn from information presented on males (see table 11.10). As the problems presented by fra(X)

females may vary from primary deficits in math to a wider range of deficits in sensory motor, speech/language, and academic areas, a decision on whether to use an integrated approach should be made on a case by case basis.

APPENDIX 11.1
Computer Information

Publishers of Computer Software to Enhance Speech and Language Development

Peal Software
P.O. Box 8188
Calabasas, CA 91302

Don Johnson Developmental
 Equipment, Inc.
P.O. Box 639
1000 N. Rand Rd., Bldg. #115
Wauconda, IL 60084-0639

Hartley Courseware, Inc.
133 Bridge St.
Dimondale, MI 48821

Edmark Corporation
P.O. Box 3903
Bellevue, WA 98009-3903

Laureate Learning Systems, Inc.
110 E. Spring St.
Winooski, VT 05404

Sunburst Communications
39 Washington Ave.
Pleasantville, NY 10570-2898

Cambridge Development &
 Laboratory, Inc.
214 Third Ave.
Waltham, MA 02154

National Special Educators Alliance Member Centers

California

Computer Access Center
2425 16th St., Rm. 23
Santa Monica, CA 90405

Disabled Children's Computer Group
2095 Rose St.
Berkeley, CA 94709

Special Awareness Computer Center
Rehabilitation Center
2975 North Sycamore Dr.
Simi Valley, CA 93065

Special Technology Center
c/o UCPA
100 View St., Ste. 108
Mountain View, CA 94041

Team of Advocates for Special Kids
18685 Santa Ynez
Fountain Valley, CA 92708

Colorado

AccessAbility Resource Center
1056 East 19th Ave.
Denver. CO 80218-1033

Illinois

Technical Aids & Assistance for the
  Disabled Center
1950 West Roosevelt
Chicago, IL 60608

Kansas

Technology Research for Special
  People
3023 Canterbury
Salina, KS 67401

Kentucky

Blue Grass Technology Center for
  People with Disabilities
898 Georgetown St.
Lexington, KY 40505-1392

SpecialLink
36 W. 5th St.
Covington, KY 41011

Louisiana

CATER-Center for Adaptive
  Technology and Education
3340 Severn Ave., Bank of the South,
  Ste. 200
Metairie, LA 70002

Michigan

Living and Learning Resource Center
Physically Impaired Association of
  Michigan
601 W. Maple St.
Lansing, MI 48906

Florida

Computer C.I.T.E.
Valencia Community College
215 E. New Hampshire
Orlando, FL 32804

Iowa

R.E.A.D.I.
318 Fifth St., S.E.
Cedar Rapids, IA 52401

Disabled Citizens Computer Center
Louisville Free Public Library
4th and York Sts.
Louisville, KY 40203

Massachusetts

Massachusetts Special Technology
  Access Center
P.O. Box J
Bedford, MA 01730

Minnesota

Pacer Center, Inc.
4826 Chicago Ave. South
Minneapolis, MN 54187-1055

Missouri

Computer Resource Center
St. Louis Easter Seal Society
1710 Mississippi Ave.
St. Louis, MO 63104

Montana

Parents, Let's Unite for Kids
1500 N. 30th St.
Billings, MT 59101-0298

Nevada

Nevada Technology Center
819 Las Vegas Blvd. South
Las Vegas, NV 89101

New York

Techspress
Resource Center for Independent
  Living
401 Columbia St.
Utica, NY 13502

Ohio

Communication Assistance Resource
  Service
3201 Marshall Rd.
Dayton, OH 45429

Tennessee

West Tennessee Special Technology
  Resource Center for the Disabled
227 McCowat
P.O. Box 3685
Jackson, TN 38303

East Tennessee Special Technology
  Access Center
Department of Special Services
  Education
325 Claxton Addition
Knoxville, TN 37966-3400

APPENDIX 11.2

Suggested Academic Materials for Use with Fragile X Children

1. Reading (sight/visually based)

    A. Logo Reading System by Marcia L. Braden, M.S.,
       219 E. St. Vrain, Colorado Springs, CO 80903
       The Logo Reading System utilizes well-known logos, traditional flash
       cards, sort cards with placements, phrase cards, and matching/fine-
       motor worksheets.

    B. Edmark Corp., PO Box 3903, Bellevue, WA 98009-3903
       The Edmark Reading Program, Level 1, is a beginning reading and

language development program recommended for use with any individual who is considered a nonreader. The program contains 227 lessons presented in five formats: prereading, word recognition, direction book, picture/phrase matching, and storybook lessons.

C. SRA (Science Research Associates), Science Research Associates, Inc., 155 N. Wacker Dr., Chicago, IL 60606

Corrective Reading Comprehension develops the reasoning processes (analogues, deductions, inductions, classification), vocabulary, and writing skills students need. Reasoning is taught, not just practiced, in carefully written lessons that foster an experience of success and self-worth.

D. Merrill Reading Series, Merrill Publishing Co., PO Box 508, Columbus OH 43216-0508

The Merrill Linguistic Reading Program motivates students to become independent readers and encourages them to learn, to know, to think, and to discover. The program offers readings in important areas such as science, health, history, mathematics, and literature.

E. Appletree—Dormac, Inc., PO Box 270459, San Diego, CA 92128-0983

Appletree is an acronym for "A Patterned Program of Linguistic Expansion through Reinforced Experiences and Evaluations." It is a language system that provides sequential procedures for construction and development of the basic sentence structures that are the foundation of verbal language. The program has six workbooks, a teacher's manual, and a pre-post test booklet.

F. Capture the Meaning—CC Publications, PO Box 23699, Tigard, OR 97223-0108

Here is an exciting new program that really *teaches* comprehension. Effective and easy to use, "Capture the Meaning: Strategies for Reading Comprehension" focuses on strategies for building comprehension. This 10-unit, 35-lesson program consists of teacher-guided instruction and practice, independent practice that includes individual and group activities, and tests—all designed to reinforce and build reading comprehension skills.

G. Reading Attainment System, 1987—Educational Design, Inc., 47 W. 13th St., New York, NY 10011

This program is specially designed to supply practice for students who fail when basal texts reach the 3–5 grade reading level. Ease in reading comes only with practice at low reading levels. This system supplies that practice and produces fluency and confidence in students for whom ordinary methods of remediation have failed. Reading skills, vocabulary skills, and thinking skills are offered in three different sets of multiquestion exercises.

2. Spelling
A. I Can Print—Pro-Ed, 5341 Industrial Oaks Blvd., Austin, TX 78735
Designed to help students develop the necessary skills to form letters, begin writing sentences, and build handwriting fluency, "I Can Print" can be used as a developmental program in kindergarten, first grade, and special education. Also designed to be used as a remedial program for older children who have already learned to write but consistently have trouble with letter formation and spacing.

3. Mathematics
A. I Can Plus & Minus—Pro-Ed, 5341 Industrial Oaks Blvd., Austin, TX 78735
A complete arithmetic program based on learning theory and practical experience, this is a beginning series that moves from an assumption of no skill by the student through 116 ordered skills, culminating in regrouping two-place subtraction.
B. Good Apple Math Book—Grimm & Mitchell, 6 Apple, Box 299, Carthage, IL 62321
Math can be fun when students discover how to apply basic skills in practical ways. Activities are based on nature, mail order catalogs, popular foods, calendars, etc. Complete instructions for a math center with 28 idea cards and four gameboards are included.

4. Social
A. I Can Behave—Pro-Ed, 5341 Industrial Oaks Blvd. Austin, TX 78735
"I Can Behave" revolves around an illustrated storybook comprising 10 stories and 125 full-page drawings. Each of the 10 stories focuses on a specific classroom dilemma ("My Turn, Your Turn"—letting others talk; "Marvin and His Mouth"—using a quiet voice). Lessons include working independently, waiting for help, doing careful work, handling classroom frustrations, and sitting still.
B. Social Skills for Daily Living—American Guidance Services, Publisher's Building, PO Box 99, Circle Pines, MN 55014-1796
"Social Skills for Daily Living" presents a proven, effective method for enhancing the social skills of mildly learning-disabled, mildly emotionally disturbed, and mildly mentally retarded adolescents and young adults aged 12–21.

References

Anonymous. 1989. Physical exercise: A simple prescription for behavior problems? *Autism Res Rev* 3:1–7.

Arnold, L. E., D. L. Clark, L. A. Sachs, S. Jakim, and C. Smithies. 1985. Vestibular and visual rotational stimulation as treatment for attention deficit and hyperactivity. *Am. J. Occup. Ther.* 39:84–91.

Arwood, E. L. 1984. *Pragmaticism: Treatment for language disorders.* Rockville, Md.: National Student Speech, Language, Hearing Association.

Ayres, A. J. 1965. Patterns of perceptual motor dysfunction in children: A factor analytic study. *Percept. Mot. Skills* 20:335–368.

———. 1972. *Sensory integration and learning disabilities.* Los Angeles: Western Psychological Services.

———. 1978. Learning disabilities and the vestibular system. *J. Learn. Disab.* 11:30–41.

———. 1979. *Sensory integration and the child.* Los Angeles: Western Psychological Services.

Ayres, A. J., and Z. Mailloux. 1981. Influence of sensory integration procedures on language development. *Am. J. Occup. Ther.* 35:383–390.

Ayres, A. J., and L. S. Tickle. 1980. Hyper-responsivity to touch and vestibular stimuli as a predictor of positive response to sensory integration procedures by autistic children. *Am. J. Occup. Ther.* 34:375–381.

Baroff, G. S. 1986. *Mental retardation: Nature, cause and management.* New York: Hemisphere Publishing, pp. 337–340.

Bates, E. 1979. *The emergence of symbols: Cognition and communication in infancy.* New York: Academic Press.

Bellman, K., and L. Goldberg. 1984. Common origin of linguistic and movement abilities. *Am. J. Physiol.* 6:915–921.

Birren, F. 1979. *Color and human response.* New York: Van Nostrand Reinhold.

Bloom, L., and M. Lahey. 1978. *Language development and language disorders.* New York: Wiley.

Bonadonna, P. 1981. Effects of a vestibular stimulation program on stereotypic rocking behavior. *Am. J. Occup. Ther.* 35:775–781.

Braden, M. 1989. *Logo reading system,* 219 E. St. Vrain, Colorado Springs, Colo. 80903.

Bright, T., K. Brittick, and B. Fleeman. 1981. Reduction of self-injurious behavior using sensory integrative techniques. *Am. J. Occup. Ther.* 35:167–172.

Brown, L., M. Branston, S. Hamre-Nietupski, F. Johnson, B. Wilcox, and L. Gruenewald. 1979. A rationale for comprehensive longitudinal interactions between severely handicapped students and non-handicapped students and other citizens. *AAESPH Rev.* 4:3–14.

Burns, E., and L. Hickman. 1989. Integrated therapy in a summer camping experience for children with fragile X syndrome. *S. I. Int. News* 17:1–3.

Caldwell, B., and D. Stedman. 1977. *Infant education: A guide for helping handicapped children in the first three years.* Durham, N.C.: Walker Publishing.

Camp, B. W., and M. S. Bash. 1981. *Think aloud: Increasing social and cognitive skills—a problem solving program for children.* Champaign, Ill.: Research Press.

Campbell, P. H., W. F. McInerney, and M. A. Cooper. 1984. Therapeutic programming for students with severe handicaps. *Am. J. Occup. Ther.* 38:594–602.

Clark, S., and L. Miller. 1978. A comparison of apparent and sensory integrative methods on developmental parameters in profoundly retarded adults. *Am. J. Occup. Ther.* 32:86–92.

Clark, F., and L. Steingold. 1982. A potential relationship between occupational therapy and language acquisition. *Am. J. Occup. Ther.* 36:42–44.

Cronister, A., R. Schreiner, M. Wittenberger, K. Amiri, K. Harris, and R. J. Hagerman. 1991. The heterozygous fragile X female: Historical, physical, cognitive and cytogenetic features. *Am. J. Med. Genet.* In press.

Dalrymple, N. 1986. *Transitional autism program.* Bloomington, Ind.: Indiana University Press.

Densom, J. F., G. A. Nuthall, J. Bushnell, and J. Horn. 1989. Effectiveness of a sensory integrative treatment program for children with perceptual motor difficulties. *J. Learn. Disab.* 22:221–229.

de Quiros, J. 1976. Diagnosis of vestibular disorders in the learning disabilities. *J. Learn. Disab.* 9:51–58.

de Quiros, J., and O. Schrager. 1978. *Neuropsychological fundamentals in learning disabilities.* San Rafael, Calif.: Academic Therapy Publications.

Ellis, E. S., and E. J. Sabornie. 1986. Effective instruction with microcomputers: Promises, practices and preliminary finding. *Focus Except. Child.* 19:1–16.

Farber, S. 1982. *Neurorehabilitation: A multisensory approach.* Philadelphia: W. B. Saunders.

Fryns, J. P. 1985. X-linked mental retardation. In *Medical genetics: Past, present and future.* New York: Alan R. Liss, pp. 309–319.

Giangreco, M. 1986. Delivery of therapeutic services in special education programs for learners with severe handicaps. *Phys. Occup. Ther. Pediatr.* 6:5–15.

Grandin, T., and M. Scariano. 1988. *Emergence labeled autistic.* Nova, Calif.: Arena Press.

Gustavson, A., M. Dawson, and D. Bonett. 1987. Androstenal, a putative human phenome, affects human (*Homo sapiens*) male choice preference. *J. Comp. Psychol.* 101:210–212.

Hagerman, R. J. 1987. Fragile X syndrome. *Curr. Probl. Pediatr.* 25:621–674.

Hagerman, R. J., and A. Smith. 1983. The heterozygous female. In R. Hagerman and P. McBogg (eds.), *The fragile X syndrome: Diagnosis, biochemistry and intervention.* Dillon, Colo.: Spectra Publishing, pp. 83–94.

Hagerman, R. J., and W. Sobesky. 1989. Psychopathology in fragile X syndrome. *Am. J. Orthopsychiatry* 59:142–152.

Hamre-Nietupski, S., J. Nietupski, P. Bates, and S. Maurer. 1982. Implementing a community-based educational model for moderately/severely handicapped students: Common problems and suggested solutions. *J. Assoc. Severely Handicap.* 7:38–43.

Hayes, R. 1987. Training for work. In P. Cohen and A. Donnellan (eds.), *Handbook of autism and pervasive developmental disorders.* New York: Wiley, pp. 360–370.

Huss, A. 1976. Touch with care or a caring touch. *Am. J. Occup. Ther.* 31:11–18.

Hutchinson, D. J. 1983. The transdisciplinary approach. In J. B. Curry (ed.), *Mental retardation: Nursing approaches to care.* St. Louis: C. V. Mosby, pp. 65–74.

Jenkins, J. R., and L. Jenkins. 1981. *Cross age and peer tutoring: Help for children with learning problems.* Reston, Va.: Council for Exceptional Children.

Jones, A., P. Currier, and L. Hickman. 1986. Pragmatics camp and offshoot programs for the adolescent language-learning disabled population. Presented to the Colorado Speech and Hearing Association, Breckenridge, Colo.

Kantner, R., B. Kantner, and D. Clark. 1982. Vestibular stimulation effect on language development in mentally retarded children. *Am. J. Occup. Ther.* 36:36–41.

Kawar, M. 1973. The effects of sensorimotor therapy on dichotic listening in children with learning disabilities. *Am. J. Occup. Ther.* 27:226–231.

Kemper, M. B., R. J. Hagerman, R. S. Ahmad, and R. Mariner. 1986. Cognitive profiles and the spectrum of clinical manifestations in heterozygous fra(X) females. *Am. J. Med. Genet.* 23:139–156.

Kemper, M. B., R. J. Hagerman, and D. Altshul-Stark. 1988. Cognitive profiles of boys with the fragile X syndrome. *Am. J. Med. Genet.* 30:191–200.

Koegel, R., M. O'Dell, and L. Koegel. 1987. A natural language teaching paradigm for nonverbal autistic children. *J. Autism Dev. Disord.* 17:187–200.

Krug, D., J. Rosenblum, P. Almond, and J. Arick. 1980. *Assessment, behavior management, and communication training program.* Portland, Oreg.: ASIEP Education.

Leckman, J. F., R. M. Hodapp, E. M. Dykens, S. S. Sparrow, D. Zylinsky, and S. I. Ort. 1989. Evidence for a specific profile of cognitive processing among fragile X males. Presented at the 4th International Workshop on Fragile X Syndrome and X-linked Mental Retardation, New York.

Levitas, A., R. Hagerman, M. Braden, B. Rimland, P. McBogg, and I. Matus. 1983. Autism and the fragile X syndrome. *J. Dev. Behav. Pediatr.* 4:151–158.

Levy, S. 1983. School doesn't last forever: Then what? Some vocational alternatives. In E. Shoper and G. Mesibov (eds.), *Autism in adolescents and adults.* New York: Plenum, pp. 133–148.

Lucas, E. V. 1980. *Semantic and pragmatic language disorders: Assessment and remediation.* Rockville, Md.: Aspen.

Luria, A. 1976. *Cognitive development: Its cultural and social foundation.* Cambridge, Mass.: Harvard University Press.

Maddux, C.D. 1984. Using microcomputers with the learning disabled: Will the potential be realized? *Educat. Comput.* pp. 31–32.

Madison, L., C. George, and J. Moeschler. 1986. Cognitive functioning in the fragile X syndrome: A study of intellectual memory and communication skills. *J. Ment. Defic. Res.* 30:129–148.

Magun, W. M., K. Ottenbacher, S. McCue, and R. Keefe. 1981. Effects of vestibular stimulation on spontaneous use of verbal language in developmentally delayed children. *Am. J. Occup. Ther.* 35:101–104.

Marks, L. 1978. *The unity of the senses.* New York: Academic Press.

McCune-Nicolich, L. 1981. Toward symbolic functioning: Structure of early pretend games and potential parallels with language. *Child Dev.* 52:785–797.

McEvoy, J., and R. McConkey. 1986. Count me in: Teaching basic counting and number skills. *Ment. Handicap* 14:113–115.

McKibben, E. H. 1973. The effect of additional tactile stimulation in a perceptual-motor treatment program for school children. *Am. J. Occup. Ther.* 27:191–197.

Meegrum, W., K. Ottenbacher, S. McCue, and R. Keefe. 1981. Effects of vestibular stimulation on spontaneous use of verbal language in developmentally delayed children. *Am. J. Occup. Ther.* 35:101–104.

Miezejeski, C., E. Jenkins, A. Hill, K. Wisniewski, J. French, and W. Brown. 1986. A profile of cognitive deficit in females from fragile X families. *Neuropsychologia* 24:405–409.

Mithaug, D., and L. Hagmeier. 1978. The development of procedures to assess prevocational competencies of severely handicapped young adults. *AAESPH Rev.* 3:94–115.

Mokros, R. J., and S. J. Russell. 1986. Learner-centered software: A survey of microcomputer use with special needs students. *J. Learn. Disab.* 19:185–190.

Montgomery, J. 1980. *Non-oral communication: A training guide for the child without speech.* Exemplary/Incentive Dissemination Project, ESEA, Title IV-C, Plavan School, Fountain Valley, Calif.

Musselwhite, C., and K. St. Louis. 1982. *Communication programming for the severely handicapped: Vocal and non-vocal strategies.* San Diego, Calif.: College Hill Press.

Nobak, C. 1975. *The human nervous system.* New York: McGraw-Hill.

Ottenbacher, K. 1982. The effect of a controlled program of vestibular stimulation on the incidence of seizures in children with severe developmental delay. *Phys. Occup. Ther. Pediatr.* 2:25–33.

Ottenbacher, K., and R. Altman. 1984. Effects of vibratory, edible and social reinforcement on performance of institutionalized mentally retarded adults. *Am. J. Ment. Defic.* 89:201–204.

Parham, D. 1988. Format for efficacy studies and some sensory integration efficacy data. *S.I. Int. News* 16(2):10–15.

Paul, R., E. Dykens, J. Leckman, M. Watson, W. Breg, and D. Cohen. 1987. A comparison of language characteristics of mentally retarded adults with fragile X syndrome and those with nonspecific mental retardation and autism. *J. Autism Dev. Disord.* 17:457–468.

Reilly, C., D. Nelson, and A. Bundy. 1983. Sensorimotor versus fine motor activities in eliciting vocalizations in autistic children. *Occup. Ther. J. Res.* 3:199–212.

Rogers, S. J., and H. Lewis. 1989. An effective day treatment model for young children with pervasive developmental disorders. *JAACAP* 28:207–214.

Rogers, S. J., J. M. Herbision, H. C. Lewis, J. Pantone, and K. Reis. 1986. An approach for enhancing the syn com and interpersonal functioning of young children with autism or severe emotional handicaps. *J. Dis. Early Child.* 10:135–148.

Sarnat, H., and M. Netsky. 1981. *Evolution of the nervous system.* New York: Oxford University Press.

Scharfenaker, S., and L. Hickman. 1989. Combined speech-language and occupational therapy and the fragile X child. *Fragile X Assoc. Mich. Newslett.* 2:4–5.

Scharfenaker, S., and R. Schreiner. 1989. Cognitive and speech-language characteristics of the fragile X syndrome. *Rocky Mount. J. Commun. Disord.* 5:25–35.

Scherer, N., and L. Olswang. 1989. Using structured discourse as a language intervention technique with autistic children. *J. Speech Hear. Disord.* 54:383–394.

Schiefelbush, R. (ed.) 1980. *Nonspeech language and communication.* Baltimore: University Park Press.

Schwartz, R., and L. Leonard. 1985. Lexical imitation and acquisition in language impaired children. *J. Speech Hear. Disord.* 50:31–39.

Scott, J. 1986. *The olfactory bulb and central pathways.* Basel: Birkhauser Verlag.

Short-DeGraff, M. 1988. *Human development for occupational and physical therapists.* Baltimore: Williams & Wilkins.

Silverman, F. 1982. *Communication for the speechless.* Englewood Cliffs, N.J.: Prentice-Hall.

Smith, C. 1985. *Ancestral voices and evolution of human consciousness.* Englewood Cliffs, N.J.: Prentice-Hall, pp. 5–93.

Sparks, R., and A. Holland. 1976. Method: Melodic intonation therapy for aphasia. *J. Speech Hear. Disord.* 41:287–297.

Sparks, R., N. Helm, and R. Albert. 1974. Aphasia rehabilitation resulting from melodic intonation therapy. *Cortex* 10:303–316.

Sternat, J., R. Messina, J. Nietupski, S. Lyons, and L. Brown. 1977. Occupational and physical therapy services for severely handicapped students: Toward a naturalized public school service delivery model. In E. Sontag, J. Smith, and N. Certo (eds.), *Educational programming for the severely and profoundly handicapped.* Reston, Va.: Council for Exceptional Children, pp. 263–277.

Stokes, T., and D. Bauer. 1977. An implicit technology of generalization. *J. Appl. Behav. Anal.* 10:349–367.

Storey, K., P. Bates, N. McGhee, and S. Dycus. 1984. Reducing the self-stimulatory behavior of a profoundly retarded female through sensory awareness training. *Am. J. Occup. Ther.* 38:510–516.

Strain, P. S. 1987. Comprehensive evaluation of intervention for young autistic children. *Top. Early Child. Spec. Ed.* 7:97–110.

Theobald, T., D. Hay, and C. Judge. 1987. Individual variation and specific cognitive deficits in the fra(X) syndrome. *Am. J. Med. Genet.* 28:1–11.

Travis, L. (ed.) 1971. *Handbook of speech pathology and audiology.* Englewood Cliffs, N.J.: Prentice-Hall.

Uma, K., H. R. Nagendra, R. Nagarathna, S. Vaidehi, and R. Seethalakshmi. 1989. The integrated tool for mentally retarded children: A one year controlled study. *J. Ment. Defic. Res.* 33:415–421.

Ungerer, J. A., and M. Sigman. 1984. The relation of play and sensorimotor behavior to language in the second year. *Child Dev.* 55:1448–1455.

U.S. Congress. 1975. Public Law 94–142, Education for All Handicapped Children Act of 1975. Washington, D.C.

U.S. Congress. 1986. Public Law 99–457, Individualized Family Service Plan. Washington D.C.

Walker, D., J. Palfrey, M. Handley-Derry, and J. Singer. 1989. Mainstreaming children with handicaps: Implications for pediatricians. *J. Dev. Behav. Pediatr.* 10:151–156.

Webb, G., J. Halliday, D. Pitt, C. Judge, and M. Leversha. 1982. Fragile (X)(q27) sites in a pedigree with female carriers showing mild to severe mental retardation. *J. Med. Genet.* 19:44–48.

Wehman, P., and J. Hill. 1981. Competitive employment for moderately and severely handicapped individuals. *Except. Child.* 47:338–345.

———. 1982. Preparing severely handicapped youth for less restrictive environments. *J. Assoc. Sev. Handicap.* 7:33–39.

Wehman, P., J. Kregel, and J. M. Barus. 1985. From school to work: A vocational transition model for handicapped students. *Except. Child.* 52:25–37.

Wetherby, A. 1986. Ontogeny of communicative functions in autism. *J. Autism Dev. Disord.* 16:295–316.

Wilbarger, P., and J. Wilbarger. 1988. Sensory affective disorders: Beyond tactile defensiveness. Presented at the Sensory Integration Workshop, Denver, Colo.

Wimmer, D. 1981. Functional learning curricula in the secondary schools. *Except. Child.* 47:610–616.

Windeck, S., and M. Laurel. 1989. A theoretical framework combining speech language therapy with sensory integrative treatment. *Am. Occup. Ther. Assoc. S.I. Sp. Int. Sect. Newslett.* 12(1).

Yoder, D. (ed.) 1982. Communication interaction strategies for the severely communicatively impaired. *Top. Lang. Disord.* 2.

Zivin, D. (ed.) 1979. *The development of self-regulation through private speech.* New York: Wiley.

INDEX

Aggression, 50–52, 316, 317, 322
Allan-Herndon-Dudley syndrome, 210, 214, 216
Alleles, 148, 160, 230, 236, 237
Amantadine (symmetrical), 304
Amniocytes, 112, 123, 124
Anthropomorphic studies, 7
Anticonvulsants, 29, 287–90, 296, 301; carbamazepine (Tegretol), 29, 287–89, 301; phenobarbitol, 289; phenytoin (Dilantin), 288, 289, 296; primidone, 289; valproic acid (Depakene), 288, 290
Antipsychotic agents, 299–301; chloropromazine, 300; clozapine, 300; extrapyramidal side effects, 299, 300; sulpiride, 300; thiordazine, 299–301
Anxiety, 40, 45, 48, 49, 51–53, 195, 292, 299, 303, 318, 323, 338, 339, 349, 353
Anxiolytic medication, 303; alprazolam (Xanax), 303; buspirone (Buspar), 303; clonazepam, 303
Aphidocolin, 102
Approach withdrawal, 40
Arithmetic deficits, 48, 179, 186, 190, 191, 353
Articulation problems, 181–83, 192, 283
Ascertainment bias, 69, 83, 126, 176, 187, 188, 241, 242, 245
Asperger syndrome, 47, 50, 55
Atkin syndrome, 55
Attention deficit hyperactivity disorder (ADHD), 15, 35, 220, 174, 285, 289, 293, 315, 358; attentional deficits, 179, 184, 329, 338, 345; hyperactivity, 15, 35, 220, 358; multimodal therapy, 285; pharmacotherapy, 290–97
Attentional deficits, 179, 184, 329, 338, 345
Autism, 33, 38–45, 52, 81, 174, 185, 193, 196, 315, 331, 341
Autistic-like features, 35–39

Bayesian analysis, 259–61
Bayley Scales, 283

Behavior modification, 284, 287
Behavior problems, 35–48, 51–55, 311–24; anger control, 317, 318; anxiety, 40, 45, 48, 49, 51–53, 195, 292, 299, 303, 318, 323, 338, 339, 349, 353; approach withdrawal, 40; autism, 33, 38–45, 52, 81, 174, 185, 193, 196, 315, 331, 341; autistic-like features, 35–39; behavior therapy, 317, 318; coprolalia, 46; depression, 53, 303, 323, 324; echolalia, 36, 40, 42, 184; hand biting, 18, 25, 35, 38, 54–55, 301, 320, 334, 359; hand flapping, 25, 35, 38, 42, 54–55, 320, 350; hyperactivity, 15, 35, 37–38, 46, 220, 358; imitation, 46, 340, 355, 356, 360; inappropriate laughter, 36; obsessivecompulsive behavior, 46, 48, 303; panic attacks, 20, 52; perseveration, 35, 38–40, 46, 53, 182, 184–86, 293, 301, 320, 337–39, 341; poor eye contact, 35, 38, 54, 55, 194, 321; psychosis, 50, 80, 300; psychotherapy, 311–24; schizophrenia, 50, 52; schizotypal features, 52, 53; schizotypy, 174; self-injurious behavior, 301, 316, 322, 331; shyness, 45, 52, 195, 323; sleeping problems, 320, 321; stereotypies, 46, 299; tactile defensiveness, 41, 184, 185, 334; tantrums, 35, 284; tics, 46, 292–93, 301
Beta-blockers, 297–99, 322; naldolol, 298, 299; pindolol, 298, 299; propanolol, 297–99
BrdU (5-Bromodeoxyuridine), 127

Calming activities, 317, 319–21, 323, 348–49, 357–58
Cardiac abnormalities, 20–21; aortic dilatation, 20; mitral valve prolapse, 3, 18, 20, 285; murmur, 285; palpitations, 20
Carpenter syndrome, 204, 214, 216
Cell cycle, 129, 132
Cerebellum, 32, 33–35; vermis, 33–35
Cerebral palsy, 28

Syndromes (*cont.*)
211, 216, 219, 222, 223; Down, 55, 81, 196, 270; Ehlers-Danlos, 28; Gerstmann, 191, 194; Juberg-Marsidi, 209, 214–17, 220; Klinefelter, 55, 270; Lujan, 55, 207, 214–16, 220; Marfan, 3, 9; Partington, 214, 216, 222; Prader-Willi, 23, 55; Renpenning, 202, 208, 212, 214–16, 221; Schimke, 206, 216, 220; Simpson-Golabi-Behmel, 204, 210, 218; Smith-Fineman-Myers, 216, 221; Soto, 22, 55; Sutherland, 212, 214–16; Thode, 211, 214–17, 219; Tourette, 46, 50, 292, 293; Tranebjaerg, 208, 211, 214–16; Turner, 174, 175, 196; Williams, 81, 196
Syntactical competence, 183
Syntax, 186

Tactile defensiveness, 41, 184, 185, 334
Tangential language, 184, 185
Tantrums, 35, 284
Tegretol. *See* Medications, carbamazepine
Temporal spikes, 29
Thode syndrome, 211, 214–17, 219
Thymidine, 70, 100, 110–13, 117, 123, 128
Thymidylate synthetase, 110
Thioridazine, 49
Tics, 46, 292–93, 301
Tissue cultures, 98–118; MEM-FA, 109, 113, 116, 117, 123; RPMI 1640, 99, 116, 117; TC 199, 99, 100, 102, 109, 113, 115–17
Topic maintenance, 185, 337
Tourette syndrome, 46, 50, 292, 293
Tranebjaerg syndrome, 208, 211, 214–16
Transmitting males. *See* Nonpenetrant (transmitting) males
Tricyclics, 292–93; desipramine, 293; imipramiane, 292
Trimethoprim, 110, 295
Tri-radial figures, 101, 104, 107–9, 128
Tuberous sclerosis, 81

Tumors, 14
Turner syndrome, 174, 175, 196
Twin studies, 81, 270

Ultrasound, 260, 269
Uracil misincorporation, 131

Vectors, 147
Vermis, 33–35
Vineland Adaptive Behavior Scale, 184, 185
Violent outbursts, 285–87, 289, 299, 354, 357, 358; pharmacotherapy, 297–303
Visual cuing, 352
Vitamin B$_6$, 296
Vocational training, 355, 356, 358, 359

Wechsler intelligence tests, 189–91
Williams syndrome, 81, 196

X-inactivation, 28, 99, 123, 126–27, 163, 232–47, 256
X-linked mental retardation, 3, 69, 71–73, 82–83, 86, 100, 121, 124, 202–23; Atkin syndrome, 204, 211–13, 215, 216; Clasped thumb, 209, 221–22; Coffin-Lowry syndrome, 203, 204, 211, 216, 219, 222, 223; Juberg-Marsidi syndrome, 209, 214–17, 220; Lujan (Marfanoid habitus), 207, 214–16, 220; Renpenning syndrome, 202, 208, 212, 214–16, 221; Schimke syndrome, 206, 216, 220; Simpson-Golabi-Behmel syndrome, 204, 210, 218; Smith-Fineman-Myers syndrome, 216, 221; Thode syndrome, 211, 214–17, 219; Trunebjaerg syndrome, 208, 211, 214–16
Xq27.2, 84
XXX, 196
XXY, 196

Yeast artificial chromosomes (YACs), 166–67